KU-622-473

Level 3

Health and Social Care Diploma

Val Michie, Caroline Morris,
Layla Baker and
Fiona Collier

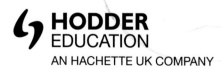

HODDER
EDUCATION
AN HACHETTE UK COMPANY

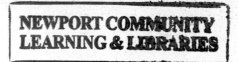

NEWPORT COMMUNITY LEARNING & LIBRARIES

Orders: please contact Bookpoint Ltd, 130 Milton Park, Abingdon, Oxon OX14 4SB. Telephone: (44) 01235 827720. Fax: (44) 01235 400454. Lines are open from 9.00 - 5.00, Monday to Saturday, with a 24 hour message answering service. You can also order through our website www.hoddereducation.co.uk

If you have any comments to make about this, or any of our other titles, please send them to educationenquiries@hodder.co.uk

British Library Cataloguing in Publication Data
A catalogue record for this title is available from the British Library

ISBN: 978 1 444 12067 7

First Edition Published 2011
Impression number   10 9 8 7 6 5 4 3 2
Year   2015 2014 2013

Copyright © 2011 Val Michie, Caroline Morris, Layla Baker and Fiona Collier

All rights reserved. No part of this publication may be reproduced or transmitted in any form or by any means, electronic or mechanical, including photocopy, recording, or any information storage and retrieval system, without permission in writing from the publisher or under licence from the Copyright Licensing Agency Limited. Further details of such licences (for reprographic reproduction) may be obtained from the Copyright Licensing Agency Limited, Saffron House, 6-10 Kirby Street, London EC1N 8TS.

Hachette UK's policy is to use papers that are natural, renewable and recyclable products and made from wood grown in sustainable forests. The logging and manufacturing processes are expected to conform to the environmental regulations of the country of origin.

Cover photo © Bloom Image/Getty Images;
Typeset by DC Graphic Design Limited, Swanley Village, Kent
Printed in Italy for Hodder Education, An Hachette UK Company, 338 Euston Road, London NW1 3BH

Contents

Acknowledgements and Author biographies

Acknowledgements

Every effort has been made to trace and acknowledge ownership of copyright. The publishers will be glad to make suitable arrangements with any copyright holders whom it has not been possible to contact.

P. 29, 56, 67, 72, 85, 119, 171, 207 References to *GSCC Code of Practice* © Copyright General Social Care Council 2010; **P. 191** Extracts from Terry Pratchett interview from www.dailymail.co.uk, www.alzheimers.org.uk; **P.191** *Living well with dementia: A National Dementia Strategy' DH 2009* Contains public sector information licensed under the Open Government Licence v1.0.

The authors and publishers would like to thank the following for the use of images in this volume.

Photo credits
1.1 © Paul Doyle/Alamy; **1.2** © CLEO Photo/Alamy; **1.4** © aceshot/Fotolio.com; **1.6** © Brad Killer/iStockphoto; **1.8** © amana images inc./Alamy; **1.10** © manley099/iStockphoto; **2.1** © 5AM Images/Fotolia.com; **2.3** © LanaK/Fotolia.com; **2.6** © naka/Fotolia.com; **2.7** © Paula Solloway/Photofusion; **3.1** © Sally and Richard Greenhill/Alamy; **3.2** © Ulrike Preuss/Photofusion; **3.5** © John Birdsall/Press Association Images; **3.6** © Ocean/Corbis; **4.1** © Paul Doyle/Photofusion; **4.3** © Joanne Obrien/Photofusion; **5.4** © Alain Machet (2nd)/Alamy; **5.6** © gwimages/Fotolia.com; **5.8** © Ocean/Corbis; **6.3** © Paula Solloway/Photofusion; **7.2** © Ocean/Corbis; **7.3** © Vehbi Koca/Photofusion; **7.4** © Monkey Business/Fotolia.com; **7.5** © RubberBall/Alamy; **7.7** © Yuri Arcurs/Fotolia.com; **8.6** © Wellcome Photo Library, Wellcome Images; **8.7** © Andrzej Tokarski/Fotolia.com; **8.8** © Medical-on-Line/Alamy; **8.9** © Steve Taylor/Getty Images; **8.10** © Indigo Images/Alamy; **8.11** © Construction Photography/Corbis; **9.3** © luchshen/Fotolia.com; **10.8** © Macduff Everton/Corbis; **11.6** © Terry J Alcorn/Getty Images; **11.8** © Geo Martinez/Fotolia.com; **12.8** © deanm1974/Fotolia.com; **13.4** © Adrian Sherratt/Alamy; **13.9** © Photosymbols, www.photosymbols.com; **13.12** © Ghislain & Marie David de Lossy/Alamy; **14.5** © Dean Mitchell/Alamy; **15.1** © AVAVA/Fotolia.com; **15.5** © JGI/Blend Images/Corbis; **15.6** © Alina Solovyova-Vincent/iStockphoto; **16.3** © Rolf Bruderer/Corbis; **16.5** © Image Source/Corbis; **16.6** © lunapiena98/Fotolia.com; **16.10** © Custom Medical Stock Photo/Alamy

Author biographies

Val Michie has an academic background in the biological sciences and in health and social welfare. Prior to becoming a Consultant in Education and Training for the Health and Care Sector in 2001, in which capacity she works with a wide range of training providers within the private, statutory and trades union sectors, she worked in medical research and then as a lecturer in FE, teaching health sciences, key skills and Health and Social Care. Her more recent role as a technical author has involved her in writing underpinning knowledge and assessment activities for a number of qualifications, including NVQs, Technical Certificates and BTECs in Health and Social Care. She is currently exploring issues related to dementia and elderly care in health and social care settings.

Caroline Morris has a background in the health service, having worked as a nurse, Registered Care Manager and, more recently, a teacher and lecturer, delivering in Health and Social Care since 1992. Caroline has provided services to OCR, Edexcel, OU and EDI as an external verifier in Public Services since 1997, and has been involved in writing materials and specifications for publishers and EDI and OCR awarding bodies. Caroline is carrying out post-graduate research in education to achieve PhD, and also undertakes inspections on behalf of BIIAB, EDI, OU and BAC.

Layla Baker is currently Subject Leader in Health and Social Care and Lead IV for BTEC courses, taught Health and Social Care for 14 years at Level 1, 2,3 and in Higher Education. She has worked in Further Education, Higher Education, 6th form college and is currently in a school teaching Key Stage 4 and 5. Layla has qualifications in BA Social Policy, Masters Health Service Studies, PGCE in Post 16 Education, QTS and is currently studying for a Masters in Teaching and Education. She has previously written textbooks and CD-roms for BTEC Firsts and BTEC Diplomas as well as learning materials for Age Concern.

Fiona Collier is a registered nurse with a varied experience within the field of Health and Social Care. In addition to her clinical skills Fiona has also worked as a teacher, trainer and internal moderator within Further Education providing work based training and education to health and social care workers. Fiona is presently working as a Consultant in Education and Training for the Health and Social Care Sector. This role involves designing, delivering and evaluating training as well as writing educational material for publishers and awarding bodies. Fiona has written the underpinning knowledge and assessments for a number of awards and qualifications including NVQs and VRQs.

Walkthrough

We want you to succeed!

This book has been designed to support the new QCF Level 3 Diploma in Health and Social Care. This qualification has replaced the previous NVQ at Level 3. It has been written with the work-based learner in mind. Everything in it reflects the assessment criteria and evidence based approach that is applied to this vocational qualification.

We've included everything you will need for the mandatory units at this level. We've also included enough of the most popular optional units to see you through a full Diploma in Health and Social Care.

In the pages that follow you will find up-to-date resource material which will develop your knowledge, rehearse your skills and help you to gain your qualification. Each unit incorporates a step-by-step guide for you to follow allowing you to work your way through each unit with materials such as activities and real life case studies.

Prepare for what you are going to cover in this unit, and prepare for assessment:

When you have read this chapter you will know how to:
- Communicate effectively
- Support individuals to communicate
- Overcome barriers to communication
- Maintain confidentiality.

Reinforce concepts with hands-on learning and generate evidence for assignments

Practice activity

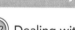 Dealing with complaints

Locate a flow chart of how complaints are dealt with. Make a copy of this for your own evidence.

Time to reflect

 Reasons for communication

- Think about all the people you communicate with. Reflect back over your day, or think about yesterday. How many people did you talk to? Why did you communicate with them?
- Consider the different reasons we communicate. Make a list of the different people you communicate with and why you communicate with them. You will be surprised!

Evidence activity

 Ineffective communication

Two friends are talking to each other but both are obviously really excited, so they are talking at the same time.

Research & investigate

 Communication needs

Think about an individual you have been supporting. How do you know the way they like to communicate and what is effective for them? Make notes on the approaches you use and how you ensure

Walkthrough

Understand how your learning fits into real life and your working environment

Case Study *contd.*

The GP knows that the absent father is HIV positive. To the best of the GP's knowledge, neither the social worker nor the health visitor are aware of this. It is also possible that Ms X is unaware.

2. In these particular circumstances, should the GP share this information with the following people, and why?

(a) Ms X

(b) the health visitor

Check new words and what they mean

Key term

Diversity means variety, particularly in relation to people. You must understand that each individual is unique.

You've just covered a whole unit so here's a guide to what assessors will be looking for and links to activities that can help impress them

Assessment summary

Your reading of this chapter and completion of the activities will have prepared you to be able to engage in personal development in health, social care or children's and young people's settings.

To achieve the unit, your assessor will require you to:

Learning outcomes	Assessment Criteria
Learning outcome 1: Show that you understand why effective communication is important in the work setting by:	1.1 identifying the different reasons people communicate See Time to reflect 1.1, p. 2
	1.2 explaining how communication affects relationships in the work setting See Evidence activity 1.2, p. 2 and p.4
Learning outcome 2: Be able to meet the communication and language needs, wishes and preferences of individuals by:	2.1 demonstrating how to establish the communication and language needs, wishes and preferences of individuals See Research activity 2.1, p. 5

The internet's great for further research. There are pointers to some of the more useful information out there for assignments

Weblinks

Skills for Health	www.skillsforhealth.org.uk
Skills for Care and Development	www.skillsforcareanddevelopment.org.uk
Care Quality Commission	www.cqc.org.uk
General Social Care Council	www.gscc.org.uk
Nursing and Midwifery Council	www.nmc-uk.org

Promote communication in health, social care or children's and young people's settings

For Unit SHC 31

What are you finding out?

This chapter is about how to identify ways of communicating with individuals on difficult, complex and sensitive issues. The unit also explores the importance of communication in such settings, and ways to overcome barriers to meet individual needs and preferences in communication.

Difficult, complex and sensitive aspects of communication include issues of a personal nature or distressing situations. They also include any situation that may pose a risk to, or is likely to have serious implications for, individuals and their families, as well as other workers.

When you have read this chapter you will know how to:

■ Communicate effectively

■ Support individuals to communicate

■ Overcome barriers to communication

■ Maintain confidentiality.

LO1 Understand why effective communication is important in the work setting

1.1 The different reasons people communicate

Communication between workers and individuals

As a worker you can provide a range of information to individuals who use services, to enable them to understand the support that is available to meet their needs. You could ask the individual for their opinions about the provision available and encourage them to make choices.

Exchanging information is important in order to develop your understanding of the needs of an individual, so that you can provide the support the client requires and improve the quality of service provision. If the information exchanged is inaccurate, mistakes can be made, for example, an individual could be prescribed the wrong medication if the GP did not know they were allergic to it. If information is not exchanged, individuals may not feel supported and workers will not be able to carry out their job roles as effectively as they could.

Developing and promoting relationships

You will establish many different relationships across the sector, some of which will be formal and others more informal. Two-way communication is required to form relationships and establish the boundaries. It will help to ensure that everyone concerned understands the purpose of the relationship and what they are aiming to achieve.

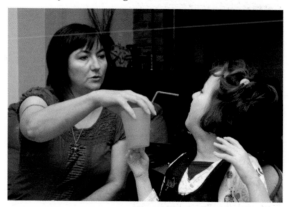

Figure 1.1

The relationships between workers and service users, and also between colleagues, have a significant impact on the ability to provide effective care and support. Respect for each other can be developed through communication.

Getting to know people by talking and listening to them will enable you to develop an understanding and awareness which will lead to stronger relationships in the longer term.

Relationships are developed between workers and service users when they communicate effectively and appropriately, and trust is established. In order to maintain effective support and achieve success, each person involved in a relationship should know clearly what their responsibilities are and what the other person's expectations are. The targets for effective communication are to form a good working relationship or partnership where each contributor is valued. This involves:

- respecting individuals' rights

- maintaining confidentiality

- considering the person's beliefs and cultural views and opinions

- supporting individuals in expressing their views and opinions

- respecting **diversity** when individuals do not behave in the same way or have the same views as you.

Key term

Diversity means variety, particularly in relation to people. You must understand that each individual is unique.

Time to reflect

1.1 Reasons for communication

- Think about all the people you communicate with. Reflect back over your day, or think about yesterday. How many people did you talk to? Why did you communicate with them?

- Consider the different reasons we communicate. Make a list of the different people you communicate with and why you communicate with them. You will be surprised!

1.2 How communication affects relationships in the work setting

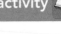

Evidence activity

1.2 Ineffective communication

Two friends are talking to each other but both are obviously really excited, so they are talking at the same time.

Describe two examples of how ineffective communication may affect individuals.

Conversations are such common, everyday events that people often think they do not require any specific or specialist skills. Some interactions will be informal, such as speaking with friends or family members. Other conversations will be more formal, for example, having a conversation with a health specialist, colleague or employer.

Communication in work settings may be complex. This means that it may have several purposes. As a practitioner, you will need to be aware that each individual has their own way of interpreting what is said. Effective communication means more than just passing on information, it means involving or engaging the other person or people with whom you are interacting.

Communicating has to be a two-way process where each person is attempting to understand and interpret, or make sense of, what the other person is saying. Often it is easier to understand people who are similar to us, for example, a person who has the same accent as us, or is in a similar situation. The decoding equipment in our brain tunes in, breaks down the message, analyses the message, understands it and interprets its meaning, and then creates a response or answer. When a practitioner is speaking with an individual they are forming a mental picture of what they are being told.

Supporting communication with individuals

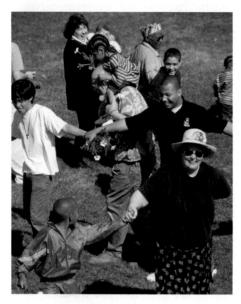

Figure 1.2

Maintaining good eye contact – focusing on the individual

Eye contact is a way of showing that the person who is listening is interested in the conversation. Eye contact will help the person you are communicating with realise that you are concentrating on what they are saying rather than on other conversations or activities that may be going on around you. Eye-to-eye contact can also help you to know how the other person is feeling. If either the individual or the practitioner is angry or upset, they might have a fixed stare that can send out that message; if they are excited or interested in someone, then their eyes will get wider. This means that when you are talking to an individual, the person can tell whether you like what you are hearing or not.

Good eye contact at appropriate times can encourage individuals to talk more openly. It conveys that you understand the individual's situation; you can put yourself in the person's position and can see things from their perspective, making it easier to provide support for them.

As a practitioner, you need to understand that eye contact conveys different meanings for people from different cultures. For example, direct eye contact is considered to be rude in some cultures and should be avoided. It is important to understand what is and what is not acceptable for the people with whom you are working. Also, some individuals may be unable or unwilling to make and/or maintain eye contact because of a disability.

Listening attentively and responding

Active listening helps to maximise the effectiveness of communication. It is important to show not only that you are listening to the individual, but that you have actually heard and understood what has been said. By responding to what has been said, you will reassure the individual and encourage them to speak more openly. Responses can include nodding, smiling, or reflecting back what has been said. Making encouraging sounds can also indicate interest and can be used to gain further information. The person who is talking is encouraged by signals which show that the listener wants to know more.

Looking interested

Using smiles and eye contact ensures that people know that you are interested in what is being said. You should display open body language, and using gestures can also be helpful. Showing a person that you are interested in what is being said encourages them to communicate fully and can improve the level of detail they are prepared to give. Showing interest also helps to develop a trusting relationship which, over a period of time, can help improve communication.

Research & investigate

 Communication methods

Investigate the range of communication methods used in a specific setting, e.g. nursery or learning disability provision, and list the benefits of each method.

Time

Communication should never be rushed, as this may make an individual feel that they are not important, or that you lack respect for them. Also, taking too much time can be seen as dragging out the conversation and can make people feel uneasy. Timing should be appropriate for the purpose of the communication and take into account the needs of the individuals involved. It is important to give individuals time to say what they want to; this ensures that they feel respected and that their personal interests have been considered fully. Individuals should not be interrupted when they are speaking, as this may make them feel that they are not being listened to properly.

Use of technology, e.g. JAWS

JAWS is a computer program that reads information on the screen and speaks it aloud through a speech synthesiser. It works with any PC to provide access to software applications and the internet. It also outputs to refreshable **Braille** displays, providing Braille support for screen readers. Where the use of technology is appropriate to assist with communication, this should be encouraged so that everyone feels actively involved and no one is struggling to hear what others are saying or is unable to present their ideas or opinions.

> ### Key term
>
> Braille is a system of writing and printing for blind or visually impaired people. Varied arrangements of raised dots representing letters and numerals are identified by touch.

> ### Evidence activity
>
> **1.2** **Your communication experience**
>
> Think about a time when you wanted to make a comment or complain about a service you received. How did you do this? How did you feel? What was the outcome? Did you need someone to help you?

Use of advocates or interpreters

An advocate is a person who tries to understand the needs and preferences of an individual and speaks on their behalf. Advocates are often needed when someone has a disability which makes it difficult for them to speak for themselves. An advocate should try and get to know the service user and develop an understanding of their culture and background, so that they can represent them accurately. The advocate should understand the person's needs and communicate these to practitioners or professionals involved with them. To ensure that they are unbiased, advocates are independent of the professional carers who work with the individual.

Interpreters can help people for whom English is not their preferred or first language. In the past interpreters may have been family members of the person in question, but this is now discouraged as far as is possible for

reasons of confidentiality. For example, a mother whose daughter was interpreting for her may not want her daughter to know that she had cancer. Interpreters communicate meaning of one spoken language to another, while translators change written material from one language to another.

There are drawbacks to using translators and interpreters, as it may sometimes be difficult to grasp the exact meaning of a message or to express the meaning in the other language. Where an interpreter is used, it is important to remember to communicate with the service user rather than the interpreter, to ensure that the individual is empowered and feels valued.

In many services, leaflets concerning health topics or health facilities are produced in several other languages in addition to English, so that people from ethnic minorities can access the information. If information is not readily available in the relevant language it will need to be translated.

Awareness of personal space and positioning

Seating arrangements and positioning should be considered carefully when communicating with others, and will depend on the circumstances and purpose of the communication. For example, if the interaction is informal and between two people, sitting next to one another, with the worker mirroring the **body language** of the client, could be most suitable. If, however, the communication is of a more formal nature, then having a table that is higher than the chairs, with chairs either side of it, may be more appropriate. The height of chairs and tables can influence communication.

> ### Key term
>
> Body language is conscious and unconscious communication through movements or attitudes of the body.

If information is to be communicated to a large audience then a lecture theatre layout would be more appropriate, as the speaker could be seen and heard by all.

Open body language

Open body language generally indicates that a person is relaxed and welcoming to others. Crossing your arms and legs can create a barrier between you and those you are communicating with. Uncrossing your legs and arms, and opening your hands indicates that you are not hiding anything from the other person. Displaying open body language is likely to lead to the development of a more trusting relationship in which the service user relates to the practitioner and is likely to communicate in a more open manner.

Leaning towards individual

Gerald Egan's 'SOLER' theory of communication indicates that leaning towards an individual when communicating with them shows interest and commitment to what is being said. It enhances the ability to listen to and, consequently, to hear what has been said. There is less likelihood of distractions interfering with the communication and increased effectiveness.

Awareness of individual's body language

Being aware of an individual's body language can help to support communication. When the individual is displaying open and positive body language it indicates that they are actively involved in the communication and are not feeling uncomfortable. If there is evidence of closed or negative body language this can indicate that there is tension, and the individual is less likely to communicate or listen to what is being said. Making allowances for body language in this way will help to improve the communication, for example, when there is tense closed body language it may be time to have a short break or give the individual the opportunity to ask questions. This could refocus the communication and improve the situation for all concerned.

LO2 Be able to meet the communication and language needs, wishes and preferences of individuals

 How to establish the communication and language needs, wishes and preferences of individuals

Research & investigate

2.1 Communication needs

Think about an individual you have been supporting. How do you know the way they like to communicate and what is effective for them? Make notes on the approaches you use and how you ensure individuals are fully consulted.

Active listening

In your role you are encouraged to use active listening techniques in order to encourage effective communication and maximise the communication process. Active listeners focus on:

■ what is being said verbally, i.e. content

■ how the person is saying it, i.e. the tone of voice

■ what is being communicated non-verbally, i.e. body language.

The use of questioning

Only about ten per cent of our communication is actually spoken, and it is very important that you make the most of your conversations with individuals and their families, as this will enable you to establish relationships and accurately identify their needs and feelings. Much of this information can be collected through careful questioning, and it is important that you consider the different techniques that might be used to accurately and effectively collect information without creating too much distress. For example, you might use:

■ *Closed questions* – e.g. 'Would you like an extra pillow, Mr Smith?' The breathless person need only reply 'Yes' or 'No'. A more complex question would need a longer answer, and cause further breathlessness and discomfort.

■ *Open questions* – e.g. 'Tell me about your family, Mr Smith.' This will enable you to start up a conversation.

■ *Process questions* – e.g. 'What did you think the doctor was saying, Mr Smith?' This type of questioning can give you an indication as to how the individual understands his or her situation.

■ *Clarification* – e.g. 'I think you said that this made you feel worse. Is that right, Mr Smith?' This is a useful way of checking or summarising the outcomes of a conversation, and shows that you are listening.

Describe the factors to consider when promoting effective communication

Evidence activity

2.2 Helping an individual

Alice is a new member of staff and speaks very quietly and slowly. Not all individuals understand her. How can you help Alice to communicate more effectively?

Communication makes the world go round. On a smaller level, communication, or being able to communicate effectively, is what gets you through each day, in both your career and personal life. No matter what your age, background or experience, communicating effectively is something that every person can achieve. It requires self-confidence, good **articulation** and knowledge of how communication can be made more effective.

Key term

Articulation is the formation of clear and distinct words when communicating through speech.

Choose the right moment and the right place. If you need to discuss something in private with a person, make sure that the choice of venue is private and that you do not feel uncomfortable about the possibility of being overheard. On the other hand, if you need to make your point before a group of people, ensure that the location is somewhere that your discussion will be audible to all who are present, to ensure that you engage everyone in the group.

Organise and clarify ideas in your mind before you attempt to communicate them. Decide on some key points and stick with these to avoid your message becoming garbled, which can happen if you feel passionately about a topic. A good rule-of-thumb is to choose three main points and keep your communication focused on those. That way, if you wander off topic, you will be able to return to one or more of these key points without feeling flustered.

2.3 & 2.4 A range of communication methods and styles to meet individual needs & How to respond to an individual's reactions when communicating

Verbal communication

Verbal communication is an important method of communication between workers and service users across the sectors. People talk to each other and have conversations regularly, receiving and giving information quickly and effectively. Ideas can be exchanged and decisions made there and then. If there is any confusion about what has been said, this can be clarified at the time so that everyone knows and understands exactly what has happened or is going to happen in the future. Service users will be able to find out about the treatment or procedures they are going to have. Instructions can be given to other workers so that they know what their duties are. Activities can be carried out and problems solved, using speech as the method of communication.

Sign language

The British Sign Language (BSL) is used by a large number of people within the UK. It is thought that nearly 70,000 people use sign language in the British Isles. The government officially recognised the BSL in March 2003. Children find sign language fascinating and, as a result, learn the signs quite easily. The BSL has a phrase, 'make your fingers count', which appeals to children. Sign language can be taught at any age and is used by many of those with hearing impairment. It is a language that has developed over hundreds of years and enables interaction between people who otherwise might experience difficulty. It may or may not be the first language of those using it.

DID YOU KNOW

It is said that as little as ten per cent of communication takes place verbally, and that facial expressions, gestures and posture form the largest part of our culture and language.

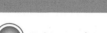
2.3 BSL and Makaton

Look up BSL or Makaton on the internet. Learn a simple sentence and then review how you did. Was it easy to use?

Body language

The non-verbal signals you use when talking to people, such as gestures, facial expressions, body positioning and movement of the body, are known as 'body language'. Body language is a way of giving messages to those with whom we are speaking, for example, smiling will convey friendliness. First impressions are often made from observing an individual's body language. A person can convey confidence or lack of confidence through their body language, which can have an impact on the effectiveness of the communication. By developing an awareness of the signs and signals of body language, you will find it much easier to understand other people and to communicate more effectively with them. Increasing understanding of body language can also help you to become more aware of the messages you are conveying to others.

There are subtle, and sometimes less subtle, movements, gestures, facial expressions and even shifts in individuals' whole bodies that indicate something is going on. The way they talk, walk, sit and stand all say something, and whatever is happening on the inside can be reflected on the outside. There are also times when mixed messages are sent – a person says one thing and their body language displays something different. This can be confusing, so it is important to understand the messages being sent to others as well as those being received.

Take care not to assume meanings, particularly when communicating with individuals from other cultures. For example, not making eye contact may, for some, be read as 'having something to hide', while others may see it as a mark of respect.

Gestures

Gestures are hand or arm movements that can portray a message to another person. Usually gestures are used to enhance the understanding of what is being said verbally, but some gestures carry their own meaning and can be misinterpreted by others. People who cannot use sign language may be able to relay a message to, or understand a message from, a person with speech impairments by using or watching gestures.

Gestures can be used to convey both positive and negative responses. For example, 'thumbs up' can mean 'OK', 'success' or even 'yes please'. Putting a hand up with the palm facing a person gives the meaning of 'stop that'. Shrugging shoulders can mean 'not sure'. However, you should be aware that these gestures can mean different things to people from different cultural groups, for example, in some cultures the thumbs-up sign can have negative connotations.

Facial expression

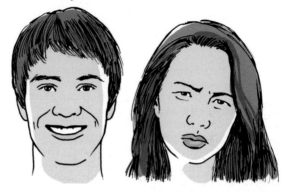

Figure 1.3

Facial expressions are used to convey meaning in communication. They can be an indication of the emotional state of the person communicating. Facial expressions include smiling, frowning, raising an eyebrow or pulling the mouth into particular shapes. A quizzical expression can show that a person has misunderstood or wants to ask a question. A sad expression can indicate that something is wrong. Facial expressions can also show pain or surprise.

Position

The position in which a person sits or stands can send out messages to those they are communicating with. Crossing your arms can mean, 'I'm not taking any notice'. Leaning back can send out messages of boredom or being relaxed, whereas leaning slightly forward is seen as positive as it shows interest in what the other person is saying. Leaning too far forward can be seen as intrusive and intimidating. Standing turned away from another person shows a lack of interest.

Dress

The way an individual dresses and the clothes they wear play an important role in the way they are perceived by others. A person's physical appearance and dress creates a definite impact on the communication process. When working in the health and social care sectors, clothing should be appropriate for the task, and for the group of people you are working with. For example, when attending a community meeting you should dress in a way that shows respect for the people who are involved in the interaction, their culture, age, gender etc. while leaving a positive impression on them.

People's appearance may make a statement about their gender, age, economic class, and often their intentions before you even speak to them. Individuals begin to recognise the important cultural clues for this at an early age. The vocabulary of dress that we learn includes not only items of clothing but also hairstyles, jewellery, makeup, and other body decoration such as tattoos. In most cultures, however, the same style of dress communicates different messages depending on the age, gender and physical appearance of the individual wearing it. Putting on certain types of clothing can change an individual's behaviour and the behaviour of others towards them. When an individual is approached by a police officer in **uniform** they may feel scared even though they know they have not done anything wrong. Their behaviour would be different if they were approached by a plainclothes police officer.

Key term

A uniform is clothing of a distinctive design worn by members of a particular group or organisation as a means of identification.

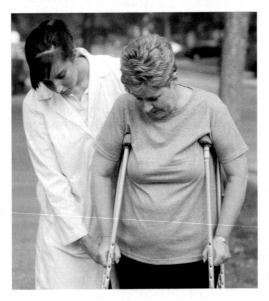

Figure 1.4

A uniform is a symbol of status and clearly identifies an individual as belonging to a

particular organisation so they can be approached with some level of confidence by service users. Confusion can occur where there are several different uniforms worn by workers. For example, the variety of different uniforms and name badges that are present within the Health Service can be very confusing. People may not know or understand which roles the uniforms are associated with. Each member of staff introducing themselves as they meet the patient can be a way of overcoming this.

When working with children it is important to ensure that they feel at ease and do not find the uniform scary. Children's workers often wear clothing the children can recognise, for example, nursery workers may wear brightly coloured polo shirts or tabards; nurses may wear uniforms with animals or pictures on them. These can create a starting point for a conversation which can be used to gain the trust of the child before giving them medication or an injection.

Some organisations prefer their staff not to wear uniforms, so that service users feel more confident when communicating with them. Social workers, youth workers and advocates are among these.

Written communication

The written word is very common and is a widely established form of communication. The rules that govern writing are very different from those that are followed for spoken language. In many services written communication is used to record personal history. In all the sectors, accuracy of the written word is extremely important. If **inaccuracies** occur when keeping formal records, a person using the services could have the wrong treatment or be given incorrect information, with disastrous results. False, inaccurate or misleading written records could result in inappropriate actions, failure to carry out the required actions or even complaints and litigation.

Key term

Inaccuracies are things that are not accurate, containing mistakes/errors.
Acronyms are words formed from the initial letters of the words in a name, e.g. NHS is an acronym for the National Health Service.

When writing information down, make sure it is clear, accurate and legible.

Evidence activity

2.4 Written communication

Review some of the daily reports you have written in your setting. Do they make sense? Have you used lots of initials or **acronyms** that others may not understand?

Communicating in writing helps services to maintain contact with other professionals within and across the sectors. Written communication is a means of giving information to others, obtaining information from others and exchanging ideas relating to a variety of aspects of the sectors involved. Some services also require that certain information is confirmed in writing, for example, when making a referral to a social services department regarding concerns about the well-being of a child, the initial referral may be taken over the phone but must be confirmed in writing. In many settings the communication policy will lay down that all written communication must be shown to the manager before it is passed on.

Copies of written communication should be stored securely so that they are accessible should they be required for future reference. In some roles written notes and records may be required for use in hearings or court cases, for example in care proceedings regarding children. It is essential that all copies of information regarding the children are kept, including jotted notes, typed-up notes, letters and records of phone calls, emails, faxes etc. and stored according to the guidelines and procedures of the organisation. Documentation that is no longer required should be destroyed using the correct procedures to ensure that confidentiality is maintained – it should not be retained or kept unsecured.

Each of the different forms of written communication has its own characteristics, but the common element relating to all recording documents is the need for accuracy and clarity. If a person reading the information cannot clearly understand the points that are being made, misunderstandings are likely to occur. The writer needs to clearly establish the purpose of writing, for example:

- Who will be reading the written information?

- What points are to be made?

- What does the writer hope to achieve?

Clear concise writing cannot be done in a hurry. You will need to learn how to express yourself clearly and effectively in writing.

Using technology/ICT

In recent years the development of electronic mail (email) has proved to be a significant form of communication. Emails can be formal or informal, depending on their purpose. The internet is also being used increasingly as a source of information for a variety of purposes.

An advantage of emails is that they provide a very quick way of interacting with other people or organisations, as answers can be received in a matter of minutes, rather than having to wait several days for a letter. A disadvantage is that on some occasions emails are lost and, as a consequence, the sender has to repeat the process. Care also needs to be taken to ensure that confidentiality is maintained. 'Secure' systems are necessary before personal confidential information can be exchanged.

Electronic forms of communication are now a well-established way of everyday life. In the health and social care and community justice settings, computers can be used for networking between one organisation and another. A GP surgery could use the computer to send information about a patient to a consultant at a hospital or to send a prescription to a pharmacy. Similarly, an internal system can enable employees within one setting to be linked with others to share information. In all situations, care must be taken to ensure that the requirements of the Data Protection Act 1998 are followed so that personal data is safeguarded and kept **confidential**.

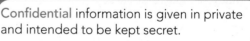

Key term

Confidential information is given in private and intended to be kept secret.

Technological aids can be used to enhance communication with people who may otherwise have difficulties. Some people may use word or symbol boards to support their speech so that a picture enhances the listener's understanding of what has been said. Others may use speech synthesisers, which replace speech either by producing a visual display of written text or by producing synthesised speech that expresses the information verbally. Hearing aids, hearing loops, text phones, text messaging on a mobile phone and magnifiers are also forms of technological communication devices. Voice recognition software can be purchased for any computer which supports the communication of individuals who find writing difficult. Computers can also be used to present information with graphics and sound.

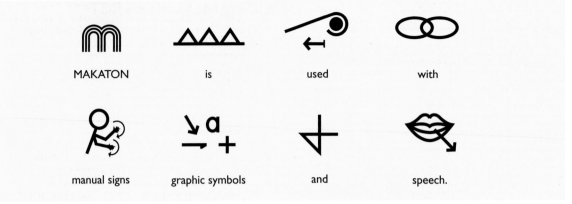

MAKATON   is   used   with

manual signs   graphic symbols   and   speech.

Figure 1.5

Makaton

Makaton is a large collection of symbols that can help people who have a hearing impairment, or who have a learning difficulty, to communicate with others. It is a system that uses signs, speech and symbols. Those using Makaton may use all three methods to help them communicate with others. Makaton uses an established set of hand movements to convey meaning. It is usually taught to children when they are young, as soon as it is realised that they have a need.

Braille

The communication system known as Braille was first introduced in 1829, by a blind man called Richard Braille. The system is one of raised dots that can be felt with a finger. For people who have limited vision or who are blind the system provides the opportunity for independent reading and writing as it is based on 'touch'. It is possible, with the correct computer software, to change the printed word into Braille and to print out using special printers.

As well as being used for reading books and magazines to satisfy the intellectual needs of people who have poor sight, Braille can be used for leaflets and handouts, for example, giving information about the person's treatment.

Evidence activity

(2.4) **Communicating about a difficult or sensitive issue**

Choose a situation where you have communicated with an individual over a difficult or sensitive issue. Produce a reflective account of how you supported communication with the individual. Include answers to the following questions: *contd.*

Evidence activity

- Why was this a difficult or sensitive situation or topic?
- How did you communicate effectively using verbal and non-verbal skills?
- How did you position yourself in relation to others?
- How well did you support the individual to communicate?
- How did you maintain a professional relationship?

LO3 Be able to overcome barriers to communication

(3.1) **How people from different backgrounds may use and/or interpret communication methods in different ways**

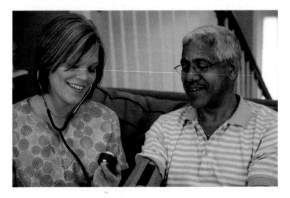

Figure 1.6

Respecting cultural preferences and differences

It is important to respect the fact that people have different cultural preferences and values, and therefore different priorities. You will need to recognise the diverse attitudes of those with whom you come into contact, and must not condemn or treat people differently if their values are different from yours.

Body language can be interpreted differently by different cultures. Certain cultures use gestures or touch much more than others, and gestures can mean different things in different cultures. In some cultures, touching someone shows understanding and empathy, but in British culture it might be considered unacceptable in a work situation. Making direct eye contact when communicating may be considered acceptable and even desirable in one culture (e.g. British), but rude and totally unacceptable in another (e.g. Greek). In order to avoid causing any offence or misunderstanding, it is worth taking time to find out about an individual's cultural background.

It is important to develop your knowledge and understanding of different cultures. For example, you should know that in some cultures, young women can only receive medical attention if they are accompanied by an older family member. Also, decisions about whether to have treatment or care are often made collectively by the senior members of the family rather than by the individual. These considerations may not at first seem to be directly linked to communicating with services users, but they do have an impact on the way people communicate and with whom.

Tips for communicating with people from different cultures include:

1. Understand the individual's values: Understand that people from other cultures might have entirely different value systems from yours. It is useful to check the person's records for information, or speak to a member of their family or a friend if appropriate or possible. Ask someone else from the same culture, either another worker or an advocate. Use reference books and/or the internet if necessary.

2. Give the appropriate amount of personal space: Different cultures have different norms regarding a person's public space (in which others can stand and converse with you) and their private space (reserved only for people who are close to you). For example, people from Arab countries do not share the British concept of 'personal space' – for them it is considered offensive to step or lean away while talking to some. Make sure you leave the correct amount of space between yourself and others when you talk to them. If you are unsure, you can always ask what the other person prefers.

3. Do not belittle their religion: Remember, most people believe passionately in their religion, and they may have different beliefs from yours. If you have trouble dealing with this, you may wish to avoid discussing the topic of religion altogether.

4. Learn to recognise physical cues: Physical gestures that are acceptable when communicating vary widely between different cultures. When people visit other countries they often miss subtle cultural cues, which leads them to misinterpret others. For example, the use of irony or the implication of a laugh may be shown only in a squinting of the eyes or a shaking of the hand, which a cultural outsider might miss.

5. Know relationship differences: Many foreigners think British relationships are superficial (with a brief, 'Hi, Jim', and never a backward glance). British people might think relationships in other cultures are too sentimental. So, know that if a person strikes you as too outspoken or withdrawn, it may be considered normal in their culture.

6. Learn about their culture: Learn about greetings, goodbye rituals, before-meal ceremonies, food and clothes. This will help you understand people from other cultures and improve your communication with them.

7. Accept that there may be lapses in communication: Even the best communicators fall short when jumping across the large gap that exists between different cultures. Humour and non-defensiveness are the best way of dealing with these situations.

8. Ask: There is no better tool for effective communication than asking a question. If something strikes you as funny or inappropriate, if you feel the other person is neglecting you or is offended, simply ask them what you can do to change the situation. Misunderstandings can create big problems unless they are discussed openly.

Asking questions to clarify points, aiding understanding

Asking the right questions without being too intrusive is an important skill to develop. It will help you to clarify the important points and understand the communication. Questions should be short and to the point. Using language and vocabulary that is easy to understand will help to avoid confusion. You should avoid asking multiple questions, as these may be difficult for the individual to answer.

Closed questions (with 'yes' and 'no' answers) should be used to gather factual information when you need to know about specific points, such as date of birth, allergies, medication being taken.

Open questions should be used where more detailed information is required, as these give the individual the opportunity to give longer answers. These questions give more of an insight into how the individual is feeling or about their views and opinions.

Using language appropriate to the individual's understanding

It is important to avoid using language that individuals do not understand, for example using adult language when working with a child would be inappropriate. Likewise, using sophisticated language when communicating with an adult with learning difficulties is not suitable. If acronyms or technical terminology are used these should always be explained, to ensure that the person understands what has been said. You should always assess the individual you are communicating with before progressing with your communication, so that the interaction is as effective as possible.

 Evidence activity

 3.1 Overcoming language barriers

Think about a time when you were on holiday or speaking to a person whose first language was not English. How did you feel? What changes did you make to your method of communication?

Needs and preferences

Individuals should always be given the opportunity to express their needs and preferences. Practitioners should not make assumptions and definitely should not make decisions on behalf of the service user unless they have been given permission to do so or are acting as an advocate for the person.

Respecting individuals' rights to confidentiality within legal and organisational procedures

Individuals have a right by law, under the Data Protection Act 1998, to have confidentiality maintained and their personal information kept private. When an individual knows and understands that their information will not be shared with others, unless it is absolutely necessary, they will feel that they can trust the person they are communicating with and will feel more at ease with them. They are likely to share more detailed information, which could result in them ultimately receiving more effective levels of care.

Ensuring own and/or others' safety

Sometimes interactions have to take place around difficult issues, or with individuals who may present a threat, or who may be vulnerable.

Organisations generally have procedures and policies to support staff in these situations. For example, there may be guidance on ensuring that workers have easy access to the door, have someone else in the room or have a panic button when interviewing individuals who may be violent or aggressive. There may be a policy regarding working with children, whereby workers should not be alone with a child, or should hold discussions in a room which has a glass door.

3.2 Barriers to effective communication

Research & investigate

3.2 Barriers to communication

You are working in setting. There is a lot of noise going on, with new staff and new service users. What barriers do you think there are?

Research how you can overcome these barriers, and produce a simple plan outlining your solutions.

Attitude of the worker

Your attitude can affect the way others communicate with you. When a worker is abrupt towards an individual, that person could feel intimidated and not want to communicate. They may feel that the worker is not interested in them and does not want to help. An insincere approach or lack of empathy may make an individual feel that they are wasting their time, and could make them reluctant to divulge personal information. A sincere and polite attitude is likely to promote more open communication from the service user.

Limited use of technology

Some individuals need technological aids to support their communication. When there is limited availability of a technology, communication may be more difficult. For example, the absence of a **hearing loop** could be a barrier to an individual who uses a hearing aid. Workers who have limited experience of using technology (e.g. computers, fax machines or other technological devices), could interfere with their ability to communicate, for example they may not be able to communicate via email or use a fax machine. This could ultimately delay messages being received and responded to, and could undermine someone's authority if they need to ask for help.

Key term

A hearing loop provides information on an induction loop system, to assist the hearing impaired by transmitting sound from a sound system, microphone, television or other source, directly to a hearing aid.

Sitting too far away or invading personal space

Sitting too far away from a person may make them feel that they are not important or that the practitioner is not interested in what they have to say. It may also mean that they need to speak more loudly, which could compromise confidentiality or make them feel uncomfortable about communicating. Invasion of personal space (getting too close) can also make people feel uncomfortable. Most people prefer to get to know someone first, and often only allow those who are close to them into their 'intimate zone'.

Emotional distress

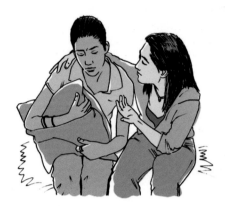

Figure 1.7 Distress

Emotional issues, especially those that cause worry or distress, can make people behave erratically and unpredictably. When individuals have serious emotional needs they can be afraid or depressed because of the stresses they are experiencing. They may lack self-awareness or appear to be shy or aggressive, which has an impact on their ability to communicate. Listening involves learning about frightening and depressing situations, which can mean that practitioners sometimes avoid listening to avoid feeling unpleasant emotions. The practitioner can become emotionally distressed by the needs of the individual and can also make assumptions, or label or stereotype others.

Practitioners may have their own emotional issues that can create barriers. The practitioner may not be able to focus or may be tired due to worrying and lack of sleep. Listening and empathising takes mental energy, which may not be available if the practitioner has their own concerns. Practitioners who believe they do not have sufficient time to communicate properly can become stressed and so create a barrier.

When individuals are depressed, angry or upset, these emotions will influence their ability to understand what is being communicated to them, and to be able to communicate their own needs. Additionally, individuals who do not trust service providers or practitioners are less likely to share information with them.

Evidence activity

(3.2) Helping those in emotional distress

Tilly is upset as she has just been told some distressing news. What can you do to help Tilly?

Not giving individuals time to say what they want to

Some individuals need more time than others to express themselves. This may be due to a lack of confidence or because they have communication difficulties. When individuals are not given the time they need to express themselves, they may feel that they are being rushed. They get annoyed when, for example, someone else finishes off their sentences for them, or they may 'clam up' and not talk at all.

Poor or unwelcoming body language

A worker who displays negative body language in the form of crossed arms or legs, using inappropriate gestures, poor facial expressions, poor body positioning or constant fidgeting creates barriers to communication.

Poor interpersonal skills

A worker who has poor **interpersonal skills** does not make an individual feel welcome. They may use inappropriate language or rely too heavily on technical terminology. Their manner and demeanour may be off putting, which can create a barrier to successful communication. If the worker is not paying attention to the individual or is not listening properly they may miss important information. It is inappropriate to then ask for this to be repeated, as it will make the individual feel that they are not being valued.

> ### Key term
>
> Interpersonal skills are the skills we use to interact with others.

Lack of privacy

Conversations should not be held in a public place where others can overhear what is being said, as this lack of privacy and can feel disrespectful. Interruptions by other people may make the individual feel intimidated and unimportant. A person is likely to communicate much more freely if they feel that what they are saying is being taken seriously and kept private.

Lack of respect for individual

An individual is unlikely to communicate if they feel that they are not being respected. Addressing someone as 'dear' or 'lovie', or invading their personal space shows a lack of respect. Any action that is going to be taken should be clearly explained before actually carrying it out, and the opinions and choices of the individual should be respected. If someone feels that they are not being respected they may withhold information which could be vital.

Stereotyping

Stereotyping means describing everyone in a particular category as being 'the same', or describing aspects of their behaviour or characteristics as 'the same'. It is an easy way of grouping people together. For example, it is stereotyping to believe that everyone over 70 years old is less mentally able or needs a walking aid, or that all children below the age of 4 are unable to make decisions for themselves. Sometimes individuals are stereotyped because of their language or the colour of their skin. Some people may assume that anyone who is not white cannot speak English, so they speak in 'broken English' to the individual without first finding out if they can speak English or if English is their preferred language.

Practitioners sometimes impose their own views and opinions on situations at work. These may be views and opinions they have learnt while growing up, or which they have assumed because they have friends who hold such opinions. A good practitioner will avoid stereotyping and labelling by making sure that they are informed and knowledgeable. They will also examine their own attitudes and values to make sure that they know themselves and are not unjustly judging others.

 3.3 Ways to overcome barriers to communication

> ## Research & investigate
>
> **3.3** Overcoming communication barriers
>
> Select a culture and investigate the language, beliefs and preferences.
>
> What aspects do you need to consider when communicating?

Respecting cultural preferences and differences

Cultural differences can influence communication. Culture is much more than just the language that is spoken, it includes the way people live, think and how they relate to each other. In some cultures children are not allowed to speak if certain adults are present. Other cultures do not allow women to speak to men they do not know. Cultural differences can sometimes make relationships difficult; therefore workers across the sectors need to make sure they prepare well for this.

You must make sure that you acknowledge culture when communicating. For example, certain hand gestures are acceptable in this country but would not be in others. To show friendliness, in one culture you may say hello with a smile on your face; in another, you may make a silent formal bow; and in a third, you may even embrace the people warmly. Looking straight into the eyes of the person you are speaking to is desirable in most conversations in this country, but would be considered rude in others. These cultures believe that looking down shows proper respect for another individual. A practitioner who feels that eye contact is important must learn to accept and respect this cultural difference.

These examples show that people of different cultures communicate differently even when they have the same motive to communicate.

It is important across the sectors for information to be made available in a person's chosen language. It may also be appropriate to employ interpreters to support individuals so that they can be actively involved in any communication and understand the support available or the procedures being carried out.

When communicating it is important to remember the following points:

■ Do not make assumptions when meeting a person – they could appear to be demanding simply because they feel insecure or because they are not familiar with their surroundings.

■ Treat a person with a same-sex partner accompanying them in the same manner as everyone else.

■ Show respect for the values of individuals.

■ Do not invade personal space – often people feel uncomfortable with this until they develop trust.

■ Acknowledge the beliefs and differences of individuals from other cultures.

■ Develop knowledge and understanding of different cultures in order to avoid making mistakes or causing offence.

Asking questions to clarify points, aiding understanding of communication

■ Ask an individual to summarise their understanding of the situation so that further explanation can be given if necessary.

■ Always ask if there is anything that is not understood – this can prevent mistakes being made or something being interpreted in the wrong way.

■ Ask questions relating to timing, place and procedures to enhance understanding.

Evidence activity

(3.3) Integration

Hamid is a new service user. He speaks little English but is keen to get to know people. How can the service, and you, help Hamid integrate?

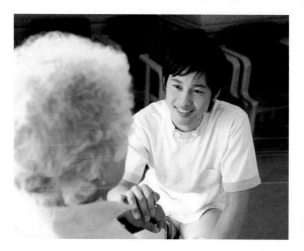

Figure 1.8

Using level appropriate to individual's understanding

■ If possible, check the approximate age of the individual before communicating with them.

■ Read through their records to find out what level of understanding they are likely to have.

■ Never use technical terminology which has not been explained to the individual.

■ Never use acronyms without explaining what they mean.

■ Do not assume that an individual will understand what you have said, or that they must have understood because they did not state otherwise.

A comfortable, safe environment

■ Make sure that the environment is at the right temperature – not too hot and not too cold.

■ Check the environment for any hazards and take precautions to reduce these risks before the communication takes place.

■ Make sure the layout of the room is appropriate for the communication to take place.

■ Make sure the environment has adequate ventilation – not too draughty or too stuffy.

■ Check suitability of seating arrangements – some people prefer chairs with arms so that they can push up to get out of them, some may prefer softer seating, and others may prefer lower/ higher chairs.

Respecting dignity and privacy

■ Ask what name the individual prefers to be called by.

■ Do not speak to the pusher of a wheelchair and by-pass the wheelchair user.

■ Involve children in conversation – do not presume they do not understand the discussions.

■ Talk to the child and ask their opinions.

■ Offer choices wherever possible.

■ Allow preferences to be expressed.

■ Use a private room where appropriate.

■ Do not discuss personal issues where others can overhear.

■ Use passwords on the computer.

■ Never disclose information over the telephone unless the identity of the caller can be established.

■ Ask people to leave the room when appropriate to respect the privacy of the individual.

■ Ask permission from the individual before sharing information with others.

■ Explain who will have access to personal information.

3.4 Demonstrating strategies that can be used to clarify misunderstandings

However you choose to send a message, you must try to ensure that those who are receiving it are aware that it is genuine and purposeful. However, there may be occasions when a message is misinterpreted because potential barriers to the communication process have not been duly considered. These might include:

■ environmental barriers

■ language barriers

■ barriers due to sensory loss

■ barriers due to physical disability

■ cultural barriers

■ barriers due to prejudice and discrimination.

Environmental barriers

A health and social care environment can be noisy, distracting and confusing at times. It is important that members of staff recognise this and reduce any background noise to a minimum. For example, how often have you seen individuals placed next to a noisy television that no one is watching? What effect do you think this will have on their ability to concentrate or to converse with others? It is also important to ensure that the environment is freely accessible, and that the placement of furniture encourages individuals to interact with each other. Notices to inform individuals of activities and events should also be placed in freely accessible locations. This will not only encourage conversation between carers and individuals, but will also encourage individuals to plan for the event, and to participate and socialise with other individuals and their families.

Language barriers

Successful communication hinges on how well you listen and respond to others. Here are some language behaviours that may hinder the communication process:

■ Dominance – if someone dominates the communication process, communicating becomes a one-way process and responses from individuals are hindered.

■ Inappropriate self-disclosure – if someone talks too much about themselves, the topic or focus of the communication changes.

■ Self-protection – individuals often protect themselves from meaningful contact by: talking exclusively about safe topics; avoiding uncomfortable issues; emotionally detaching themselves from the topic of conversation.

■ Swearing – such language may be powerful, but it usually turns others off.

■ Using jargon – people often use words that belong exclusively to their area of expertise.

■ Judging others – as a health and social care worker it is important that you do not impose your own value judgements on others. Avoid telling others that their ideas or opinions are bad or wrong. Simply say, 'I disagree.'

■ Patronising – condescending words, tone or behaviour, will make individuals and their families feel angry and defensive.

■ Pressurising – using threats, implied or explicit, to persuade someone.

■ Being insensitive – being callous or unaware of your own feelings and the feelings of others.

Sensory Loss

Some older people may have difficulty communicating because of poor eyesight or hearing. You can assist individuals who have visual impairment by making sure that their eyesight is tested regularly, that their spectacles are clean and worn properly, and that their possessions are kept in the same, familiar place. You could also learn the correct way to guide and assist a partially sighted person while they are walking, and find out what visual aids are available in your nursing home, such as large-print books and newspapers or talking books. When communicating with visually impaired individuals, it is important that you:

■ let them know you are nearby in a quiet and unhurried manner

■ introduce yourself by name

■ use appropriate forms of touch to initiate and them sustain the conversation

■ ask the individual what form of communication suits them best

■ allow the individual to take your arm before you lead them around

■ treat the person as an individual, and never assume that all visually impaired people have the same communication needs.

You can support individuals with hearing impairment by making sure that their hearing is tested regularly, that a hearing aid, if they wear one, is clean and worn properly, and that the battery is not flat. You can also learn the correct way to replace a hearing aid battery, or talk to colleagues about how the hearing-impaired use sign language. You can also find out what aids are available, such as flashing lights instead of telephone bells or door bells. When communicating with hearing-impaired individuals, it is important that you:

■ speak clearly, listen carefully and respond to what is said to you

■ minimise any distractions, e.g. noisy television

■ make sure any aids to hearing are working

■ use written forms of communication that are appropriate

■ use signing, where appropriate, by involving a properly trained interpreter.

Evidence activity

3.4 Ineffective communication

Describe two examples of how ineffective communication may affect individuals.

3.5 Explaining how to access extra support or services to enable individuals to communicate effectively

If problems with communication are identified, there is a range of services which can be accessed. Never presume that you or anyone else can be heard, understood and responded to, without first thinking about the person involved. Ensure that you are supporting someone to communicate as effectively as possible by working with them to overcome as many challenges and barriers as possible. It may be necessary to access additional support or services to help make communication better, or clearer. People may have problems in communicating with others due to:

■ intellectual impairment leading to problems comprehending and processing information

■ sensory difficulties (hearing, vision)

■ problems in understanding social interaction (e.g. autism)

■ speech problems (e.g. articulation problems)

■ others not listening or not valuing what they are trying to communicate.

Many different professionals may be involved in this, but a person's motivation and efforts are equally important. Key experts likely to be encountered include speech and language therapists to help with communication problems, advocates, interpreters and clinical psychologists to help with problems affecting mental processes and emotions.

Health professionals need to:

- ■ take time and have patience
- ■ value what is being communicated
- ■ recognise non-verbal cues
- ■ find out about the person's alternative communication strategies if verbal communication is difficult (e.g. their typical non-verbal cues, use symbols, sign language)
- ■ explain things clearly in an appropriate way (verbally and with pictures etc.)
- ■ be prepared to meet the person several times to build up rapport and trust
- ■ use the knowledge and support of people's carers.

Research & investigate

(3.5) Support mechanisms

Think about the support mechanisms available. Carry out research into two of these and identify their key features.

LO4 Be able to apply principles and practices relating to confidentiality

(4.1) Explain the meaning of the term confidentiality

What is confidentiality?

Confidentiality means that personal and private information obtained from or about an individual must only be shared with others on a 'need-to-know' basis. Information given to a worker should not be disclosed without the person's informed permission. Confidentiality is an important principle in health and social care because it provides guidance on the amount of personal information and data that can be

disclosed without consent. A person disclosing personal information in a relationship of trust reasonably expects his or her privacy to be protected, i.e. they expect the information to remain confidential. The relationship between health and social care professionals and their patients/clients centres on trust, and trust is dependent on the patient/client being confident that personal information they disclose is treated confidentially.

However, confidentiality can be countered when there is a public interest in others being protected from harm.

Case Study

(4.1) Confidentiality

Ms X lives with her two children in a small market town. She is to have a minor operation and arrangements need to be made for the care of her children while she is in hospital and convalescing.

Arrangements for the care of the children are being discussed at a case conference by Ms X and the family's GP, social worker and health visitor. The elder child's school will be informed of the final arrangements. Various pieces of information are known to the four people at the case conference, although not each piece of information is known by each individual. The privacy of interests of Ms X, her children and their absent father may be different.

Here are some criteria that can influence whether or not information is disclosed or shared:

- ● confidence that the recipient of the data will handle it responsibly
- ● the need for consent to disclosure and respect for refusals to consent
- ● the accuracy, relevance, and pertinence of the data.

1. Can you think of any other considerations?

   It is not always easy to decide which pieces of information should be shared. Consider the following:

   contd.

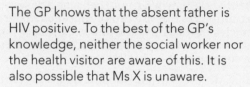

Case Study *contd.*

The GP knows that the absent father is HIV positive. To the best of the GP's knowledge, neither the social worker nor the health visitor are aware of this. It is also possible that Ms X is unaware.

2. In these particular circumstances, should the GP share this information with the following people, and why?

   (a) Ms X

   (b) the health visitor

   (c) the social worker

3. As a health or social care professional it is vital that you apply the principles of confidentiality. Inappropriate disclosure of information can have a significant negative impact on people's lives. What could be the impact of disclosure in this situation?

4.2 Ways to maintain confidentiality in day-to-day communication

Maintaining confidentiality

Maintaining confidentiality is a very important aspect of building trust between a client and a worker. Without trust, communication is less likely to progress between two or more people. This involves honouring commitments and declaring conflicts of interest. It also means making sure that the policy which relates to ways of communicating with people is followed.

The right to confidentiality means that a person's notes must not be left lying around or stored insecurely (e.g. left in a car). Computerised information relating to the person should only be accessed by those who have the authority to do so, so it should be password protected and the password given only to authorised staff. Conversations with clients should not be so loud that others can hear and, if the content of the conversation is personal, the interaction should be in a room where others are not present and the door is closed. People have the right not to be spoken about in such a way that they can be identified.

There are occasions when a worker may have to break confidentiality. Such situations arise when:

- a person is likely to harm themselves
- a person is likely to harm others
- a child or vulnerable adult has suffered, or is at risk of suffering, significant harm
- a person has been, or is likely to be, involved in a serious crime

It must also be remembered that other professional workers will need to have specific information on a need-to-know basis and, in these circumstances, information may have to be passed to others.

Ways to maintain confidentiality

- Safe storage of information so that people who should not see the information cannot gain access to it.
- The use of passwords for computer logon.
- Only giving information on a need-to-know basis.
- Not passing on information without the relevant permission.
- Only using the information for the intended and agreed purpose.
- Adhering to relevant legislation relating to data protection and accessing personal files.

The most common ways in which confidentiality can be breached

- Notes left in an unattended area.
- Failure to ask whether information may be disclosed to others.
- Discussions in public areas about service users.
- Failure to log off the computer system.
- Allowing others to know and use your password.
- Leaving information on a VDU screen which can be seen by the public.
- Failure to establish a person's identity before giving them information.
- Holding conversations, including on the telephone, in a public area.
- Leaving personal and private information in a car.

Evidence activity

(4.2) Maintaining confidentiality

A client's cousin has telephoned from Australia asking for an update on their family member's health. They say that due to the distance, they will not be able to get over to visit for a long time so they should be given the information.

What action do you take and why?

Legal requirements

The approach of courts of law to record keeping tends to be that 'if it is not recorded, it has not been done'. Workers across the sectors have both a professional and a legal duty of care to their clients, so their record keeping should be able to demonstrate:

■ a full account of their assessment and the care that has been planned and provided

■ relevant information about the condition of the patient/client at any given time

■ the measures taken by the worker to respond to their needs

■ evidence that the worker has understood and honoured their duty of care, that all reasonable steps have been taken to care for the patient/client and that any actions or omissions on the part of the worker have not compromised their safety in any way

■ a record of any arrangements that have been made for the continuing care of a patient/client.

Organisational policies

All organisations have their own policies and procedures regarding recording and reporting of information to make sure that all practitioners observe the regulations that apply to them. Confidentiality is an essential component of an accessible service. Some users of services bring issues with them and provide personal details in order for practitioners to help them. By being assured that their information is going to be recorded, stored and shared appropriately, individuals feel more able to disclose information that they may not have been previously happy to discuss. Some people feel intimidated by, or reluctant to talk about, their issues. Young people, refugees and offenders, for example, may feel especially vulnerable.

Users of services need reassurance that they will not be judged, and that anything they tell workers will not be shared with others without the client's knowledge and consent. The few exceptions to this are usually outlined in the policies the organisation follows. In order for policies to operate successfully, there needs to be commitment from all the staff.

Many different organisational policies refer to responsibility in relation to recording and reporting of information, including:

■ Confidentiality Policies

■ Health and Well-being Policies

■ Information Governance Policies

■ Health and Safety Policies

■ Child Protection Policies

■ Assessment, Recording and Reporting Policies

■ Codes of Conduct and National Standards Frameworks relating to practitioners across the sectors, which also apply within organisations.

Research & investigate

(4.2) Confidentiality procedures

Select a source user group and find out the confidentiality precedures which apply.

Meet the needs of individuals

Only information required to meet the individual's specific needs should be recorded and reported. Information that is not relevant should not be recorded at all. For example financial information would not be relevant to a patient who has been admitted to hospital for an operation; however, it may be needed to determine an individual's ability to pay for adult social care services. Information describing personal characteristics such as age, gender, disability, ethnicity, religion and sexual orientation should only be used to support the provision of high-quality care to meet individual needs. This information can be used to meet the requirements of legislation, regulations and policies and to demonstrate good practice.

The Caldicott Principles were developed for the NHS in relation to the recording and sharing of personal information. These principles can easily be applied to any organisation or setting. The Caldicott Standards are based on the Data Protection Act 1998 principles.

The Caldicott Principles

1. Justify the purpose(s) of using confidential information

Every proposed use or transfer of patient-identifiable information within or from an organisation should be clearly defined and scrutinised, with continuing uses regularly reviewed by an appropriate guardian.

2. Do not use patient-identifiable information unless it is absolutely necessary

Patient-identifiable information items should not be included unless it is essential for the specified purpose(s) of that flow. The need for patients to be identified should be considered at each stage of satisfying the purpose(s).

3. Use the minimum necessary patient-identifiable information that is required

Where use of the patient-identifiable information is considered to be essential, the inclusion of each individual item of information should be considered and justified so that the minimum amount of identifiable information is transferred or accessible as is necessary for a given function to be carried out.

4. Access to patient-identifiable information should be on a strict need-to-know basis

Only those individuals who need access to patient-identifiable information should have access to it, and they should only have access to the information items that they need to see. This may mean introducing access controls or splitting information flows where one information flow is used for several purposes.

5. Everyone with access to patient-identifiable information should be aware of their responsibilities

Action should be taken to ensure that those handling patient-identifiable information – both clinical and non-clinical staff – are made fully aware of their responsibilities and obligations to respect patient confidentiality.

6. Understand and comply with the law

Every use of patient-identifiable information must be lawful. Someone in each organisation handling patient information should be responsible for ensuring that the organisation complies with the legal requirements.

Caldicott Guardians are senior staff in the NHS and social services appointed to protect patient information to ensure that it is used for the purposes intended, meeting the individual needs of the patients in their care.

Evidence activity

4.2 The Caldicott Principles

What is the impact of the Caldicott Principles on service delivery?

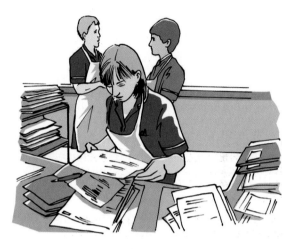

Figure 1.9

Procedures and practices

Across the sectors there are different procedures and practices that may be expected to be followed within each organisation.

Every organisation must have a policy that explains the procedures to be followed for sharing information. The policy should clearly state:

■ which senior managers have the responsibility to decide about disclosing information

■ what to do when action is required urgently

■ how to make sure that information will only be used for the purpose for which it is required

■ procedures to be followed to obtain manual records

■ procedures to be followed to access computer records

■ arrangements for reviewing the procedures.

Relevant legislation relating to data protection, accessing personal files and medical records

Data Protection Act 1998

Data Protection Act 1998 governs access to the health records of living people. It became effective from 1 March 2000, and superseded the Data Protection Act 1984 and the Access to Health Records Act 1990, though the Access to Health Records Act 1990 still governs access to the health records of deceased people. The Data Protection Act 1998 gives every living person the right to apply for access to their health records.

The Data Protection Act protects people's rights to confidentiality and covers both paper and electronic records. The act provides individuals with a range of rights, including:

■ the right to know what information is held on them and to see and correct this information

■ the right to refuse to provide information

■ the right that data held should be accurate and up to date

■ the right that data held should not be kept for longer than is necessary

■ the right to confidentiality – information should not be accessible to unauthorised people.

The Data Protection Act 1998 is not confined to health records held for the purposes of the National Health Service (NHS). It applies equally to the private health sector and to health professionals' private practice records. It also applies to the records of employers who hold information relating to the physical or mental health of their employees, if the record has been made by or on behalf of a health professional in connection with the care of the employee.

Access to Medical Reports Act 1988

This Act gives guidelines covering requests from employers or insurance companies wanting medical reports on individuals. For example, the individual's specific consent has to be given before a medical report can be written for employment or insurance purposes. The individual also has the right to see the report before it is passed to the employer or insurance company; they can then request alterations to be made and refuse permission for the report to be sent. For example, a GP could not give information about an individual's medical history to an insurance company without a consent form signed by the individual stating that they agree to their personal information being given. The consent form would include a statement saying that the individual did or did not want to see the report before it was sent to the insurance company.

Other legislation

Other appropriate legislation may include:

■ Crime and Disorder Act 1998

■ Criminal Procedures and Investigations Act

■ Human Rights Act 1998

■ Freedom of Information Act 2000

■ Children Act 2004

4.3 The potential tension between maintaining an individual's confidentiality and disclosing concerns

English common law makes provision for a confidential relationship and the duty of confidence. The Data Protection Act 1998 and Human Rights Act 1998 have introduced enforceable rights for service users about how the information they provide is used. The Data Protection Act has restrictions on storing personal data in all formats, written and electronic. The Human Rights Act 1998 emphasises respect for private life and strengthens the hand of those advocating increased privacy for the individual. Due to these Acts and the duty of confidentiality there is a potential conflict between protecting the privacy and confidentiality of individuals and protecting the public, and a duty of care to the service user.

Confidentiality can be breached:

■ To protect children at risk of significant harm as defined by the Children Act 1989.

■ To protect the public from acts of terrorism as defined in the Prevention of Terrorism Act 1971.

■ As a duty to the Courts.

■ Under the Drug Trafficking Offences Act 1986.

■ Section 115 of the Crime and Disorder Act 1998 gives public bodies the power, but not a duty, to disclose information for the prevention or detection of crime.

■ To ensure the service provides a duty of care in a life-threatening situation, for example serious illness or injury, suicide and self-harming behaviour. This includes when a service user continues to drive against medical advice when unfit to do so. In such circumstances relevant information should be disclosed to the medical advisor of the Driver and Vehicle Licensing Agency, without delay.

■ To protect the service provider in a life-threatening situation, for example calls to police regarding a violent service user. There is government guidance about the issue of violence against staff, which can be accessed via the Department of Health website. **www.doh.gov.uk/violencetaskforce**

Research & investigate

 (4.3) Maintaining confidentiality

Find out about tensions there may be when maintaining confidentiality in a specific setting of your choosing.

What procedures need to be followed and why?

Risks involved in information sharing

Whenever and wherever information is shared there are always going to be **risks** involved, whether the information is shared verbally or in written format.

Key term

Risks, in this context, are things that may cause loss of or damage to information.

Risks to individuals

Information could be passed on to people who should not have access to it. If unauthorised people gained access to the personal details, medical or financial information this could be used fraudulently by others. The identity of the individual could be used by someone else to take money from them or to pretend they are the individual for a variety of reasons. The individual could be put at risk themselves. The information may not be passed on accurately and this could result in their welfare or care needs not being met.

When to disclose confidential information, what to disclose and who to

When information is shared, the full details surrounding the collection of the information may not be explicit. Practitioners receiving the information may not fully understand the individual's circumstances. There could be confusion over when it is appropriate to share confidential information, how much of the information can be shared and who the information should be shared with. Ethical dilemmas can create issues in this way, for example when a 15 year old goes to see her GP because she is pregnant, should the girl's parents be informed? Services should include guidance on this in their confidentiality policy to ensure that all workers are following the same procedures and are absolutely clear about these issues.

Risks to practitioners

Practitioners may not understand the information that has been shared and could make mistakes. The accuracy of the information shared may lead to misinterpretation by the practitioner which could mean they cannot carry out their role effectively, such as when and where to provide the care required. Practitioners may, inadvertently, break confidentiality without realising what they have done by including too much detail in the information they share or, when receiving information, sharing it with others who did not need to know.

Importance of accuracy of records

All records that are kept must be accurate, as others may need to use them and mistakes can be made as a result of the wrong information being recorded. Workers should always read through the information they have recorded to check that it is accurate. There are a number of reasons why accuracy is particularly important:

It may be a legal document

A legal document may be required to be used as evidence in a court of law. If the information is not accurate the evidence recorded could cause many issues. For example, if it were to be used for criminal proceedings, the person may not be able to be prosecuted or, if there was a claim that malpractice had been carried out in the care provided to an individual, the records may not support the evidence given and a worker could be sued, when in fact they had not done anything wrong.

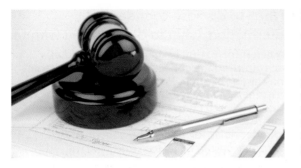

Figure 1.10

If it is a medical record

Medical records have to be accurate to ensure that the needs of the individual are met. When an individual sees a care professional regarding their medical care, the records of their previous treatment and care may need to be referred to to ensure that any changes or progression of their care meets their needs. This may not be possible if there are any inaccuracies in the records that have been made. It is also important to remember that individuals have the right to see their medical records under the Access to Medical Records Act and may be annoyed if the information is not accurate or points have been made that are insensitive or judgmental.

Misinterpretation of illegible drug dosage could be fatal

On drugs charts used in hospitals and nursing homes the dosage the individual is prescribed must be accurate and legible. If this is not the case, individuals could easily be given too much of the medication which could have fatal consequences. Too little of the medication could result in their health deteriorating and their needs not being met.

Currency, accuracy, validity and reliability

All records that are kept should be current (up to date), accurate, valid and reliable.

Accuracy of information is essential to ensure that mistakes are not made and the needs of individuals are met. In health, up-to-date information about a patient's condition is crucial. In children and young people's care settings, accurate details of children's allergies might be essential. In adult social care, accurate contact information for next of kin may be necessary, and any care plan changes must be recorded clearly.

Assessment summary

Your reading of this chapter and completion of the activities will have prepared you to be able to engage in personal development in health, social care or children's and young people's settings.

To achieve the unit, your assessor will require you to:

Learning outcomes	Assessment Criteria
Learning outcome **1**: Show that you understand why effective communication is important in the work setting by:	(1.1) identifying the different reasons people communicate See Time to reflect 1.1, p. 2
	(1.2) explaining how communication affects relationships in the work setting See Evidence activity 1.2, p. 2 and p.4
Learning outcome **2**: Be able to meet the communication and language needs, wishes and preferences of individuals by:	(2.1) demonstrating how to establish the communication and language needs, wishes and preferences of individuals See Research activity 2.1, p. 5

Learning outcomes	Assessment Criteria
Learning outcome 2: Be able to meet the communication and language needs, wishes and preferences of individuals by:	(2.2) describing the factors to consider when promoting effective communication See Evidence activity 2.2, p. 6
	(2.3) demonstrating a range of communication methods and styles to meet individual needs See Evidence activity 2.3, p. 7
	(2.4) demonstrating how to respond to an individual's reactions when communicating See Evidence activity 2.4, p. 9 and 10
Learning outcome 3: Be able to overcome barriers to communication by:	(3.1) explaining how people from different backgrounds may use and/or interpret communication methods in different ways See Evidence activity 3.1, p. 12
	(3.2) identifying barriers to effective communication See Evidence activity 3.2, p. 13
	(3.3) demonstrating ways to overcome barriers to communication See Evidence activity 3.3, p. 15
	(3.4) demonstrating strategies that can be used to clarify misunderstandings See Evidence activity 3.4, p. 17
	(3.5) explaining how to access extra support or services to enable individuals to communicate effectively See Research and investigate activity 3.5, p. 18

Learning outcomes	Assessment Criteria
Learning outcome **4**: Be able to apply principles and practices relating to confidentiality by:	**(4.1)** explaining the meaning of the term confidentiality See Case study 4.1, p. 18
	(4.2) demonstrating ways to maintain confidentiality in day-to-day communication See Evidence activity 4.2, p. 20 and 21
	(4.3) describing the potential tension between maintaining an individual's confidentiality and disclosing concerns See Research activity 4.3, p. 23

Good luck!

Web links

Community Care	www.community-care.co.uk
Royal National Institute for the Deaf	www.rnid.org.uk
Royal National Institute of the Blind	www.rnib.org.uk
Social Care Sector Skills Council	**www.skillsforcare.org.uk**
Health Care Sector Skills Council	www.skillsforhealth.org.uk
Skills for Justice Sector Skills Council	www.skillsforjusticce.com

For Unit SHC 32

What are you finding out?

Personal development is not just to do with education or training and the development of skills and interests. It is also about developing a better understanding of yourself, your values, beliefs and experiences, and how they impact on your behaviour. And it is about learning what motivates you to learn, so that you can achieve your full potential.

Personal development is important because life without change would be a pretty dull existence. The thought of change can be unwelcome – 'I am quite comfortable as I am, thank you.' But in order to handle new challenges, achieve a better quality of life, become accomplished in our work, we need to move out of our comfort zone, reflect on our experiences and … change, even if it is just a minor adjustment. As Mark Twain said, 'Twenty years from now you will be more disappointed by the things you didn't do than by the ones you did do. So throw off the bowlines. Sail away from the safe harbour. Catch the trade winds in your sails. Explore. Dream. Discover.'

Personal development is stimulating and energising. It opens doors, in our personal lives and at work. The reading and activities in this chapter will help you to:

■ Understand what is required for competence in your work role

■ Reflect on your work practice

■ Be able to evaluate your performance at work

■ Be able to agree a personal development plan

■ Be able to use learning opportunities and reflective practice to contribute to personal development.

LO1 Understand what is required for competence in your work role

1.1 The duties and responsibilities of your work role

Work in the health and social care sector covers a multitude of job roles, from **ancillary workers** and office staff, such as domestics, electricians and receptionists, through to senior management, such as chief executives and owner-managers of private care providers. There is a multitude of organisations, professional journals and newspapers that describe job roles within health, social care and children's and young people's settings. Descriptions will include the entrance requirements for each role, such as qualifications, skills and personal qualities; the professional development and career pathways associated with job roles; hours of work and rates of pay, and so on.

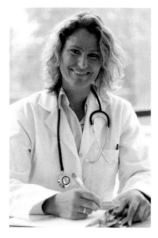

Figure 2.1 A multitude of job roles

Key term

Ancillary workers in health and social care are staff who do not provide hands-on care. Being responsible means being accountable for your actions and being prepared to improve.

The internet is a good starting point for exploring roles within the health and social care sectors. Websites you may find interesting include:

- healthcare careers:
www.connexions-direct.com/jobs4u

- social care and counselling:
www.connexions-direct.com/jobs4u

- Community Care:
www.communitycare.co.uk/jobs/search

- Skills for Health:
www.skillsforhealth.org.uk

- Skills for Care and Development:
www.skillsforcareanddevelopment.org.uk

- Directgov: www.direct.gov.uk

No doubt you applied for your current job role because the job description caught your eye and you thought you would enjoy the duties and responsibilities involved.

- Duties are the tasks or activities you are paid to carry out. They are listed in your job description and contract of employment.

Research & investigate

(1.1) Fancy a change?

- Think about a couple of jobs in a health or care setting that you'd like to be in now, instead of your current role. Research as much information as you need in order to decide whether either of the jobs would be appropriate for you, for example, you could search the internet or visit your local Connexions office or Jobcentre.

- What do you think? Are you suited for each or either role? Would you enjoy either or each of them?

- Responsibilities are to do with the qualities that underpin the way you work, for example that you are **responsible**, reliable, dependable, conscientious and trustworthy; that you conduct yourself as required and demonstrate respect, consideration and maturity; that you comply with policies, procedures and codes of practice as relevant to the care setting.

Evidence activity

(1.1) Duties and responsibilities of your work role

This activity enables you to demonstrate your knowledge of your own work role.

Write a job description for your work role, which outlines your duties and responsibilities.

Time to reflect

(1.1) How do you measure up?'

- Compare the job description that you wrote for Evidence activity 1.1 with the official description for your job role. How do they compare?

- Are you carrying out your duties as required, and do you conduct yourself in a responsible manner?

1.2 Expectations about your work role as expressed in relevant standards

The Care Quality Commission (CQC) is the health and social care regulator for England. Its aim is to ensure high-quality care for everyone in hospital, in a care home and at home, in other words that care:

- is safe

- has the right outcomes, for example that people get the right treatment and that they are well cared for

- is a good experience for the people who use it, their carers and their families

- helps to prevent illness and promotes healthy, independent living

- is available to those who need it when they need it

- provides good value for money.

Ofsted carries out a similar role to the CQC in that it regulates children and young people's care and education services in England.

People who use health and care services have a right to expect, and health and care service providers have a responsibility to deliver, high standards of care. One of the priorities of Ofsted and the CQC is to improve services by eliminating poor-quality care. It does this by inspecting services and comparing what it finds with the standards it expects. Inspection results and quality ratings are published, enabling service providers to compare their performance with others, to see where improvement is needed, and to learn from each other about what works best.
www.cqc.org.uk; www.ofsted.gov.uk

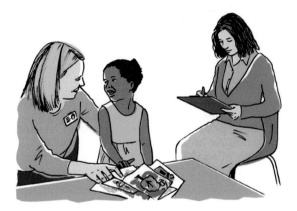

Figure 2.2 Inspection

In addition to the standards monitored by Ofsted and the CQC during inspections, the Care Standards Act 2000 requires providers of health and care services to ensure that care provision is fit for purpose and meets the assessed needs of people using the services. These requirements are written into national minimum standards (NMSs) by the Department of Health, for example, NMS for Independent Health Care, NMS for Care Homes for Older People and NMS for Children's Homes. Although NMSs are specific to individual health and care settings, all describe how a worker is expected to demonstrate competence in their work role.

Codes of practice set out the criteria against which providers are assessed by Ofsted and the CQC. They also describe the standards of conduct and practice within which workers must carry out their activities and ensure that what they do is competent and consistent with the values of their employer. Codes of practice are specific to work roles, for example, codes of practice for social care workers and employers (General Social Care Council, GSCC); codes or standards of conduct, performance and ethics for nurses and midwives (Nursing and

Midwifery Council, NMC), and the Code of Conduct and Practice for Registered Teachers (Greater Teaching Council for England, GTC). www.gscc.org.uk; www.nmc-uk.org; www.gtce.org.uk

National occupational standards (NOS) are benchmarks of performance and provide the means for assessing how well someone can do a job. They are work-related statements of the ability, knowledge, understanding and experience that an individual should have in order to carry out key tasks competently and effectively. The Health and Social Care (HSC) NOS and the Children's Care Learning and Development (CCLD) NOS have been compiled by the **Sector Skills Councils**: Skills for Care, Skills for Health, and the Children's Workforce Development Council.

Key term

Sector Skills Councils (SSC) are employer-led organisations that work to boost the skills of their sector workforces.

Research & investigate

1.2 Standards and best practice

1. Look at the most recent inspection report for your workplace. What is its overall quality rating?

2. In what ways does it suggest or expect the performance of your workplace to improve? How do these suggestions or expectations impact on your work role?

3. Sum up how the NMS for your work setting impact on your work role.

4. Sum up how the Codes of Practice for your work role impact on your work role.

5. What abilities, knowledge, understanding and experiences do the NOS for one of your key areas of work say you need to be able to carry it out competently and effectively?

Evidence activity

(1.2) Expectations of your work role

This activity enables you to demonstrate your understanding of the expectations of your own work role as expressed in relevant standards.

Identify three of your key duties and responsibilities. For each:

- describe how relevant national minimum standards, codes of practice and national occupational standards say you should perform your work

- explain why it is important to conform with the national minimum standards, codes of practice and national occupational standards.

LO2 Be able to reflect on practice

(2.1) The importance of reflective practice in continuously improving the quality of service you provide

Some of the most important personal development skills we can acquire are the ability to reflect on our actions and experiences, to learn from them and the ability to adapt our behaviour accordingly. These are of equal importance in a professional development scenario.

Reflective practice is the process that enables us to achieve a better understanding of ourselves, our knowledge and understanding, our skills and competencies, and workplace practices in general. It involves:

- thinking critically about our behaviour, i.e. the skills and competences with which we perform work activities and the personal beliefs and values that underpin our performance

- assessing how our behaviour impacts on our thoughts and feelings and on the thoughts and feelings of the individuals we work with

- evaluating whether that impact was good or bad, for example, was the activity an all-round success or did it provoke physical or emotional discomfort or dissatisfaction?

- reviewing how things might be done differently, for example, by having a different approach or carrying out activities in a different way

- planning for that change.

Engaging in critical reflective practice can be difficult. It challenges our comfortable assumptions about ourselves. However, it is very important for improving quality of service. Through reflective practice:

- We become more self-aware. Being self-aware goes hand-in-glove with having a raised awareness of others and an increased sensitivity to their needs and perception of how we care for them.

- We are able to identify problematic work practices, monitor standards and consider alternative approaches and activities in the pursuit of best practice.

- We have the opportunity to consider our and others' learning and development needs, thereby ensuring competent practice and improved quality of service.

- We have an opportunity to explore and deal with any negative feelings or anxieties associated with our work and, as a result, develop a more positive attitude and improved relationships.

Evidence activity

(2.1) The importance of reflective practice

This activity enables you to demonstrate your understanding of the importance of reflective practice in continuously improving the quality of service provided.

Explain why engaging in critical reflective practice is so important to your ability to continuously improve the quality of service you give to the people you work with.

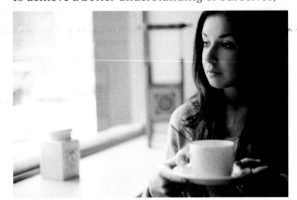

Figure 2.3 Reflection

Demonstrate the ability to reflect on your practice

There are two main types of reflection:

1. Reflection *on* action is reflecting on an activity after it has happened. Reflecting *on* action allows you to learn from what has happened – learning from experience. For reflection *on* action to make any difference to your practice, you have to make a commitment to *take action* as a result. In other words, you have to be prepared to move out of your comfort zone!

2. Reflection *in* action is reflecting on an activity while it is happening. Reflecting *in* action allows you to make changes to an activity while it is happening, usually because something unexpected or unwanted happens. Reflection *in* action requires you to think on your feet, quickly – learning on the job.

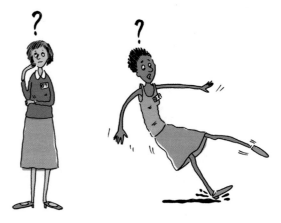

Figure 2.4 Reflection on action and reflection in action

Practice activity

2.2 The ability to reflect on your practice

This activity gives you an opportunity to practise demonstrating your ability to reflect on your work practice.

Identify an activity that you carried out recently. Complete the table below to show that you are developing the skills of reflective practice.

Activity: _____	
Area to reflect on:	Your reflections:
1. Think critically about your behaviour while carrying out the activity, for example: What were you doing? What were you trying to achieve? How were you feeling when you started the activity? What were you thinking about at the time? What influenced the way you did the activity? Where were you? Why were you in that place? Who else was there? What were they doing?	
2. Assess the impact of your behaviour, for example: How did the activity make you feel? How did the activity make you behave? Why did you behave as you did? What were the consequences of your behaviour for yourself? What were the consequences of your behaviour for others? How did others feel? How do you know this?	*contd.*

Practice activity *contd.*

Area to reflect on:	Your reflections:
3. Evaluate the impact that the activity had, for example: Did the activity achieve what it was meant to achieve? What went well? What did you do well? What did others do well? What went wrong or did not turn out as it should have done? In what way did you or others contribute to this? Whose interests seem to be served by the way the activity was carried out?	
4. Review how the activity could be changed, for example: Could you have done things differently? Could others have done things differently? How else could the activity be carried out? What would be the consequences of making these changes?	
5. Plan for change, for example: How will you carry out the activity next time?	

2.3 Describe how your values, belief systems and experiences may affect your working practice

We ascribe a value to something that we respect and admire or that we feel has worth. Tangible things like cars and jewellery have an economic value. On the other hand, we also appreciate less tangible things, such as qualities like health and happiness, and family and friends we hold dear –even though we cannot put a price on qualities and people, we value them. Values are very personal – different people value the same thing differently.

A belief system is a set of beliefs, ideas and principles about what is right and wrong, true or false. Like values, beliefs, ideas and principles are very personal. One person's religious and political beliefs will be different from another's; their ideas about, for example, how to dress, what to eat and how to behave, will vary; and their principles or views about what is right and wrong, just and decent, will also differ. Our belief systems underpin the way we live.

Everyone has a unique identity because of the unique mix of personal and social factors that make them who they are. Genetic influences contribute to our physical make-up and, to a certain extent, our personalities, likes and dislikes and so on, but social factors, in

particular our experiences, have a significant effect on who we are and the way we view life. Despite their identical genetic make-up, even identical twins have a different take on life because of their different experiences.

You are unlikely to agree with the values and belief systems of all the people you work with, and you will not share many of their experiences. However, best practice involves putting your own values, beliefs and experiences to one side and respecting, promoting and responding positively to those of the people you work with. Allowing your own values, beliefs and experiences to influence the way you work with people will prevent you seeing them as individuals and taking their individual needs into account. A lack of respect for others' values, beliefs and experiences threatens their right to fair treatment, and a disregard for their individual needs is neglect.

Time to reflect

(2.3) Who do you think you are?

1. Think about a time when you felt that you had been unfairly judged, perhaps ridiculed for your beliefs, questioned about your sense of value or made to think that your experiences didn't count for anything. How did this treatment make you feel?

2. Now think about whether, in your personal life, you ever judge people unfairly because of their values, beliefs and experiences.

   - Why do you treat them unfairly?

   - Do you think you have any right to judge people like this?

   - How do you think you would have made them feel?

   - How could you change the way you treat people who have values and beliefs with which you do not agree or who have different experiences from you?

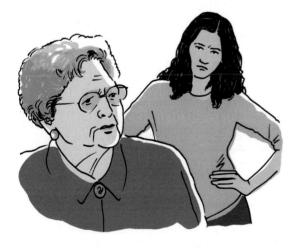

Figure 2.5 Respect? What's that?

Case Study

(2.3) Dorothy and Jessica

Dorothy is an elderly resident at the care home where Jessica works. She has a wealth of life experiences – she served as a nurse during World War II (WWII) and not only had the opportunity to nurse a number of very interesting people, but also got to travel through Europe. She has been a committed Christian since her early childhood, which she spent in South East Asia where her mother and father were missionaries. Her husband was killed in action during WWII and as a consequence, and much to her disappointment, she has no children. She is also a staunch Conservative.

Jessica is 23 years old. She worked in a supermarket when she first left school, but the proximity of the care home to where she lives and the opportunity to swap shifts suits her better as it allows her, as a single parent, to play a more active role in bringing up her little boy. She is divorced from her husband because of the pressure he put on her to conform to his cultural background, including to embrace his religion and social customs. She has no religious beliefs but, because of her father's influence, is a loyal trade unionist.

Jessica doesn't enjoy working with Dorothy. She has no time for her 'happy clappy sermonising' and stories about what she got up to in the war, and makes unkind remarks about her politics and the reasons she doesn't have any children. As a result, Dorothy feels lonely and neglected; she has no confidence in Jessica as a care worker and is frustrated and angered by her lack of respect.

1. What do you think lies behind Jessica's unkind treatment of Dorothy?

2. How might the tensions between the two women be resolved?

Evidence activity

(2.3) The effect of values, beliefs and experiences

This activity gives you an opportunity to demonstrate your knowledge of how your values, belief systems and experiences may affect your working practice.

Identify two or three individuals with whom you work whose values, beliefs and experiences are different from your own.

1. In what ways are their values, beliefs and experiences different from yours?

2. Describe how you respond to them as a consequence and how your response impacts on your ability to work with them to meet their needs.

LO3 Be able to evaluate own performance

 ### (3.1) Evaluate your own knowledge, performance and understanding against relevant standards

As you read in the introduction to this chapter, personal development is not just to do with education or training and the development of skills. However, development in these areas is very important if you are to become a knowledgeable, competent and insightful worker and hope to make your way up the career ladder.

How would you assess your knowledge, performance and understanding at the moment? Obviously you feel it is in need of developing or you wouldn't be reading this! To someone who doesn't work in the health and care sector or use its services, you might already appear to be rather clever. Complimentary though that may be, it is not a valid measure of your abilities. In order to show that you are indeed knowledgeable, competent and insightful, you need to meet the standards set by the various organisations that have an interest in boosting the skills of the health and care sector workforces.

Case Study

(3.1) Charlotte

Charlotte Brown recently started working as a domestic at Tiny Tots Playgroup because, according to her mother, 'She absolutely loves children, is so good with them, she's always buying them presents – they love her to bits.'

1. Do you think Mrs Brown's assessment of her daughter's performance has any value? Explain your answer.

2. How would you suggest that Charlotte evaluate her performance?

As you will remember, standards describe what is expected of a worker regarding their knowledge, understanding, conduct and competence. Whichever setting you work in, be it health, social care or with children and young people, there are national minimum standards, codes of practice and national occupational standards setting out the standards that are required and expected of you at work and, indeed, by which you can measure yourself.

It is important that you do measure or monitor your knowledge, understanding, conduct and competence, for your own personal and professional development and also for the health, safety and well-being of the people you work with. To do this, you need regularly to reflect on and evaluate:

■ your knowledge and understanding, for example, are you confident that you have a clear and up-to-date knowledge and understanding of: codes of practice and legal issues that apply to your work; your level of responsibility and to whom you are **accountable**; what you are expected to do, why you have to do it, when and who with? And are you clear about the degree of **autonomy** you have for managing you own activities?

■ your attitudes and behaviour, and how they impact on your work and the people you are working with

■ your values, beliefs and experiences, and whether they affect your work and the people you are working with

■ your skills, how safely and effectively you use them and whether they need improving

■ the outcome or results of the activities you carry out.

Key terms

Being accountable means having to answer to someone for your actions.
Autonomy means being independent and self-reliant.

Practice activity

(3.1) Self-evaluation

This activity enables you to practise evaluating your knowledge, performance and understanding against relevant standards.

In Evidence activity 1.2 you were asked to describe how relevant NMSs, codes of practice and NOS say you should carry out three of your key duties and responsibilities. Build on your learning from that activity by evaluating or assessing how well you perform these duties and responsibilities in terms of your knowledge and understanding of them and your competence or ability at carrying them out.

1. Does your knowledge, performance and understanding meet the expectations of the standards? If so, how?

2. Is there room for improvement? In what ways?

(3.2) Demonstrate the use of feedback to evaluate your performance and inform your development

You read above that it is important for you to regularly reflect on and evaluate your performance. It is also a good idea to seek feedback from others, including your line manager or supervisor, colleagues, other professionals, the individuals you work with and their friends and family. Feedback from others is useful because they can offer a viewpoint on your work that you may not see for yourself.

Your line manager or supervisor is a very important source of feedback as they are ultimately responsible for your work and conduct. Feedback from a line manager or supervisor should happen during appraisal and should be constructive, that is, positive and helpful. Negative feedback is destructive and doesn't promote personal development and change. Appraisals are an opportunity for you to reflect on your work practice and behaviour, talk about your strengths and plan for change in areas that are weak and need developing. You will read about personal development plans later.

Feedback from colleagues and other professionals is equally important and usually takes place on the job, perhaps over a coffee, or at any time when it is appropriate to make a comment on or discuss your performance. Welcome feedback, ask for it, and accept any criticism with a positive attitude to show that you are intent on doing your best and learning from your mistakes. Having a positive attitude and being willing to learn will encourage you to reflect on what you have been told. It will also help you deal with any negative comments and complaints and keep them in perspective.

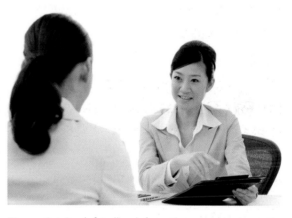

Figure 2.6 Seek feedback from the people you work with

Feedback from the people you work with is probably the most important advice to take on board. Your relationship with them is a partnership, and partnership working demands a mutual show of respect. However, in order to receive respect you have to demonstrate that you value other people's opinions, choices and suggestions about the way you support and care for them. Encourage their respect for you by seeking feedback about your performance and behaviour and actively listening to what they have to say.

As with reflective practice, for feedback to make any difference to your practice, you have to be prepared to act on it and make changes. Think about the feedback you are given. You may not agree with the changes you are asked to make, for example you may be asked to do something in a way that you feel is inappropriate, is not within your level of responsibility or would compromise health and safety. In situations like this, talk with your supervisor or line manager. However, most feedback will be positive and changes you are asked to make will be well within your capability.

Practice activity

3.2 **Demonstrate use of feedback to evaluate your performance and inform your development**

This activity enables you to practice using feedback to evaluate your performance and inform your development

Ask your superior/line manager, a colleague and an individual with whom you work for feedback on two or three aspects of your work. Think carefully about what they tell you.

■ What changes do you think you need to make in response to their feedback that would promote your development? Are you able to make these changes? If yes, how will they enhance your performance and promote your development?

■ If you're not able to make the changes requested, why not? How should you deal with this feedback?

LO4 Be able to agree a personal development plan

4.1 **Identify sources of support for planning and reviewing your development**

Personal development planning is a process that involves reflecting on your knowledge, understanding, attitudes and behaviour, work practice and achievements, and planning for your personal and career development. It aims to help you understand what and how you are

learning, and to review, plan and take responsibility for your own development. Personal development planning will help you:

■ become a more effective, independent and confident learner

■ understand how you learn and apply your learning to different situations, thereby developing in your job role, both as a person and a practitioner

■ set personal goals and evaluate and review your progress towards achieving them

■ develop a positive attitude to learning and self-development throughout your life.

Personal development planning is a structured and supported process. You read earlier that it is wise to seek feedback from others because they can offer a perspective on your work that you may not see for yourself. Similarly, it is a good idea to seek support from others when you are planning and reviewing your development.

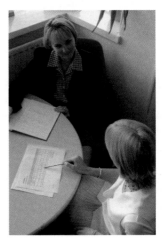

Figure 2.7 Formal supervision

There are a number of support systems, both formal and informal, set up specially to help you plan and review your development. Supervision is something which you are probably very familiar with. Appraisals and performance reviews are an example of formal supervision in that they are planned, carried out according to official workplace policy and conducted in private. They are an opportunity for you and your line manager or supervisor to get together to:

■ assess your performance against relevant standards and agreed **outcome-based performance indicators**

■ discuss your knowledge, understanding and achievements, including what you have learnt and achieved since your last appraisal/review, your personal attitudes and conduct, and your learning and personal development needs

■ exchange views about your work practices – your strengths and how you can improve; your concerns and how they might be dealt with; how you would like your career to develop; what you need to do to further your development and the support you need to meet your professional development needs

■ agree a date for a further get together, to ensure that your development is continuously reviewed.

Key term

Outcome-based performance indicators are a method of measuring the degree to which outcomes are achieved.

Research & investigate

4.1 Formal supervision in your workplace

Check out how often formal supervision (appraisal or performance review) should take place at your workplace, when and where your next appraisal or performance review will take place, and who will carry it out with you.

To be successful, appraisals and performance reviews should be used as the basis for making and reviewing your personal development plan. You will read about personal development plans shortly.

Informal supervision, while not quite as structured as appraisals and performance reviews, is a very useful source of support. Informal supervision takes place on the job, by someone who is trained in supervisory skills or who has the relevant experience. The role of your supervisor is to observe your performance, assess your knowledge and understanding and make recommendations about your learning and development needs in a relaxed but professional manner. For informal supervision to be effective, you need to be open to and prepared to act on suggestions and criticism; but you also need to feel comfortable with any comments and suggestions you receive about how to change. If you have any concerns at all about what your supervisor requests of you, you must talk things through and seek alternative ways of moving forward.

Other important sources of support for personal development within your workplace include the individuals and colleagues you work with on a

day-to-day basis. They will be aware of your skills and developmental needs and happy to help you develop your care and team-working skills if they know you will accept their support with a positive attitude and act on their advice. If, however, you are antagonistic to criticism and respond with belligerence, they will think twice before giving any advice, however thoughtful their intentions.

Time to reflect

4.1 How do you respond?

Think about the last two or three times you were given feedback on your attitude, behaviour or performance.

● How did you respond?

● Why did you respond in that way?

● Do you think you need to change the way you respond to feedback?

Your organisation may employ a Staff Development Officer, who can map your development needs with appropriate training courses and opportunities for **mentoring** and **coaching**. It may employ a training officer or an NVQ assessor, each of whom have a responsibility to help you assess your learning and development needs and support you in having them met. You may also have a colleague who is a trade union learning representative, whose function is to refer you to appropriate learning opportunities. And, of course, staying knowledgeable about your duties and responsibilities and the standards and codes of practice that relate to your job role will ensure that you constantly assess and review your performance and think about ways to develop.

Key terms

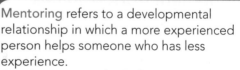

Mentoring refers to a developmental relationship in which a more experienced person helps someone who has less experience.
Coaching is a method of directing, instructing and training a person or group of people, to help them achieve some goal or develop specific skills.
Introspection means examining your own thoughts and feelings.

Sources of support for planning and reviewing your development outside of your workplace include organisations, such as: Connexions, which supports young people living in England who want advice on getting to where they want to be in life; your local College of Further Education, which will assess your current skills and abilities and refer you to a learning programme that will meet both your personal and career development needs; websites, such as Connexions and the Careers Advice Service, many of which can help you self-assess your current circumstances.
www.connexions-direct.com;
www.careersadvice.direct.gov.uk

There is no excuse for sitting there and letting the world pass you by! Do not be disappointed in 20 years by the things you do not do now.

Evidence activity

 Identifying sources of support

This activity enables you to demonstrate your knowledge of sources of support for planning and reviewing your development.

Make a list of the supervision and support systems, both at and outside your workplace, which you can access to help you plan and review your personal and professional development.

4.2 Demonstrate how to work with others to review and prioritise your learning needs, professional interests and development opportunities

Planning and reviewing our personal development alone can be quite difficult. For example, routine work practices can become a habit and we do not consider them in terms of our strengths and weaknesses. We may not realise that our knowledge falls short of what it should be. How can we know that there is more to learn unless it is pointed out to us? Facing up to our shortcomings can cause anxiety, especially if we didn't achieve at school and were made to feel a failure. You should avoid such **introspection** at all costs. And although planning is key to achievement, some of us just

aren't planners – we are happy to take what life throws at us without any thought for the future.

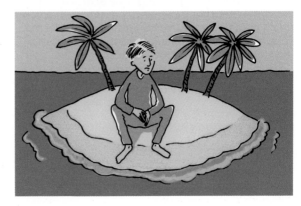

Figure 2.8 No man is an island

In the previous section you read about some of the support systems available to help you develop. Hopefully you can see the benefit of using support for this purpose. This section aims to show you how to work with other people to review and prioritise your learning needs, professional interests and development opportunities.

Your own reflective practice and feedback from your line manager, supervisor, colleagues and the individuals you work with should, if you are receptive to criticism, identify a wealth of areas for improvement. It is important to know that that 'criticism' and 'needing to improve' do not necessarily mean that your current learning and performance is poor. There is always room for improvement: even brain surgeons and astrophysicists can do better! However, to prevent being swamped by a sea of changes, it is important to be able to prioritise your learning and development needs, in other words, to first address those that are most in need of improvement.

Sometimes it is obvious in which direction you need to develop, and prioritising learning and development needs is easy. For example, if your half-yearly appraisal indicates that you lack knowledge and understanding about dementia care, but the majority of people you work with are not affected, and that you still do not follow health and safety procedures, despite agreeing six months ago that you would follow them to the letter, it would seem obvious that your priority would be to put H&S procedures into practice without delay. If you do not do this, there could be an accident and your employment might be terminated. Or should your priority be to improve your knowledge and understanding about dementia care? After all, the population is ageing and the number of people presenting with **Alzheimer's disease** is rapidly increasing.

Key term

Alzheimer's disease is a progressive disease that affects the brain and causes dementia. An advocate is someone who speaks up on behalf of an individual so that their views are heard, their rights promoted and any problems they have can be solved.

As this example demonstrates, prioritising can be difficult, and personal development pathways are often dictated by the needs of the workplace and the people using its services. However, all development is valuable, so be willing to develop in ways that you perhaps weren't expecting, and be receptive to development opportunities which you hadn't given much thought to. Explore. Dream. Discover!

Research & investigate

(4.2) Staff development in your workplace

Check out the priorities that your workplace has for staff development.

Why has it prioritised staff development in this way?

Willingness to learn and improve is key to personal development, but sometimes it is easier to show willing in a private, supportive appraisal situation than it is to the individuals and colleagues and other professionals who you work with on a day-to-day basis. As you read earlier, these people will be very conscious of your strengths and weaknesses – your practices and behaviours have a first-hand impact on them. But if you are on the defensive and antagonised by their judgment of you, they will be deterred from pointing out areas of your practice that need particular attention, potentially holding back your development, not to mention jeopardising your relationship with them.

Finally, do not forget the family and friends of the people you work with and any **advocates** that speak on their behalf. They have a wide-ranging knowledge and understanding of the people you work with and are therefore in an excellent position to let you know whether you are meeting their needs appropriately and which areas of your practice need especial attention.

Practice activity

(4.2) Demonstrate how to work with others to review and prioritise own learning needs, professional interests and development opportunities

This activity enables you to practice demonstrating how to work with others to review and prioritise your learning needs, professional interests and development opportunities.

Identify 3 people who you know would be willing to give you feedback on your performance at work. They should include at least one individual with whom you work and one colleague.

- Ask them what they think you need to prioritise as regards development of your skills, knowledge, attitude and behaviour, the way you do your work.

- Ask them what development opportunities they think you might benefit from, for example learning programmes and training courses you might undertake, mentoring or coaching.

- Now reflect on the way you responded to their comments and suggestions. Were you a willing or a reluctant listener? Did you take on board what they said with good grace or were you on the defensive?

- If you were unenthusiastic about their comments and suggestions, why? Does this mean that you aren't prepared to engage in personal development, that you have no ambition? On the other hand, if you heard them out with good grace, well done!]

(4.3) Demonstrate how to work with others to agree your personal development plan

Your personal development plan (PDP) is the document that identifies your present situation regarding your learning and understanding, competences, attitudes and behaviour. It identifies your expectations and ambitions for the future and plans how you might fulfil them and reach your full potential. So far, the aim of this chapter has been to encourage you to reflect on your practice, and to alert you to the people and systems available to support you in reviewing your development and prioritising your learning needs. This section looks at how you can use that information to agree your own personal development plan.

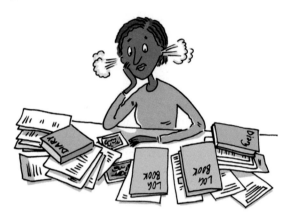

Figure 2.9 Preparing to agree your PDP

You are most likely to draw up your PDP with the support of your line manager during an appraisal or performance review. Planning for such a meeting is an opportunity for you to show responsibility for your own development and your capacity to reflect and plan. Therefore, before the meeting, consider and be prepared to discuss the following points:

■ what you do now , what you enjoy doing and what you and others think you do well

■ what you do not enjoy doing and how you and others think you could improve

■ your ambitions and expectations, including how you would like to develop in your role

■ what you think you need to learn and what development opportunities you need to access in order to develop in your role, improve your practice, fulfil your expectations and achieve your ambitions

■ how you think this learning and development could be achieved, including any support and guidance you think you would need

■ when you would like to have completed the learning.

Having celebrated your strengths and explored the learning and development opportunities available to you, you can start to plan. Planning involves setting goals, for example, to demonstrate competence in the use of health and safety procedures, or to improve your knowledge and understanding about dementia care. Goals are relatively long term – it might take a couple of months to brush up on H&S procedures and a couple more to demonstrate convincingly that you use them effectively; a dementia care learning programme might involve six months of study. Sometimes it can be difficult to commit to self-development that does not have immediate results.

Goals become less overwhelming and are more easily achieved if they are broken down into smaller, shorter-term sub-goals or objectives. An objective describes a short-term, specific, measurable, achievable and realistic outcome within a period of time that is moving toward achieving the long-term goal. Smart, intelligent planning for development uses SMART objectives:

■ Specific – setting specific, well-defined objectives helps you to know exactly what is expected of you, and helps your line manager to monitor and assess your development.

■ Measurable – objectives need to be to be measurable, otherwise how would you know whether you had achieved them?

■ Achievable – there is no point in planning an objective if it is not within your capabilities or if time and personal constraints will not allow you to follow it up. Do not set yourself up to fail!

■ Realistic – objectives need to be realistic, relevant and reasonable, in other words they should support or underpin the development you wish to achieve. They should also be rewarding and enjoyable.

■ Time specific – objectives need to have timescales. Time constraints give you a boundary or time limit in which to achieve the objective. They add an appropriate sense of urgency and help you measure your achievement.

Having planned your objectives, you need to discuss and agree any support you think you will need. Being able to identify your support needs and ask for support demonstrates maturity and a desire to learn. For example, will you need time off or to change your working hours to attend workshops, training courses, a learning programme at college or to complete an **e-learning** programme? Do you need the help of a coach or mentor, someone to **work-shadow** or additional supervision? Would you benefit from access to a computer at work, a range of textbooks and professional journals? Would it help you to have experience of working with a different **user group**, to accompany colleagues on visits, to go to meetings that you wouldn't normally be expected to attend, or to meet with other professionals to find out about their job roles, skills and competencies?

4.1 Help!

Think about a goal you would like to achieve, either at work or in your personal life.

- What support do you think you would need?

- Who would give it to you?

Key terms

E-learning is the use of technology to enable people to learn at their convenience.

A user group is a group of people who have similar health and social care needs.

Work shadowing involves observing a professional in their workplace to get a taste of what their job involves.

Learning style is the way a person takes in, understands, expresses and remembers information, in other words, the way they learn best.

Finally, as with any formal supervision situation, you need to set a date to review your personal development plan. For review to be effective, it needs to be a regular and honest assessment of:

■ Whether you have achieved your objectives in the time set. If not, perhaps they were insufficiently clear or specific, not very enjoyable to pursue, too demanding of your time, or too ambitious and not appropriate to your capabilities or **learning style**. Use review to re-formulate or re-invent your short-term objectives and the way you aim to achieve them, without losing sight of your goal. Do not give up!

■ How the learning and development opportunities you undertook have actually affected your practice. You will read more about this in the next section.

■ Whether the support mechanisms you requested were appropriate and useful. If yes, in what ways were they useful? In what other ways could you use them? If they proved to be of little use, why? In what other ways do you feel you need support?

■ How well you feel you are progressing towards your long-term goals. Do not forget to celebrate your achievements!

4.3 Demonstrate how to work with others to agree own personal development plan

This activity enables you to practice demonstrating how to work with others to agree own personal development plan.

Produce a check list for a colleague who is new to working in the health and care sector that will guide them in developing their personal development plan.

LO5 Be able to use learning opportunities and reflective practice to contribute to personal development

5.1 Evaluate how learning activities have affected your practice

Learning is most effective if you use your preferred learning style. Learning styles are simply different ways of learning, and include visual, auditory and kinaesthetic.

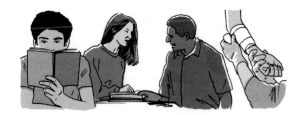

Figure 2.10 Different learning styles

Visual learners learn best through seeing, for example, they need to see somebody's body language and facial expression to fully understand an interaction. They learn best from visual displays such as diagrams, illustrated textbooks, DVDs, flipcharts and handouts, and they usually take notes during a class or training session, to help them absorb the information.

Evidence activity

5.1 **Evaluate how learning activities have affected practice**

This activity enables you to demonstrate how learning activities have affected your practice.

Think about five learning activities you have participated in that were intended to develop your work practice, and complete the table below to show how your practice has been affected as a result.

Learning activity	Learning style: visual/auditory/kinaesthetic	Effect on your practice
1.		
2.		
3.		
4.		
5.		

■ What do you conclude about your learning activities, i.e. which have had the greatest impact on your work?

■ How can you apply this conclusion to your future learning and development?

Auditory Learners learn best through listening, for example, they enjoy discussions, talking things through and listening to what others have to say. They are good at 'reading between the lines', for example, they are alert to tone of voice, pitch, speed and other nuances of speech. Written information does not inspire them to learn.

Kinesthetic learners learn through doing, through a hands-on approach. They need activity and find it hard to sit still for long periods.

While we have a preference for one style of learning, our adaptability ensures that we do learn using a variety of methods. But learning is most effective – and enjoyable – when it suits the learner's individual learning style.

We cannot rely on having our learning styles satisfied by other people and institutions – there is an expectation that we each will take responsibility for our own development. Seek out learning activities that you will enjoy and that will most benefit the way you do your work.

5.2 **Demonstrate how reflective practice has led to improved ways of working**

You looked at reflective practice earlier on in this chapter, and were given an opportunity to explain its importance in improving the service you provide as well as demonstrate your ability to reflect on your work practices. This section asks you to identify how your work has improved as a result of reflective practice.

The reflection process requires you to think critically about the following and how each affects your work:

■ your personal beliefs, values and experiences

■ your awareness of, attitude to and relationships with the people with whom you work

■ your skills, competences and work practices and whether they meet and maintain expected standards and codes of practice

■ your and others' training and development needs

■ any negative feelings or anxieties you have about your work.

Your personal beliefs, values and experiences will have a damaging effect on the people you work with if your behaviour implies that you think yours are more important and that you are disrespectful of theirs. A lack of respect flies in the face of best practice; in addition, a damaged relationship frustrates effective communication and discourages feedback. And, as you know, if you do not receive feedback from the people you work with, who encounter your behaviour first hand, you won't know how to improve your practice.

It is important to reflect on whether your and others' skills, competences and work practices meet and maintain expected standards and codes of practice. If incompetence is not challenged and if standards are allowed to slip, the people you work with may be subject to abuse and neglect and the organisation you work for taken to task by the Care Quality Commission and Ofsted, the bodies that regulate and inspect health and social care services and children and young people's services respectively. Reflection enables you to identify learning and development needs in order that skills, competences and work practices continuously improve.

Reflective practice is also an opportunity for you to think about any negative feelings or anxieties you have about your work. None of us can be expected to enjoy every aspect of our job role; neither can we be expected to be able to deal with everything a job throws at us. Identifying our concerns can be therapeutic and help us cope. In addition, articulating them to someone in authority may mean that we can be relieved of the tasks that cause concern. Either scenario helps ensure improved practice.

Practice activity

5.2 **Demonstrate how reflective practice has led to improvement**

This activity enables you to practise demonstrating how your reflective practice has led to improved ways of working.

☐ Identify three work practices that are carried out at your workplace and about which you have spent time reflecting. Describe how you think each could be improved.

☐ Discuss your ideas for improvement with your line manager or supervisor.

☐ If agreed, put your ideas for improvement into practice. How effective are the changes?

 Time to reflect

5.2 How are you getting on?

Most of the activities in this chapter have asked you to think about the effects of your behaviour and work practices on other people. This one looks at how you are affected.

- Are there any aspects of your job role or other people's work practices or behaviours that you do not enjoy or cannot cope with?

- How do you think things could be improved in order for work to become more enjoyable and manageable for you?

- Who can you talk to about your concerns and suggestions for improvement?

5.3 Show how to record progress in relation to personal development

Your personal development plan is an ongoing record of your strengths, goals and objectives, learning and development needs and achievements. In other words, it is a record of your progress in relation to your personal and professional development.

Why record personal and professional development, especially when time is at a premium and doing the learning can seem more important than noting down what you have learned? Recording is important for a number of reasons:

■ it helps you reflect and review

■ it reminds you of what you have learnt

■ it helps you build your CV and provides information for potential employers

■ it provides the framework for appraisals and promotion boards

■ it is a regulatory requirement for some professions

■ it provides evidence when you need to prove competence, for example, when applying for **professional registration**.

Key term

Professional registration is a requirement for employment for a number of professionals. It demonstrates that you have met standards of competence and is a requirement for employment of a number of professionals.

Records of personal development should include information such as:

■ what you have learnt and when, how you learnt it and any evidence that verifies your learning

■ evidence to show how your learning has developed your practice, for example, corroborative statements from your line manager, colleagues and the people you work with

■ how you have used support and in what ways you found it useful

■ how well you feel you are progressing towards your long-term goals

■ how your learning needs are developing.

Your records can take the form of a simple learning journal or logbook, on paper or in a computer file. You can use a ring-binder to store evidential statements, course notes, certificates, reading lists and lists of books, articles etc. that you have read and that have helped you. More formal personal development action plans and portfolios of evidence record learning in a more organised way, for example they might include summaries of evidence, personal references and cross-referencing of learning. Alternatively, you

could use an online system, which will provide a set format guiding you in what to record and when to update your record. However you choose to record your development, make it fit with your circumstances, the expectations of your employer and any regulatory requirements you have to comply with.

When thinking about how to record your personal development plan, bear in mind issues of confidentiality. If you refer by name to the people you work with, you must ensure confidentiality as per your organisation's legal requirements. You might also want to bear in mind the location of your records and their accessibility. You need to update your records regularly, but you also need to be able to take them with you if you change jobs.

Practice activity

(5.3) Show how to record your progress

This activity enables you to practise showing how to record your progress in relation to your personal development.

Create your own personal development plan, find an online pro-forma or get hold of one that is produced by your workplace. Start using it to keep a record of your personal development, updating it as regularly as you think appropriate or your workplace policy requires.

Assessment summary

Your reading of this chapter and completion of the activities will have prepared you to be able to engage in personal development in health, social care or children's and young people's settings.

To achieve the unit, your assessor will require you to:

Learning outcomes	Assessment Criteria
Learning outcome **1**: Show you understand what is required for competence in your work role by:	describing the duties and responsibilities of your work role See Evidence activity 1.1, p. 28
	explaining expectations about your own work role as expressed in relevant standards See Evidence activity 1.2, p. 30

Learning outcomes	Assessment Criteria
Learning outcome 2: Be able to reflect on your practice by:	(2.1) explaining the importance of reflective practice in continuously improving the quality of service See Evidence activity 2.1, p. 30
	(2.2) demonstrating the ability to reflect on practice See Practice activity 2.2, p. 31
	(2.3) describing how your own values, belief systems and experiences may affect your working practice See Evidence activity 2.3, p. 34
Learning outcome 3: Be able to evaluate your own performance by:	(3.1) evaluating your own knowledge, performance and understanding against relevant standards See Practice activity 3.1, p. 35
	(3.2) demonstrating the use of feedback to evaluate your performance and inform your development See Practice activity 3.2, p. 36
Learning outcome 4: Be able to agree a personal development plan by:	(4.1) identifying sources of support for planning and reviewing your development See Evidence activity 4.1, p. 38
	(4.2) demonstrating how to work with others to review and prioritise your learning needs, professional interests and development opportunities See Practice activity 4.2, p. 39
	(4.3) demonstrating how to work with others to agree your personal development plan See Practice activity 4.3, p. 41

Learning outcomes	Assessment Criteria
Learning outcome 5: Be able to use learning opportunities and reflective practice to contribute to personal development by:	**5.1** evaluating how learning activities have affected your practice See Evidence activity 5.1, p. 42
	5.2 demonstrating how reflective practice has led to improved ways of working See Practice activity 5.2, p. 43
	5.3 showing how to record progress in relation to personal development See Practice activity 5.3, p. 44

Good luck!

Weblinks

Government Careers Advice website	www.careersadvice.direct.gov.uk
Healthcare Careers	www.connexions-direct.com/jobs4u
Social Care & Counselling careers	www.connexions-direct.com/jobs4u
Community Care Careers	www.communitycare.co.uk/jobs/search
Skills for Health	www.skillsforhealth.org.uk
Skills for Care and Development	www.skillsforcareanddevelopment.org.uk
Government website (public services)	www.direct.gov.uk
Care Quality Commission	www.cqc.org.uk
Ofsted	www.ofsted.gov.uk
General Social Care Council	www.gscc.org.uk
Nursing and Midwifery Council	www.nmc-uk.org
Greater Teaching Council for England	www.gtce.org.uk

Promote equality and inclusion in health, social care or children's and young people's settings

For Unit SHC 33

What are you finding out?

Britain has a worldwide reputation for tolerating people's differences. It has a 2,000-year history of welcoming people from other lands and **cultures**; as far back as 1700, it was a haven for religious **refugees**; and today, anti-discrimination and human rights legislation is in place to ensure that people are treated equally and fairly regardless of their differences. But despite our perceived even-handedness, the media is awash with reports of racial abuse, child neglect, the **social exclusion** of older people and people with disabilities, **homophobia**, exploitation of immigrant workers, and so on, all of which demonstrate injustice and have dire consequences. You may be familiar with such small-minded behaviour in your local community, maybe at home, or even worse, in your workplace, where people need care, not cruelty. The reading and activities in this chapter will help you to:

■ Understand the importance of diversity, equality and inclusion

■ Be able to work in an inclusive way

■ Be able to promote diversity, equality and inclusion.

LO1 Understand the importance of diversity, equality and inclusion

1.1 Diversity, equality and inclusion

Diversity

Diversity means variety. For example, your local high street or shopping mall has a diversity of shops, restaurants, banks and bars; football teams have a diversity of roles, including full back, goalkeeper, centre forward and winger; and we live in a diverse society, where people vary in a multitude of ways, including in their age, sex, **sexual orientation**, physical characteristics such as height, weight and skin colour, ability, personal experiences and personal attributes, such as beliefs, values and preferences.

Care settings reflect the diversity of the population at large. Residents in a care home for elderly people – men and women, heterosexual and homosexual – may range in age from 60 to

> ### Key terms
>
> Culture is to do with the characteristics of particular group or society.
> A refugee is someone who flees to escape conflict, persecution or natural disaster.
> Social exclusion means exclusion from the mainstream of society.
> Homophobia means fear or dislike of homosexual people and homosexuality.

well into their ninth decade. Each will have their own set of personal experiences and, in locations with an immigrant community, may hail from a variety of different countries. And preferences, for example for food and music, will vary from one person to another, as will attitudes, for example to staff and fellow residents, beliefs, for example political ideas and religious faiths, health status and physical and intellectual ability. The same goes for child care settings and hospital wards – a nursery caters for children and a hospital ward for in-patients, but the children and the patients using the service will have a wealth of different – diverse – characteristics, experiences and personal attributes.

Key term

Sexual orientation means sexual preference, for someone of the same or the opposite sex or both.

Personal space is the region surrounding a person that they regard as psychologically theirs.

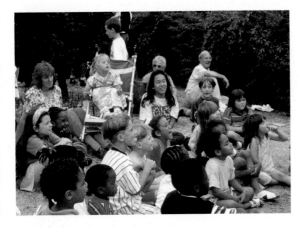

Figure 3.1 Diversity

Apart from differences in age, sex and gender, physical characteristics, ability, experiences and personal attributes, people also differ in respect of their:

■ diet, for example different health conditions mean that some people have specific dietary needs, and vegetarians and vegans can't take medication that is derived from animals.

■ religious faith, for example some religions have specific requirements with respect to diet and method of worship, others require the use of running water to maintain personal hygiene, the right hand for eating and the left for personal cleansing after using the toilet, and so on.

■ need for modesty and dignity, for example some people aren't comfortable being touched or seen undressed by someone of the opposite sex or that they don't know; and different people have different ideas about how to be addressed when being spoken to.

■ communication, for example different physical and mental health conditions require the use of different methods of communication; some people express their fear, pain and grief freely and openly whilst others are more reserved; and different people have different ideas about the extent of their **personal space**.

Time to reflect

(1.1) How different?

● Think about your family, friends and colleagues. In what ways do they demonstrate diversity?

● Now think about the people that use the service your workplace provides. No doubt they are similar in that they each belong to a particular service user group, for example they are all children, elderly people, people with a disability or people with a similar health condition. Do you assume, therefore, that they must therefore be similar in just about every other way? If so, does your behaviour towards them reflect your assumption?

Working with and getting to know a diverse range of people – service users, patients, their friends and family, colleagues and other professionals – enables health and social care workers to develop their knowledge and understanding of different ways of thinking and living and the reasons for different behaviours. As a consequence, tolerance of and respect for others develop, both of which are essential for meeting diverse – and individual – needs. And having their differences acknowledged and understood helps people to develop a sense of belonging.

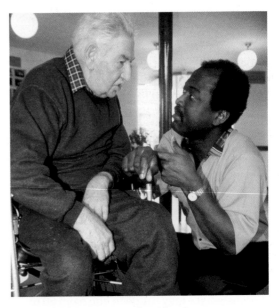

Figure 3.2 Meeting needs with tolerance

In addition, learning about different ways of thinking and living can be life-enriching. We become more open-minded to new experiences, opportunities and challenges, and are able to develop new relationships. As a result we grow as human beings and are able to achieve our full potential.

Evidence activity

 Diversity

This activity enables you to demonstrate your understanding of the importance of diversity.

Think about three health and social care settings, for example a youth club, a mother and baby clinic and a day care centre for people with learning disabilities.

1. In what ways might the individuals attending each setting be different from one another?

2. Why is it important that each setting has a diverse range of service users?

Equality

Equality is about treating people fairly, regardless of their differences, by ensuring that they have access to the same life opportunities as everyone else, i.e. that they have equal opportunities. Life opportunities include:

■ Housing. Warmth and shelter are basic human needs.

■ Education and employment. Just about everybody is capable of learning, and education not only enables us to find employment, it helps us to realise our full potential as human beings.

■ Transport, without which we couldn't get to work, to the shops, to see friends and family, to GP and hospital appointments, and so on.

■ Health and social care, which all of us need at some point in our lives.

■ Having enough money to buy a decent quality of life and not live in poverty.

■ Being able to buy **goods and services**, in person, by telephone or online using cash, cheques, credit or debit cards or **electronic transfer.**

Key terms

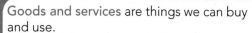

Goods and services are things we can buy and use.
Electronic transfer is a payment made automatically, usually over the internet, from a bank or savings account.
A perpetrator is someone who does something wrong.

Life opportunities

Some people need extra help to access life opportunities. For example, having a physical or sensory disability can impact on gaining an education, a job, using public transport, getting to the doctors; and being elderly or mentally ill can affect an individual's ability to maintain a decent standard of living, buy goods and services, speak up for themselves and have others listen to them. For this reason, equality is also about giving people help, providing them with appropriate services, so that they are not disadvantaged or treated less fairly than anyone else.

Research & investigate

 Equal opportunities

Select a service user group, for example children with learning difficulties, and find out what support services are available to prevent individuals within the group being disadvantaged or treated less fairly than anyone else.

People are disadvantaged for many reasons, but usually because they are different with respect to their:

■ Appearance. Racial harassment and attacks are usually acted out on people whose appearance, for example their skin colour and style of dress, is different from that of the **perpetrator.**

■ Sex. Men are still more likely to be better paid than women and to reach the top of the career ladder, and some jobs are still perceived and advertised as being 'women's' or 'men's' work.

■ Sexual orientation. Gays and lesbians remain subject to physical and verbal abuse.

■ Age. Older people often describe themselves as invisible, undervalued and a burden because of the way society treats them.

■ Ability. A general lack of understanding about the needs of people with physical or mental disabilities results in them finding it very difficult to make the most of life's opportunities.

Imposing disadvantage on people can prevent them from entering into the everyday life of their community and of society. In other words they can become socially and financially excluded.

Case Study

 1.1 Disadvantage

Anna is 6 years old and uses a wheelchair. She has cerebral palsy, misses a lot of school and has frequent appointments at hospital, many of which she is unable to attend. She lives with her mother, Jane, who is single and unable to work due to her caring commitments. Jane finds caring for Anna, getting her to school and the trips to hospital quite exhausting. She doesn't drive and receives no help other than social security benefit payments.

In what ways are Anna and Jane being disadvantaged?

Evidence activity

 1.1 Equality

This activity enables you to demonstrate your understanding of the importance of equality.

Think about Anna and Jane's situation in the case study above. Explain why it is important that they are not disadvantaged, that they are treated fairly.

Inclusion

You read above that having our individual differences acknowledged and understood helps us to develop a sense of belonging, or inclusion; and that disadvantaging people because they are different in some way leads to their becoming excluded. It follows, then, that inclusion is about accepting everyone, regardless of difference. It is also about getting rid of intolerance of

differences and providing help and support where appropriate.

Why inclusion? Because any organisation or institution, including local authorities, health service providers, educational establishments, the police service, voluntary organisations and workplaces, that supports and promotes inclusion demonstrates that it values everything about the people involved within it. Inclusion nurtures a sense of well-being and of confidence in one's own identity and abilities. And it ensures that everyone can achieve their potential and take their rightful place in society.

Research has shown that certain factors reduce the likelihood of developing a sense of belonging and living a happy and productive life.

The Government uses research findings like this to help service providers identify people most at need of help and deliver improved and more personalised services, i.e. ones that meet specific, personal needs. **www.cabinetoffice. gov.uk/social_exclusion_task_force.aspx**

Evidence activity

 1.1 Inclusion

This activity enables you to demonstrate your understanding of the importance of inclusion.

Think about the health and care services that you identified above as aiming to reduce social exclusion. Explain how an individual would benefit from using each service.

 1.2 The potential effects of discrimination

A prejudice is an attitude or way of thinking based on an unfounded, unreasonable pre-judgement of an individual, particular group of people or situation, rather than on a factual assessment. Prejudices can be positive or negative. If we are positively prejudiced towards someone, we think well of them. On the other hand, if we are negatively prejudiced against someone, we tolerate them less. In the main, negative prejudices develop against people who are different in some way. Discrimination happens when we act out our negative prejudices.

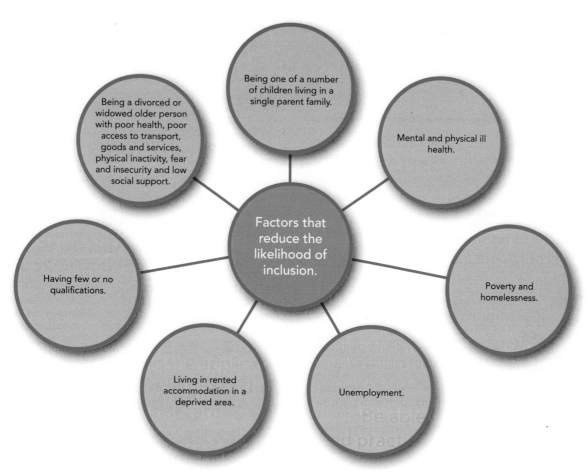

Figure 3.3 Factors that reduce the likelihood of inclusion

Time to reflect

(1.2) Prejudice?

- Do you have any negative prejudices? If so, describe how you let them affect the way you treat people.

- Do you think acting out negative prejudices like this is an acceptable way to behave?

Discriminatory behaviour results in unfair, unjust treatment. The people most likely to be discriminated against are those who are different in respect of their:

■ Age. Age discrimination, or ageism, isn't only targeted at elderly people – youngsters can also be on the receiving end of bullying, harassment and undeserved criticism.

■ Sex. Men and women continue to be treated unfairly in certain walks of life, in particular in the workplace. Discrimination based on sex is known as sexism.

■ Nationality, ethnic background, religion. Some people consider themselves superior to those from different backgrounds and faiths. The victimisation, or bullying or harassment of people for such reasons is known as racism.

■ Ability. **Barriers** that prevent disabled people from accessing the same opportunities as able-bodied people and the ignorant acting out of negative prejudices against physically or intellectually disabled people, for example through name-calling and damage of their property, is known as disablism.

■ Size. Some of us are guilty of judging people by their size and treating them unfairly as a result. This behaviour is known as sizeism.

■ Financial status. Discrimination against people on the grounds of their income, for example treating people living in poverty as inferior, is known as povertyism.
www.jrf.org.uk

Key term

A barrier is any condition that makes it difficult to make progress or achieve an objective.

There are two forms of discrimination, direct and indirect. Direct discrimination occurs when someone is intentionally treated unfairly, for example harassment on the basis of skin colour or religion. Indirect discrimination occurs when rules or guidelines meant to apply to everyone unintentionally affect one group of people more than others. For example, a company policy requiring everyone to work night shifts indirectly discriminates against single parents or people who care for elderly relatives, and menus that fail to offer a selection of food indirectly discriminates against people with specific dietary needs or preferences.

Case Study

1.2 Direct and indirect discrimination

The Head at St Horror's High is brushing up on appearances. She has brought in a new ruling that forbids both staff and pupils to wear anything on their heads and female staff and pupils to wear trousers. Any individual that fails to comply will be publicly challenged.

What sort of discrimination does this situation illustrate?

Discrimination takes place in a variety of settings, for example within educational establishments, where learners may not be given support and encouragement if it's assumed that their disability or advancing years affects their ability to learn; in the workplace, when people are persecuted on the basis of their skin colour or sexual preference; in housing, when landlords refuse to let their property to someone because of their refugee status or ethnic background; and in health and social care, when people are denied access to care on the basis of where they live – the **postcode lottery**.

Key term

The postcode lottery is the unequal availability of services in different parts of the country.

You read earlier that injustice towards people has dire effects. Discrimination is an injustice, not just for the victim but also for their family and friends, those who inflict the unfair behaviour and society as a whole. The short-term effects on an individual can include intimidation, humiliation, resentment and anger. The long-term effects can cause feelings of inferiority, loss of confidence and self-worth, distrust and fear of others, isolation and, eventually, social exclusion.

Discrimination can also deny people an opportunity to acquire an education, find employment, live in decent housing and access services. Victims and their families become sucked into deprivation, marked by insufficient income to buy a decent standard of living, the break-up of families and friendships, exposure to crime, homelessness and physical and emotional ill health. Children growing up in deprivation are not motivated to do well at school, which means they find it harder to gain employment. In the long term, discrimination results in cycles of deprivation for whole groups in society.

Evidence activity

1.2 The potential effects of discrimination

This activity enables you to demonstrate your knowledge of the potential effects of discrimination. Imagine that you are different in one of the ways that make people liable to experience unfair and unjust treatment. Describe how being discriminated against might affect you.

1.3 Promoting equality and supporting diversity through inclusive practice

Inclusive practice is about the attitudes, approaches and strategies taken to ensure that people are not excluded or isolated. It means supporting diversity by accepting and welcoming people's differences, and promoting equality by ensuring equal opportunities for all.

Inclusive practice is best practice. Health and social care workers demonstrate inclusive practice by working in ways that recognise, respect, value and make the most of all aspects of diversity. Having a sound awareness of and responding sensitively to an individual's diverse needs supports them in developing a sense of

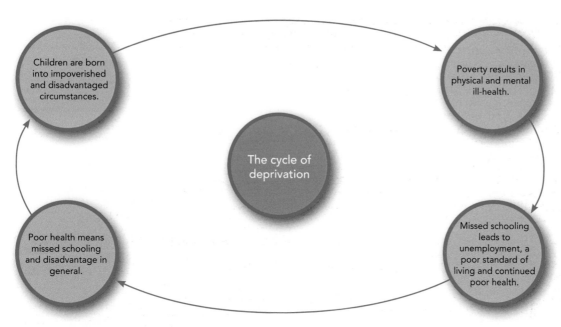

Figure 3.4 The cycle of deprivation

belonging, well-being and confidence in their identity and abilities. And it helps them to achieve their potential and take their rightful place in society.

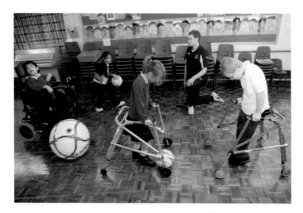

Figure 3.5 A sense of belonging, well-being

In addition, inclusive practice involves having an understanding of the disastrous impact that discrimination, inequality and social exclusion can have on an individual's physical and mental health. Having such an understanding ensures appropriate, personalised care and support, thereby enabling an individual to develop self-respect and maintain a valued role in society.

Because people who fail to support diversity or promote equality are usually entirely unaware of their attitudes and the impact of their behaviour, inclusive practice involves reflecting on and challenging one's own prejudices, behaviours

and work practices. It also involves challenging those of colleagues and other service providers, with a view to adapting ways of thinking and working and to changing services to build on good practice and to better support diversity and promote equality. You will read about this shortly.

 Evidence activity

1.3 **Inclusive work practice**

This activity enables you to demonstrate your understanding of the importance of inclusive practice.

Explain how inclusive practice promotes equality and supports diversity.

LO2 Be able to work in an inclusive way

 2.1 The application of legislation and codes of practice relating to equality, diversity and discrimination to work roles

Legislation

As you know, discrimination is an injustice and has devastating effects. The UK has in place numerous pieces of legislation (laws), rules, regulations, guidance documents and statutory codes of practice, all of which are intended to promote diversity, ensure equality and end discrimination. In other words, they are in place to promote everyone's right to fair and equal treatment, regardless of their differences.

You may be familiar with the following anti-discriminatory Acts of Parliament and regulations:

◼ **The Human Rights Act 1998**. This covers many different types of discrimination, including some that are not covered by other discrimination laws. Rights under the Act can be used only against a public authority, for example, the police or a local council, and not a private company. However, court decisions on discrimination usually have to take into account what the Human Rights Act says.

◼ The **Equal Pay Act 1970** (amended 1984). This says that women must be paid the same as men when they are doing the same (or broadly similar) work, work rated as equivalent under a job evaluation scheme, or work of equal value.

◼ The **Sex Discrimination Act 1975** (amended 1986). This makes it unlawful to discriminate against men or women in employment, education, housing or in providing goods and services, and also in advertisements for these things. It's also against the law, but only in work-related matters, to discriminate against someone because they are married or in a civil partnership.

◼ **Race Relations Act 1976** (amended 2000). This states that everyone must be treated fairly regardless of their **race**, nationality, or ethnic or national origins.

◼ **Disability Discrimination Act 1995**. This states that a person with a disability must not be treated less fairly than someone who is able-bodied.

◼ **Employment Equality (Religion or Belief) Regulations 2003**. This says it is unlawful to discriminate against people at work because of their religion or belief. The regulations also cover training that is to do with work.

◼ **Employment Equality (Age) Regulations 2006**. This says it is unlawful for an employer or potential employer to discriminate against you at work because of your age.

Key term

Race refers to the grouping of people on the basis of various heritable characteristics, such as skin colour.

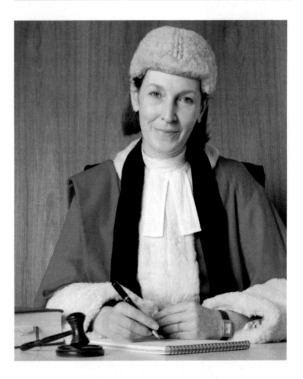

Figure 3.6 Upholding the law

Other pieces of legislation that protect the rights of people who use care services include:

◼ **The NHS and Community Care Act 1980**. This protects the rights of older and disabled people to receive care at home and in the community in ways that take account of their choices.

◼ **The Residential Care and Nursing Homes Regulations 2002**. This protects the rights of people living in care homes.

◼ **The Children Act 2004.** This protects children's rights by requiring local authorities to be flexible in meeting children's needs.

◼ **Health and Social Care Act 2008.** This Act established the Care Quality Commission (CQC), whose remit is to protect and promote the right of people using health and social care services in England to quality care and to regulate its provision. CQC took over the roles of the Healthcare Commission, Commission for Social Care Inspection and the Mental Health Act Commission in March 2009. **www.cqc.org.uk**

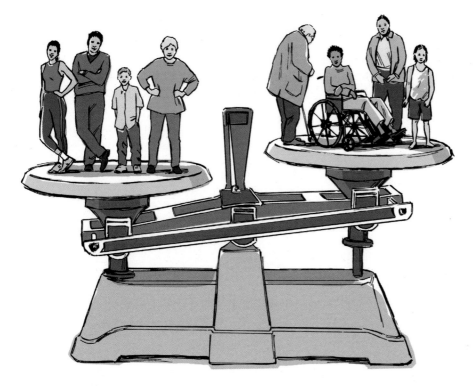

Figure 3.7 Rough justice

These pieces of legislation have helped us move forward on equality, but in 2009, women were still earning, on average, 23% less per hour than men; less able but better-off children were overtaking more able, poorer children at school by the age of six; people with disabilities were still more than twice as likely to be out of work than able-bodied people; and one in five older people was unsuccessful in getting quotations for motor insurance, travel insurance and car hire.

Research & investigate

A breach of rights

Talk to people and research the media, for example the press, TV and radio, for instances of where there is a belief that rights have been breached. Describe the rights that have been breached and the legislation that has been contravened.

To make Britain fairer and strengthen and streamline the current anti-discrimination laws, the Single Equality Bill, which the Government plans to come into force between Autumn 2010 and Spring 2011, will bring different types of discrimination within one piece of legislation. It will also provide understandable, practical guidance for employers, service providers and public bodies to ensure that rights to fair treatment are promoted for everyone. **www.equalities.gov.uk**

Health and social care providers are obliged to incorporate legislation relating to equality, diversity and discrimination into their policies and procedures. Workplace procedures dictate best practice regarding how work activities must be carried out, and they must be followed. Anything else would be a contravention of the law, in this case the breaching of an individual's right to fair treatment.

Time to reflect

Learn from your mistakes

- Can you honestly say that you always follow workplace procedures?

- Think about the consequences of failing to follow procedures... How might this bad practice impact on the people you work with and on yourself?

Codes of Practice

In England and Wales, the General Social Care Council (GSCC) is responsible for ensuring that standards within the social care sector are of the highest quality. It has developed Codes of Practice for all care workers that include information on how to protect and promote the rights of individuals using the service. The Codes of Practice provide a guide to best practice and set out the standards of conduct that workers are expected to meet. They are also recommended reading for examining your own practice and seeking out areas in which you can improve.

Code of Practice 1

As a social care worker, you must protect the rights and promote the interests of individuals and their carers. This includes 'Promoting equal opportunities for service users and carers' (1.5) and 'Respecting diversity and different cultures and values' (1.6). **www.gscc.org.uk**

Health care workers also have an obligation to protect the rights and promote the interests of patients. For example, the Nursing and Midwifery Council (NMC) code or Standards of conduct, performance and ethics for nurses and midwives states that, 'You must not discriminate in any way against those in your care'. **www.nmc-uk.org**

At the time of writing (February 2010), there is no statutory provision for the regulation of Health Care Support Workers working in the UK. However, NHS Scotland's Code of Conduct for Health Care Support Workers in Scotland states that they should 'treat all patients in the same way. It is the duty of public bodies and their employees to promote equality. Personal feelings about patients must not interfere with the standard of your work. By law, you must provide all patients with high-quality care which reflects their individual needs, whatever their race, sex, sexuality, age, religious belief or disability. This means that you owe patients a 'duty of care' and they can expect a 'reasonable' standard of care from all workers.' www. healthworkerstandards.scot.nhs.uk

Time to reflect

2.1 Examine your own work practice

- Are you familiar with any Codes of Practice or the standard of conduct required of you in your work role?
- When did you last remind yourself of the standard of conduct required of you?
- Can you honestly say that your work practice always meets expected standards of conduct?

Evidence activity

2.1 Rules, regulations and inclusive work practice

This activity enables you to demonstrate your understanding of the need to apply anti-discriminatory legislation and codes of practice to your work.

Explain how legislation and codes of practice relating to equality, diversity and discrimination apply to your own work role.

2.2 Interaction with individuals that respects their beliefs, culture, values and preferences

Much has been said so far of people's differences with regard to age, sex and sexual orientation, race and ability. You have also read that people vary in personal attributes such as beliefs, culture, values and preferences.

We develop our beliefs, values and preferences throughout our lives. As very small children we are dependent on close family and carers. It is their role to direct and shape our thoughts and behaviour and encourage and reward those that meet **cultural** customs, traditions and expectations with respect to manners, respect, what makes for right and wrong and so on. As we grow and become increasingly exposed to society at large, our preferences, attitudes, values and beliefs develop as a result of new experiences and the influence of factors such as **role models, peer groups,** education, religious institutions and the media. The personal attributes we develop throughout our lives promote the development of our **identity** and the way we want others to see us. They make us the individuals we are.

Key terms

A **role model** is someone who serves as an example and whose behaviour is copied by others.
A **peer group** is a group of people of similar age and sharing the same social status.
Identity is the individual characteristics by which a person is recognised or known.

Time to reflect

 Who are you?

- Think about the influences on your development, from as far back as you can remember until now. Who and what have they been and who and what are they now?

- How would you describe yourself now, in terms of beliefs, values and preferences? And how would you like others to see you?

- What cultural customs, traditions and expectations have been handed on to you by your family? Which of them have you abandoned or rejected and why?

Beliefs are ideas or principles that we think are true. They may be religious, for example, Christianity, Islam and Judaism; **secular**, for example, humanism; and political, for example, socialism, communism and feminism. Beliefs underpin the way we live, for example, beliefs concerning animals' rights mean that vegans will not consume meat or meat products of any description. The Human Rights Act 1998 protects our right to choose what to think and believe and to be free to express or act out our beliefs as we wish.

Key term

Secular means not concerned with religion. Abuse is cruel or inhumane treatment.

We ascribe a **value** to something that we respect and admire or that we feel has worth. Tangible things like cars and jewellery have an economic worth. On the other hand, health and happiness are qualities we appreciate, as are the family and friends we hold dear, even though we can't put a price on qualities and people. Other things we value, although to different degrees given that we are all different, are codes of behaviour, such as the following:

■ moral code, which is to do with behaviour that is right and decent

■ ethical code, which is to do with behaviour that is principled, fair and just

■ code of conduct, which is to do with standards of behaviour.

The Human Rights Act 1998 protects our right to freedom of conscience, in other words, to decide for ourselves what to respect and value, and what is right, decent, fair and principled.

Preferences are highly individual. They develop and change throughout our lives and having a preference enables us to make an informed choice. For example, a child might choose a milky drink whereas an elderly person might prefer a cup of tea; people from different cultural backgrounds, for example Aboriginal and Inuit people have entirely different preferences for dress, as do the Skinhead and Goth youth sub-cultures; someone who finds it increasingly difficult to swallow would choose to change to a liquid diet; and not until they have experienced the delights of chocolate might someone choose to eat it!

Research & investigate

 What takes your fancy?

Talk with two or three of the people you work with to explore:

- What they believe in, what they value, and their preferences, for example, for food and drink, TV programmes, dress, reading material, activities, when to have a bath/shower, other people, etc.

- Their culture, in other words the customs and traditions they are expected to follow.

- Whether they think their needs are being met in a way that pays regard to their beliefs, values, individual preferences and cultural background.

The General Social Care Council (GSCC) Codes of Practice for Social Care Workers and Employers directs social care workers to treat each person as an individual; to respect and, where appropriate, promote their individual views and wishes; and to support their right to control their lives and make informed choices. The Nursing and Midwifery Council (NMC) Standards of conduct, performance and ethics for nurses and midwives reflect this thinking by stating that health care workers should listen to the people in their care and respond to their concerns and preferences.

Whilst a health or care worker might not agree with the beliefs and values of the people they work with, nor share their preferences, inclusive work practice involves respecting and promoting:

■ the right to freedom of thought and religion, i.e. their beliefs

■ the right to freedom to express their beliefs as they wish

■ the right to freedom of conscience, i.e. to personal values and a sense of right and wrong

■ personal preferences.

Care work that doesn't demonstrate inclusive practice, for example, denying someone the opportunity to worship in the way that their religion dictates or to choose what to eat or wear, is oppression. Oppressive behaviour denies people their freedoms and is a form of **abuse**.

Case Study

 Cavalier Care Home

Cavalier Care Home provides residential accommodation for elderly people in need of personal care and support. The cultural and social make-up of residents and staff is very varied but the manager has no time for religious belief; she is a staunch follower of her local MP; she is intolerant of what she calls 'food faddies'; she is dismissive of complaints about clothing being shared on the grounds that it isn't sufficiently well labelled; and she has no procedures in place to protect valuables.

If you were asked to advocate on behalf of the residents at Cavalier Care Home, what would you tell the manager?

Practice activity

 Interaction and inclusive work practice

This activity gives you an opportunity to practise becoming competent at inclusive working.

Revisit your findings for the Research and investigate activity 'What takes your fancy?', where you were asked to explore the beliefs, values, preferences and cultural background of two or three of the people you work with and to find out whether they think their needs are being met appropriately.

contd.

Practice activity *contd.*

■ Talk to these people again to find out how they think your interactions with them could change in order for you to show respect for their individual beliefs, values, preferences and cultural background.

■ Put their suggestions into practice. If you have any difficulties, get help from a colleague or your supervisor.

■ Monitor improvements in your practice by checking with each individual that you are indeed showing respect for their beliefs, values, preferences and cultural background. In other words, that you are developing inclusive work practices.

LO3 Be able to promote diversity, equality and inclusion

Everyone that works in care must demonstrate their ability to promote diversity and equality and to challenge discrimination against people using care services, their carers, families and fellow-workers.

 Actions that model inclusive practice

The following suggestions aim to help you ensure that your work is inclusive, in other words that it promotes equality and diversity, does not discriminate and shows respect for beliefs, cultures, values and preferences.

Be aware of your own thinking and attitudes and how they affect your work. If, for example, your interactions with people are affected because you label or stereotype them, or hold a negative prejudice against them, you are likely to be accused of discrimination.

We all use labels to describe people, usually according to their appearance or behaviour, for example elderly people are often labelled as 'old dears' or 'old codgers'. However, labelling can be damaging because the label blinds us to the many other characteristics of the person concerned. The 'old dear' might in fact be a lovely old lady but she may also have been a brain surgeon or a fighter pilot and would be most offended by your disrespectful description of her!

We all tend to stereotype people. Stereotyping is about grouping together people who share one or two characteristics, again usually to do with their appearance or behaviour. The result is that we assume all the people in the group are the same in every way – we lose sight of their individuality. Thus while a lot of children do wet the bed, they don't all; and those that do are in the minority.

A negative prejudice is a negative attitude based on a pre-judgement of a person or situation. People who are negatively prejudiced hold biased, rigid feelings and beliefs, usually about particular groups of people such as benefit claimants and single parents. Their feelings and beliefs are unreasonable and are not based on facts – the great majority of benefit claimants and single parents are, in fact, genuinely in need.

Time to reflect

 What did you say?

- What labels and stereotypes do you use? Are they a fair way of describing people? Do you let them affect the way you work with people? How would you feel if you were labelled or stereotyped such that your individuality was glossed over?

- Do you have any negative prejudices? If so, why? Are they fair? Do you let them affect the way you work with people? How would you feel if people let their negative prejudices affect their interactions with you?

Similarly, if your attitude towards someone's beliefs, cultural background, values and preferences is dismissive or patronising, you will come across as being unconcerned about them and their individual needs, which will bring into doubt your ability to fulfil your **duty of care**. Keep your prejudices to yourself and maintain a positive attitude towards everyone, regardless of their differences. Be warm, welcoming and respectful in your approach and show people that you value them for who they are.

Key term

Duty of care is the requirement of a service provider to take reasonable care with respect to the interests of others, including protecting them from harm.

Get to know the people you work with, by talking to them, their friends and family, and to your colleagues and other professionals who know them; and read and digest their life histories as noted in their care plans. Find out about their cultural backgrounds and beliefs, what they value, what they like and dislike; and learn from their experiences. Increasing your understanding of why people think and behave as they do will enable you to support them appropriately in exercising their rights and meeting their needs.

Make sure that you know and follow your workplace's policies and procedures with regard to promoting equality and diversity; and that you follow the relevant Minimum Standards and Codes of Practice for the setting in which you work. The guiding principles contained in these documents serve to ensure that anti-discriminatory laws are observed. By embracing them in your work, you not only promote the rights of those you work with, you protect yourself.

Model your work on the Principles of Care, which are the gold standard for promoting inclusive work practice. They require you to:

■ Show respect, regardless of an individual's age, sex, sexual orientation, race and ability, and with regard to their beliefs, culture, values and preferences. Embrace differences and learn from them.

■ Support individuals in retaining their cultural dignity, such as how they to choose to dress, maintain their personal hygiene, cope with intimate medical procedures, and so on

■ Ensure individuals are not disadvantaged but can access equal opportunities, for example, by making sure that they receive help and support appropriate to their needs

■ Let an individual's personal preferences shape the way you work with them

■ Respect the need to maintain confidentiality of personal and sensitive information, for example, political beliefs and sexual orientation. Some people choose to keep such information private.

Research & investigate

 What makes people tick?

Talk to someone you work with who has a different cultural background from you about their beliefs, values, preferences, way of life, expectations, customs and traditions. Compare what they have to say with your perspective on things. Have you learnt anything? Would you recommend your colleagues to research cultural differences? If so, why?

Finally, maintain an up-to-date knowledge of best inclusive practice techniques; recognise when you need help with regard to your attitude, understanding of diversity and inclusive work practice; know where to get help, for example from colleagues, your line manager or supervisor, professional journals and training opportunities; be open to feedback, from colleagues and the individuals you work with; and be prepared to change.

 Practice activity

3.1 **Actions that model inclusive work practice**

This activity gives you an opportunity to practice becoming competent at promoting diversity, equality and inclusion.

Make a note of all the things that you do and could do that promote equality, diversity and inclusion. Keep a diary to show when you put them into practice and how doing so benefits the people you work with.

3.2 Supporting others to promote equality and rights

If you put everything that you have so far learned and understood about promoting equality, diversity and inclusion into practice, you will be well on your way to demonstrating the competences that this unit sets out. Your learning and understanding and your developing ability to reflect on ways of working should also have raised your awareness regarding the way that your colleagues, other professionals and the individuals you work with promote equality and rights. This section aims to help you support those others in promoting equality and rights.

You read earlier that letting labelling, stereotyping and negative prejudices affect the way you interact with people is a form of discrimination. Take the label 'single mother'. What does it conjure up for you? Many people believe that single mothers have intentionally become pregnant, to be housed and to take advantage of the benefits system. Their use of the label denotes a negative prejudice and implies that single mothers are less than equal, not as good, undeserving. As a result, single mothers are liable to be held in contempt. Such behaviour is discrimination and therefore a breach of rights.

The 'single mother' label also demonstrates a lack of respect for individual differences, for example, it doesn't take into account the myriad of different reasons why a woman with children is on her own. Is she divorced or widowed, did her partner desert her or is he or she working away from home? Is it a characteristic of her cultural background that mothers and fathers live separately? Did she make a conscious choice to have children and bring them up on her own? Everyone is different, and grouping people together on the basis of a single, shared characteristic, in this case being single with children, does not acknowledge their differences; in addition, because the label has negative connotations, it marginalises and excludes people who may be very needy.

Lead by example. If it is apparent that you don't accept the use of labels to describe individuals, and if in your work you acknowledge and respond to their individual differences, you may influence others such that they too promote equality and rights and work in an inclusive way.

As you know, being dismissive of an individual's beliefs, culture, values and preferences shows a lack of concern and brings into doubt an ability to care; it also questions any commitment to promotion of their rights, in particular to express their beliefs as they wish and to make personal choices. Health and care workers have a responsibility to **provide a high standard of care**, to protect the rights and promote the interests of the people they work with. Anything else would be **neglect**.

Key term

Neglect is lack of attention and due care.

Again, lead by example. If you are interested in, respect and are responsive to people's personal attributes, it will show in the satisfaction you get from work and others will want to imitate you.

In addition to leading by example, you should be prepared to support the equality and rights of individuals you work with by advocating on their behalf. Many people, for one reason or another, don't have the capacity to make their own voices heard, for example they may be frightened or lack the confidence to speak up for themselves; they may be ill, confused, not able to communicate effectively; and many people are just simply not aware of their rights. Training to be an advocate will ensure you know how to give appropriate support and also that you know where to find help that is out of your remit, such as organisations that have a specific expertise in championing and defending equality and human rights.

Case Study

 Mrs Singh

Mrs Singh is 87. She is in a busy hospital ward having had a stroke and is dressed in a backless hospital gown. The stroke has affected her speech and also her mobility, so she has to remain in bed. Her background dictates that she must not eat meat, that she needs to shower every morning and that she needs to keep covered in order to retain her modesty. None of these needs are being met, because she is unable to communicate them and because the staff on the ward are constantly under pressure to complete routine activities. To them she is simply 'the stroke in bed 7', not a person with her own individual set of needs. She is becoming very agitated and hasn't eaten for over 24 hours. Her family feels that her right to quality care is being breached.

Do you agree with this assertion? If so, how would you change things?

Research & investigate

 Personal and professional development

Check out training that will qualify you as an advocate and start to build a resource of statutory and voluntary services that offer advocacy and organisations that have an expertise in championing and defending equality and human rights and to which you could refer the people with whom you work.

Be prepared to talk with others about their behaviour if you feel it fails to promote equality and rights. If you are uncomfortable discussing such issues or you feel you don't have the appropriate communication skills, report your concerns to your supervisor. And of course, be open to feedback about your own work practices, and if you feel that the feedback is appropriate, act on it!

Practice activity

 Supporting others to promote equality and rights

This activity gives you an opportunity to practice becoming competent at supporting others to promote diversity, equality and inclusion.

Make a note of instances when you feel that others fail to promote equality and rights. Build on your notes with suggestions as to how you might support them to improve their practice. Keep a diary to record when you put your suggestions into practice and how doing so benefits everyone concerned.

3.3 ## Challenge discrimination in a way that promotes change

Talking to people about discrimination does not ensure that they will change their **mindset** and, as a consequence, their behaviour. Similarly, the existence of legislation, policies and procedures and Codes of Practice does not guarantee that people using services receive fair treatment and that their rights are upheld. If attitudes and behaviours are to change, discrimination needs to be challenged effectively. This section aims to alert you to ways that discriminatory practice can be challenged in a way that promotes change.

Key term

A **mindset** is a state of mind that affects an individual's attitude and behaviour and their ability to make decisions.

Achievement of a qualification in Health and Social Care at level 3 will allow you to work without direct supervision or on your own; and, depending on your workplace requirements, in a senior or supervisory capacity. The personal and professional skills associated with gaining a level 3 qualification include the ability to ensure that staff you're responsible for abide by workplace policies and procedures and Codes of Practice, including those that relate to anti-discriminatory practice. Thus one of your priorities is to develop communication skills that enable you to challenge discrimination assertively, that is, in a positive, encouraging yet firm manner such that behavioural change comes about. Challenging behaviour in an aggressive, hostile way promotes antagonism and destroys goodwill, making it very difficult to change established bad practice. And sitting on the fence, observing discriminatory practice but doing nothing about it, condones and promotes bad practice.

Example of an Equality and Diversity Policy.

You will have the following responsibilities:

1) to always behave in a way that is supportive and consistent with the aims of this policy;
2) to promote equality and diversity, challenging discrimination where/whenever it occurs;
3) you must not unfairly discriminate, bully, harass and/or intimidate in any area of your work or encourage others to do so;
4) if you suspect that unfair discrimination, bullying/harassment/intimidation are taking place you should report it to a relevant manager;
5) support colleagues, service users or carers who make a complaint of discrimination, bullying/harassment;
6) to co-operate with any measures introduced to promote equality and diversity in the workplace.

Can I complain if I feel this policy is not being implemented properly?

Yes. If you feel that the Trust is not taking its responsibility to promote equality and diversity seriously, is not implementing this policy in the way described or feel that you have been discriminated against in the application of any of the Trust's employment policies or procedures you have the right to complain and should use the Trust's Individual Grievance Procedure.

Figure 3.8 Challenging discrimination

Another tried and tested method of challenging workplace discrimination and making change happen is by analysing the reasons why a worker behaves in a discriminatory way. For example, were they brought up in an environment where labelling, stereotyping and negative prejudice were normal behaviours and therefore not questioned? Is their thinking negatively influenced by the media, which still has a tendency to present elderly people as a burden, youngsters as trouble-makers and poor people as benefit spongers? Were they themselves discriminated against and, as a result, feel it to be normal behaviour – they know no better? Having an opportunity to explore issues openly, privately and where there is no risk of accusation, for example, during an appraisal, allows people to question their behaviour and make appropriate changes. The advantage of exploring behaviour during an appraisal is that required changes can be agreed and recorded and their success measured.

Informal discussions, during a coffee break or as part of a training session, provide useful opportunities to reflect on the dire effects of discrimination. Most people using health and care services are liable to have experienced discrimination at some time or another. Indeed, their experience of discrimination may be the reason they are in need of care now. Talking through these issues, especially with people who have been victims of discrimination, and imagining how it must feel to experience unfair, unjust treatment, can have powerful effects on thinking and behaviour.

Time to reflect

(3.3) Changing the mindset …

It's possible that you may have behaved in an unfair, discriminatory way at some time or other. It may not have been intentional, but… Reflecting on the reasons for our bad behaviour can help us to overcome our gremlins. We learn to forgive ourselves, put our mistakes behind us and move on. And moving on means behavioural change.

- Think about the reasons why you have treated – or maybe continue to treat – some people unfairly. How can you change your thinking so that you don't discriminate against them in the future?

The Government has put in place a number of initiatives and resources that can be accessed to tackle discrimination. Public Service Agreements (PSAs) play an important role in building services around the needs of citizens and improving their delivery. Within each PSA is a set of **outcome-based performance indicators**, against which services can be measured. PSA 15 focuses on the disadvantages individuals experience because of their **gender**, race, disability, age, sexual orientation, religion or belief. The actions it requires service providers to prioritise are:

■ to reduce the gender pay gap

■ to tackle barriers due to gender, disability or age that limit people's choice and control in their lives

■ to increase participation in (inclusion) public life by women, ethnic minorities, disabled people and young people

■ to reduce discrimination in employment due to gender, race, disability, age, sexual orientation, religion or belief

■ to reduce unfair treatment at work, college or school, and when using health services and public transport due to gender, race, disability, age, sexual orientation, religion or belief.

Key terms

Outcome-based performance indicators are a method of measuring the degree to which outcomes are achieved.
Gender is to do with the socially-constructed concepts of masculinity and femininity.

A reduction of barriers that discriminate against people who use care services is measured according to how well they perceive their ability to make choices, control their lives and live independently. A reduction of discrimination against people who use health services is measured according to the dignity and respect with which they perceive they have been treated. Health and social care service providers are required to seek feedback from the people using their services and make improvements as necessary. And they are inspected to ensure that they comply with the required standards and that, if necessary, a change in service delivery has actually taken place.

Check that your workplace has procedures in place for measuring discriminatory practice, for example, through the use of questionnaires, complaints and comments forms, meetings with service users, their family and friends; that feedback regarding people's views and experiences is sought; that the feedback collected is analysed to check for discriminatory practice; that, if necessary, changes in behaviour and work practices are made; and that feedback regarding views and experiences demonstrates that behaviour has actually changed and is having a positive effect.

Evidence activity

(3.3) Challenging discrimination in a way that promotes change

This activity enables you to demonstrate your knowledge of how to challenge discrimination in a way that promotes change.

Describe how to challenge discrimination such that people actually change their behaviour.

Assessment summary

Your reading of this chapter and completion of the activities will have prepared you to demonstrate your learning and understanding of and competence at promoting equality and inclusion in your workplace.

To achieve the unit, your assessor will require you to:

Learning outcomes	Assessment Criteria
Learning outcome **1**: Show you understand the importance of diversity, equality and inclusion by:	explaining what is meant by diversity, equality and inclusion See Evidence activities 1.1, 1.2 and 1.3, pp. 49 and 50.
	describing the potential effects of discrimination See Evidence activity 1.2, p. 52.
	explaining how inclusive practice promotes equality and supports diversity. See Evidence activity 1.3, p. 53.

Learning outcomes	Assessment Criteria
Learning outcome **2**: Show you can work in an inclusive way by:	(2.1) explaining how legislation and codes of practice relating to equality, diversity and discrimination apply to your work role See Evidence activity 2.1, p. 56.
	(2.2) showing interaction with individuals that respects their beliefs, culture, values and preferences. See Practice activity 2.2, p. 58.
Learning outcome **3**: Be able to promote diversity, equality and inclusion by:	(3.1) demonstrating actions that model inclusive practice See Practice activity 3.1, p. 60.
	(3.2) demonstrating how to support others to promote equality and rights See Practice activity 3.2, p. 61.
	(3.3) describing how to challenge discrimination in a way that promotes change. See Evidence activity 3.3, p. 63.

Good luck!

Weblinks

Social Exclusion Task Force	www.cabinetoffice.gov.uk/social_exclusion_task_force.aspx
Joseph Rowntree Foundation	www.jrf.org.uk
Government Equalities Office	www.equalities.gov.uk
Equality and Human Rights Commission	www.equalityhumanrights.com
National Minimum Standards	www.dh.gov.uk
Care Quality Commission	www.cqc.org.uk
General Social Care Council	www.gscc.org.uk
The Nursing and Midwifery Council	www.nmc-uk.org
NHS Scotland	www.healthworkerstandards.scot.nhs.uk

For Unit SHC 34

What are you finding out?

This chapter introduces ways to address the dilemmas, conflicts or complaints that may arise where there is a duty of care.

It also covers ensuring that individuals feel safe, valued and respected, and is about offering as much choice and independence as possible, and having the opportunity to evaluate and reflect upon the key factors involved in service delivery.

The ability to change things is important, and ensuring that individuals have an awareness of and access to a robust complaints system is crucial and will be explored in this chapter.

When you have read this chapter you will understand:

■ How duty of care contributes to safe practice.

■ How to address conflicts or dilemmas that may arise between an individual's rights and the duty of care.

■ How to respond to complaints.

LO1 Understand how duty of care contributes to safe practice

What is duty of care?

Duty of care is the requirement to exercise a level of care towards an individual to avoid injury to that individual or their property. It is based on the relationship of the different parties, the negligent act or omission and the reasonable likelihood of loss to that individual.

A negligent act is an unintentional but careless act which results in loss. Only a negligent act will be regarded as having breached a duty of care. Whether an act is negligent can only be considered in the context in which it happened.

In Scotland this area of the law is called **delict**, while in England, Wales and Northern Ireland it is called the law of **tort**. Delict and tort differ from the law of contract. Contracts generally specify the duties of each of the parties and the remedy if these duties are breached. When the parties enter into a contract, they obtain specific rights and certain duties. In delict or tort these duties operate through the nature of the parties' relationship regardless of the contractual obligations.

Key terms

Delict is a concept of civil law in which a wilful wrong or an act of negligence gives rise to a legal obligation between parties, even though there has been no contract between the parties.

Tort is any wrongdoing for which an action for damages may be brought.

Liability is the state of being legally obliged and responsible.

Although much of the law of delict and tort has been developed by the courts, there are also now a number of statutory rules which apply, for example to employment, disability discrimination, health and safety, data protection and occupier's liability.

Research & investigate

 Duty of care

Ask your manager or senior in charge what they understand by 'duty of care'. How do they ensure they are meeting these requirements? Have they experienced any breaches of this duty?

Does a duty of care exist?

This depends on the relationship between the parties. A duty of care is not owed to everyone, only to those who have a suitably close relationship. There is no **liability** if the relationship between the parties is too remote. Closeness in this context, of course, also implies a professional relationship or responsibility.

Is there a breach of that duty?

Liability only arises if the action breaches the duty of care and causes a loss or harm to the individual which would have been reasonably foreseeable in all the facts and circumstances of the case.

In a social care context, a duty of care will usually exist where the social care worker has some professional or work responsibility for delivering a service to an individual. A breach would arise where a negligent act or omission to act resulted in harm to that individual and the harm was foreseeable.

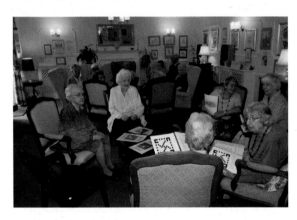

Figure 4.1 A care centre

 ## What it means to have a duty of care in own work role

Your duty of care

As a care worker, you have a duty:

■ to take reasonable care for your own health and safety, and for the health and safety of others, while at work

■ to follow reasonable directions given by, or on behalf of, the employer on issues related to health or safety

■ to use relevant safety equipment provided for your use

■ to report a workplace accident to the employer as soon as practicable after it occurs.

As a care worker you must not:

■ intentionally or recklessly interfere with or misuse safety equipment provided by your employer

■ intentionally create a risk to the health or safety of another at your workplace.

 ## Time to reflect

1.1 Duty to individuals

What do you think your duty to individuals is?

Does it match up with the expected duty of care?

In 1932 a court was asked to consider a case involving snails that had found their way into a glass of ginger beer! The woman who consumed the ginger beer suffered from nervous shock as a result of seeing the snails in the bottom of her glass and, in a landmark case, she brought an action against the publican who had served her the drink. She was able to establish that the publican owed her a duty of care and that he had breached that duty of care by unwittingly allowing the snails to get into her glass. After great deliberation, the court upheld the unfortunate woman's claim and the doctrine of duty of care was born. Since 1932 the courts have been full of people claiming that a duty of care was owed to them by someone, that the person has been negligent in observing that duty of care and has, as a result, breached it. That 1932 case has led to a society in which there is a huge amount of litigation, where, for example, councils are being sued for failing to put up signs that warn of pending dangers, publicans for allowing intoxicated people to drive off from their premises, and homeowners when a trespasser trips over an object left in an awkward place in their own home.

 ### Case Study

1.1 Did Heidi follow the duty of care?

On a ward there has been one staff nurse and one Health Care Assistant (HCA) short on the day shift for two weeks. For the last three days there has been a further Health Care Assistant missing due to sickness.

contd.

Case Study *contd.*

The one remaining day shift HCA, Heidi, tries her best but by the end of the first day is aware that even with help from the nurses, it is impossible to carry out even the minimum of necessary duties to a basic standard. She speaks to the ward sister about her concerns and is assured by her they are trying to get cover, but is told that with support from the nurses, it should be possible to keep going for a couple more days.

On the third day Heidi makes a mistake. She gives a drink to a patient who was designated 'Nil by Mouth' as they were to be operated on later in the day. Heidi is warned that she faces a serious investigation. She is very upset.

It is clear that the sister should have acknowledged her responsibilities under the NMC Code of Professional Conduct and have made greater efforts to get immediate cover. Heidi should have been able to raise her concerns formally if nothing happened when they were raised informally. However, Heidi cannot be blamed if others failed in their duty of care. Clinical governance should mean the focus of any investigation is at least as much on the staffing shortages and why they weren't tackled as on one mistake by the HCA.

1.2 How duty of care contributes to the safeguarding or protection of individuals

Health and social care professionals have a duty of care to ensure the safety and well-being of service users. Most professions have set out good practice guidelines. Not following these guidelines may amount to abuse or neglect. All health and social care professions have identified certain principles and ways of working as 'good practice'. Being aware of what 'good practice' means can help you to identify abuse or neglect.

Health authorities, including primary care trusts and mental health trusts, and local authority social services are legally responsible for all the staff they employ. This includes making sure that appointed staff have the necessary qualifications and skills to carry out their roles, and that there is no reason to believe that staff could pose a risk to others. This involves following up references and checking with the Criminal Records Bureau that prospective staff have no criminal convictions which may affect their work. Health authorities and social services departments should ensure that staff receive the ongoing supervision, training and support needed to carry out their work. A health authority or local authority is liable if a member of their staff is found guilty of professional misconduct.

Research & investigate

1.2 Good practice

Find out what is meant by 'good practice' in your workplace.

How do people ensure they work to this at all times?

Health and social care services as a whole are regulated by a national regulatory agency, the Care Quality Commission. This agency inspects health and social care services to check that standards are being met.

Most health and social care professions are also regulated by independent agencies relevant to their profession, such as the General Medical Council for doctors, and the Nursing and Midwifery Council for nurses. The General Social Care Council's code of practice requires all social care workers to '(bring) to the attention of your employer or the appropriate authority resource or operational difficulties that might get in the way of the delivery of safe care.' **www.gscc.org.uk**

In order to be allowed to do their jobs, workers in these professions have to be registered with their regulatory agency. An individual who is found guilty of professional misconduct, whether through abuse or neglect, will be disciplined by their specific professional agency or regulator.

Over the past two decades the idea of choice has become important to the health and social care professions, and to the government departments that make policies impacting on these sectors. It is now widely accepted that individuals should be able to make informed choices about the most suitable treatments for themselves. However, a patient does not have a legal right to demand a particular treatment, and complete choice does not always happen in practice, for example, the preferred treatment may not be available within an individual's local area.

Empowerment and duty of care

A crucial aspect of relationship building in your job role is making sure that people are able to make choices and take control over as much of their lives as possible. This is known as empowerment.

One of the difficulties in trying to work out when a duty of care exists is that courts always have the benefit of hindsight. Whether a duty of care is owed or not very much depends on the facts of the matter, including the positions of the people involved. For example, an expert giving advice to a non-expert can be expected to have a duty of care to the non-expert. The expert is considered to have superior knowledge and the non-expert rightfully expects to be able to rely on that superior knowledge. The expert thus assumes a duty of care in giving the advice and, if that advice is given negligently and without care, then he or she can expect a court to find that the duty of care has been breached.

Many people who receive care services are not able to make choices about what happens in their lives. This might be due to many factors, for example their physical ability, where they live, who provides care and the way services are provided.

Individuals who are unable to make choices and exercise control may also suffer from low self-esteem and lose confidence in their own abilities. There are other factors which may impact on self-esteem, including the degree of encouragement and praise a person is given from important people in their lives; the amount of satisfaction people get from their jobs and whether they have positive and happy relationships with friends and family.

Self-esteem has a major effect on people's health and well-being. Individuals who have a positive and confident outlook are far more likely to be active and interested in the world around them than those lacking confidence and belief in their own abilities. Therefore it is easy to see how this can affect an individual's quality of life and their overall health, safety and well-being.

Evidence activity

Choice

Explain how you think duty of care offers choice to individuals.

How would you feel if there was not a choice in the services you were receiving?

How do you think others will feel?

Often individuals are told the level of support they will be given and when it will be given. Services have limited budgets and resources which have to be managed in order to deliver services efficiently and effectively. They obviously try to consider and take account of the needs of the individuals, but here lies a tension, as resource and budget constraints must be adhered to. It is your role to try and ensure that your practice empowers individuals as far as possible.

LO2 Know how to address conflicts or dilemmas that may arise between an individual's rights and the duty of care

2.1 Potential conflicts or dilemmas that may arise between the duty of care and an individual's rights

Consequences of breaching a duty of care

Historically, a breach of a duty of care, once it has been proved, generally leads to damages being awarded to the injured party. In the United Kingdom, damages tend to be awarded only to **compensate** the injured party for their actual financial loss. In the United States, however, the level of damages awarded is often much greater. In courts in the United States juries are able to penalise defendants in cases where a duty of care has been breached by awarding what is called exemplary damages. The reasoning behind such awards is that they will discourage others from breaching their duty of care and set examples of the outcomes of poor practice.

Key term

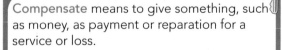

Compensate means to give something, such as money, as payment or reparation for a service or loss.

It is important that rights are supported by:

■ making sure that all staff understand the organisation's policies and guidelines relating to the rights of individuals

■ ensuring that individuals are made fully aware of the organisation's complaints procedures

■ discussing choices and preferences with individuals

■ ensuring that professional colleagues are made aware of an individual's choices and preferences

■ supporting individuals to maintain their rights and independence

■ refusing to participate in discriminatory or prejudicial behaviour.

The duty of care in childcare may involve conflicts in some situations. Issues related to the duty of confidentiality about children and their parents are an example.
A dilemma may arise which would normally require complete confidentiality, but which if not disclosed to parents of other children may put those children at risk. This would then be a breach of the duty of care to the other children. A decision to observe one duty could result in a breach of the other, and it is not always the case that one duty automatically has priority over the other. These situations require discussion, and advice and direction should be sought either from the employer or the sponsoring service or from a legal advisor.

There is no doubt that people working in health and social care are at risk of claims for breaches of duty of care. Employers and self-employed carers must ensure that they carry adequate insurance and comply with its terms. In addition, it is critical that carers comply with all obligations under any sponsored scheme or employment contract, a contract with a carer and any licensing body.

Research & investigate

(2.1) Conflicts and dilemmas

Find out what dilemmas you may encounter in your work place. How are these worked through and a resolution agreed?

(2.2) 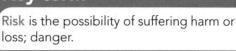 How to manage risks associated with conflicts or dilemmas between an individual's rights and the duty of care

Risk is part of everyday life and is evident in everything we do. Often it is the element or risk that allows us to grow and learn, and it is against these conditions that guidance has been developed across the sectors. Each area of health and social care has different issues with regard to consent, capacity, service involvement and areas of risk.

Key term

Risk is the possibility of suffering harm or loss; danger.

The concept of 'risk', its relevance and effect (both potential and actual) on individuals' and groups' lives in terms of their behaviour and outlook, has become increasingly important and much debated in modern society. Risk is complex and multi-dimensional, definitions and perceptions can vary across and within societies and/or cultures, and are frequently historically and event specific. Indeed, there is a growing body of literature within many academic disciplines exploring perceptions of risk: what 'risk' and 'risky behaviour' is and how this is managed in everyday life. Risk has also gained credence and prominence in the area of policy and practice, especially social policy. This growth has mirrored an increasing emphasis on personalisation and choice in the welfare state in general and social care in particular.

But it is important to recognise that the health and social care sector is large and disparate; there are many different perspectives to consider, including those of service providers, potential and actual service users and their relatives and carers. Moreover, perceptions of risk and views on what might constitute acceptable practice in appraising and assessing potential risks are likely to differ between different groups of professionals and the support they provide to different groups and informal carers in areas such as mental health, disability and older age.

Evidence activity

(2.2) Risks

Look around your workplace. What can you see that you think could be a risk? Is it the behaviour of someone or how the service is delivered?

Make a note of the risks you identify and of how you think you could reduce them.

2.3 Where to get additional support and advice about conflicts and dilemmas

Health and social care services usually involve the individual having contact with a number of staff. This could include frontline staff, a manager, volunteers, the local authority complaints manager, and inspectors and regulators as well as contract monitors. This creates a complex interaction of roles which can be confusing for the individual. It is therefore important to try to reduce duplication, but it is also important that staff are not confined to rigid roles that detract from a holistic approach to services. For example, in domiciliary services, even though the service might be monitored by both inspectors and a contract monitor, good practice might entail domiciliary staff being trained to spot possible abuse or changes in the well-being of an individual that might trigger the need for a care plan review. If domiciliary staff are not trained to do this it increases risk to the individual and wastes a resource that might reduce that risk. The same argument could be seen to apply to contract monitoring staff.

There is a legal underpinning to this argument in that if a local authority becomes aware – or ought to be aware – of risks to an individual they are likely to have a duty of care and obligations under the Human Rights Act 1998, and potentially under *No Secrets* guidance, to take action, whether or not a breach of contract is involved.

Evidence activity

2.3 Hierarchy of roles

In your workplace, ask about the hierarchy of roles. Who is responsible for what? Do you think the individuals you provide care for know all of this?

Draw a diagram or map illustrating key roles and functions.

On-going discussions, self-evaluation, **critique** of practices and professional development will help to ensure that policies and procedures are thorough, up to date, understood by all and most importantly that they translate into sound daily practice. In addition, establishing relationships with individuals, carers and relatives where there is open communication and where they are encouraged to ask questions and voice concerns will result in a shared care experience which is better for carers, parents and most importantly the individual concerned.

Figure 4.2

Key term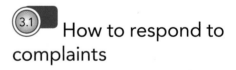

A **critique** is a critical discussion of a specified topic.

LO3 Know how to respond to complaints

3.1 How to respond to complaints

What is a complaint?

A complaint is an expression of dissatisfaction about employees' actions, lack of actions or the standard of service provided. A complaint could be one of the following:

■ An expression of unhappiness about the service provided.

■ Action or lack of action by the organisation affecting an individual or group.

■ An allegation that the organisation has failed to observe proper procedures.

■ An allegation that there has been an unacceptable delay in dealing with a matter or about how an individual has been treated by a member of staff.

Within the health and social care sector a complaint is an expression of dissatisfaction that requires an investigation and a response. Complaints that are to be dealt with under the NHS and Social Care Complaints Procedure need to be made by complainants. Where there is doubt as to whether a complaint is a 'formal' complaint or a concern, the 'complainant' should be asked whether they wish the matter to be dealt with through the Primary Care Trust (PCT) NHS complaints process leading to a formal response from the Chief Executive.

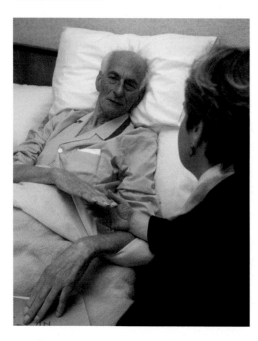

Figure 4.3

The benefits of complaints

From 1 April 2009, there is a single approach to dealing with NHS complaints. It gives organisations the flexibility they need to deal with complaints effectively. It also encourages a culture that seeks and then uses people's experiences to make services more effective, personal and safe.

Prevention is most definitely better than cure in relation to complaints. A well-organised setting with sound and effective procedures in place covering a wide range of service delivery and safety expectations will receive fewer complaints. Good communication with people ensures they have the information they need as they enter the setting and during their time with you. Policies regarding health and safety, patient care and so on will all help the smooth running of your setting. They will also reduce the likelihood of misunderstandings or dissatisfaction leading to complaints.

The legal framework

The legislation applies to NHS bodies, statutory or independent providers of NHS care (primary, secondary and tertiary care) and local authorities that provide adult social services. The new regulations came into force on 1 April 2009 and the law requires organisations to:

■ Publicise their complaints procedure.

■ Acknowledge receipt of a complaint and offer to discuss the matter within three working days.

■ Deal efficiently with complaints and investigate them properly and appropriately.

■ Write to the complainant on completion of a complaint investigation, explaining how it has been resolved, what appropriate action has been taken, and reminding them of their right to take the matter to the Health Service Ombudsman if they are still unhappy.

■ Assist the complainant in following the complaints procedure, or provide advice on where they may obtain such assistance.

■ Ensure that there is a designated manager for complaints.

■ Have someone senior who is responsible for both the complaints policy and learning from complaints.

■ Produce an annual report about complaints that have been received, the issues they raise, and any matters where action has been taken or is to be taken to improve services as a result of those complaints.

If the complaint involves two or more organisations, the person complaining should get a single, coordinated response. The Department of Health has produced a guide 'Listening, Responding, Improving' which provides a practical resource that complaints managers and their teams can use to help design excellent customer care systems locally and to support clinical and administrative staff in implementing change. http://www.opsi.gov.uk/stat.htm

People wishing to make complaints:

■ must do so within 12 months of an incident happening or of becoming aware of the matter complained about

■ can choose to complain to a commissioner instead of the service provider.

Research & investigate

 Dealing with complaints

Have any complaints been dealt with at your work setting? What process was used?

The Health Service Ombudsman – 'Principles of Good Complaints Handling'

From 1 April 2009 the Health Service Ombudsman takes over responsibility for investigating NHS complaints that can't be resolved locally, and the new approach to complaints is based on the Health Service Ombudsman's Six Principles of Good Complaints Handling. In summary, good complaint handling means:

1. getting it right
2. being customer focused
3. being open and accountable
4. acting fairly and proportionately
5. putting things right
6. seeking continuous improvement.

It is important that workers have a thorough understanding of their organisation's complaints procedure and their role in this. On occasions, it might be appropriate for the worker to assist the service user to initiate a complaint, particularly if the service user has no knowledge of the complaints procedure or if the service user is disadvantaged by language or disability. In this situation the worker may be acting as an 'advocate'. The *GSCC Code of Practice* refers to this activity as:

'3.1. Helping service users and carers to make complaints, taking complaints seriously and responding to them or passing them on to the appropriate person.'

Complaints about rights may also be made by workers. This is known as 'whistle blowing'. For example, the GSCC Code of Practice encourages social care workers to:

'3.2 Use established processes and procedures to challenge and report dangerous, abusive, discriminatory or exploitative behaviour and practice.'

The GSCC Code of Practice also encourages social care workers to:

'3.4. Bring to the attention of your employer or appropriate authority operational difficulties

that might get in the way of the delivery of safe care.'

'3.5. Inform your employer or appropriate authority where the practice of colleagues may be unsafe or adversely affect standards of care.'

Practice activity

 Codes of practice

Look for the GSCC Code of Practice. How does it impact on your role? Write down what you think you need to do to follow the Code.

Dealing with conflict and disputes

Any situation that involves close and prolonged contact with others has the potential to create conflict and disputes.

It is important that health and social care workers remain non-judgemental in their attempts to resolve disputes between individuals. If you encounter this situation, as a worker you should:

■ Remain calm and speak in a firm, quiet and controlled voice.

■ Be quite clear that neither verbal nor physical abuse will be tolerated.

■ Listen attentively to both sides of the argument, without any interruption.

■ Identify ways in which a compromise might be achieved without either party losing face.

■ Be clear that compromise is the only means to achieving a resolution.

3.2 The main points of agreed procedures for handling complaints

The complaints arrangements for health and social care have been reformed. Reports frequently identified that some complaints took too long to resolve and services did not systematically try to learn from the important feedback that complaints offer. In addition, there is strong evidence that some people do not complain because they either do not know how to or believe doing so will not result in any action.

Since 1 April 2009, a single complaints system covers all health and adult social care services in England. These revised arrangements will encourage an approach that aims to resolve complaints more effectively and ensure that opportunities for services to learn and improve are not lost. The Department of Health's new system for handling complaints about adult social care services aims to secure a first on two fronts.

Not only does it mean there will be a single process to deal with both health and social care-related complaints but the new legislation promises to deliver a more customer-focused approach. In addition the introduction of a single complaint route removes the difficulties many people claim they encounter navigating separate complaint systems for health and social services.

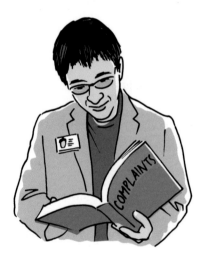

Figure 4.4

The new arrangements have three main components:

1. First, new regulations that enable local organisations to develop more flexible and responsive complaints handling systems that focus on the specific needs of the complainant, seek to reach speedy local resolution, facilitate coordinated handling of across-boundary complaints, and learning from people's experiences to help improve services.

2. Second, the introduction of a single local resolution stage, replacing the tiered stages prescribed by the old local authority social care regulations.

3. Third, a new single system for independent review by the Parliamentary and Health Service Ombudsman for healthcare.

Who is a complaint made to?

Complaints can be made to the organisation providing care, for example to a hospital or GP surgery, or direct to the commissioning body, usually the PCT or social services. If a PCT or social services receives a complaint about a provider, and they consider that they can deal with the complaint, they must seek consent from the complainant so that they can send details of the complaint to the provider. On receiving consent, the details must be sent as soon as possible. If, however, the PCT or social services consider it more appropriate for the provider to answer the complaint, and the complainant consents, the complaint can be passed to the provider for a response.

Complainants must choose at the outset whether to make a complaint to a primary care provider or the PCT. A complainant who makes an initial complaint to a provider and who does not agree with the provider's response cannot then seek a review from the PCT. Complainants who are dissatisfied with the response they receive from a primary care provider can refer the complaint to the Ombudsman.

If a complaint is made to any responsible body (the first body) which considers that the complaint should have been made to another responsible body (the second body), and the first body sends the complaint to the second body, the second body can respond to the complaint as if it had received it first. The second body must acknowledge the complaint within three working days.

The complaints procedure excludes:

■ complaints made by one NHS body against another

■ complaints made by employees in relation to their work for an NHS body

■ complaints that were first made orally and which were resolved to the complainant's satisfaction within one working day

■ complaints about the same subject matter as a complaint that has previously been made and resolved

■ complaints alleging failure by a public body to comply with a request for information under the Freedom of Information Act 2000

■ complaints about care solely provided by the independent healthcare sector, which has its own procedures.

If a responsible body considers that it is not required to consider a complaint, it must inform the complainant in writing of the decision and the reasons for it.

Practice activity

(3.2) Dealing with complaints

Locate a flow chart of how complaints are dealt with. Make a copy of this for your own evidence.

The complainant

Complainants should normally be current or former patients or nominated representatives, which can include a solicitor or a patient's elected representative, for example an MP. Never assume that someone complaining on behalf of a patient has authority to do so. The investigation of a complaint does not remove the need to respect a patient's right to confidentiality. Patients over the age of 16 whose mental capacity is unimpaired should normally complain themselves. Children under the age of 16 who are able to do so may also make their own complaint.

If someone other than the patient makes a complaint, you will need to make sure they have authority to do so. If patients lack capacity to make decisions for themselves, the representative must be able to demonstrate sufficient interest in their welfare and be an appropriate person to act on their behalf. This could include a partner or relative or someone appointed under the Mental Capacity Act 2005 with lasting power of attorney. If the power of attorney covers the person's welfare, this could include making complaints at a time when that person lacks capacity. In certain circumstances, the regulations impose a duty upon the responsible body to satisfy itself that a representative is an appropriate person to make a complaint. For example, if the complaint is about a child, the responsible body must satisfy itself that there are reasonable grounds for the representative to make the complaint, and not the child concerned. If the patient is a child or a patient who lacks capacity, the responsible body must also be satisfied that the representative is acting in the best interests of the person on whose behalf the complaint is made. If the responsible body is not satisfied that the representative is appropriate, it must not consider the complaint and must give the representative reasons for the decision in writing.

Time limits

The regulations require a complaint to be made within 12 months from the date on which the matter occurred, or from when the matter came to the attention of the complainant. The regulations state that a responsible body should consider a complaint outside that time limit if the complainant has good reason for not making the complaint within that limit and, despite the delay, it is still possible to investigate the complaint fairly and effectively. It is often the practice to consider complaints made outside the time limit if it is possible to investigate them. If there are any difficulties, for example if the relevant information is no longer available, it would be advisable to discuss this with complainants as soon as possible so they know what steps, if any, can reasonably be taken to investigate a complaint outside the time limit. While the regulations do not set timescales for the procedure itself, they do require a timely, appropriate response. If a response is not provided within six months from the date the complaint was made, or a later date if one was agreed with the complainant, the complaints manager has to write to the complainant and explain why it is delayed. The complaints manager must ensure the complainant receives a response as soon as possible.

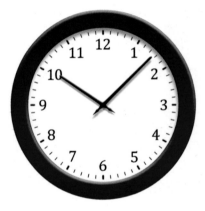

Figure 4.5

Disciplinary and criminal procedures

The complaint's procedure is a means for addressing patient complaints and does not have a disciplinary function. Inevitably some complaints will identify matters that suggest a need for disciplinary investigation. This might result in action via local procedures or referral to the practitioner's regulatory body. Complainants have no role in decisions to initiate disciplinary investigations (though they can refer serious concerns directly to the GMC, NMC or other regulatory body). Disciplinary procedures are confidential between an employer and employee, or a contracting body and a contractor, and complainants have no right to know the details or the outcome of such procedures.

In very rare cases a complaint might relate to a matter under police investigation.

Negligence claims

The regulations do not require a complaint to be stopped if there is a claim for negligence. If complainants are provided with a response setting out full details of the investigation and conclusions reached, this may help them and their legal adviser to decide whether there has been negligence.

Relevant legislation and guidance

The Local Authority Social Services & NHS Complaints (England) Regulations 2009 – came into force on 1 April 2009 and introduce a revised procedure for the handling of complaints by local authorities, in respect of complaints about adult social care, and by NHS bodies, primary care providers and independent providers in respect of provision of NHS care. The regulations align adult social care and health complaints processes into a single set of arrangements. These Regulations revoke the National Health Service (Complaints) Regulations 2004 and the National Health Service (Complaints) Amendment Regulations 2006.

Children Act 1989/2004 – provides a statutory basis for social care complaints.

Data Protection Act 1998 – governs the protection and use of person identifiable information (personal data). The Act does not apply to personal information relating to the deceased.

The Human Rights Act 1988 – Article 8.1 provides that 'everyone has the right to respect for his private and family life, his home and his correspondence.' Article 8.2 provides that 'there shall be no interference by a public authority with the exercise of this right except as in accordance with the law and if necessary in a democratic society in the interest of national security, public safety or the economic well-being of the country for the prevention of crime and disorder, for the protection of health or morals, or for the protection of the rights and freedoms of others.'

The Freedom of Information Act 2000 – the Act creates rights of access to information (rights of access to personal information remain under the Data Protection Act 1998) and revises and strengthens the Public Records Act 1958 and 1967 by reinforcing records management standards of practice.

Assessment summary

Your reading of this chapter and completion of the activities will have prepared you to demonstrate your learning and understanding of the principles of safeguarding and protection in health and social care.

To achieve the unit, your assessor will require you to:

Learning outcomes	Assessment Criteria
Learning outcome **1**: Understand how duty of care contributes to safe practice by:	**1.1** explaining what it means to have a duty of care in own work role See Research and investigate activity 1.1 p. 65.
	1.2 explaining how duty of care contributes to the safeguarding or protection of individuals See Research and investigate activity 1.2 p. 67 and Evidence activity 1.2 p. 68.

Learning outcomes	Assessment Criteria
Learning outcome **2**: Know how to address conflicts or dilemmas that may arise between an individual's rights and the duty of care by:	**2.1** describing potential conflicts or dilemmas that may arise between the duty of care and an individual's rights See Research and investigate activity 2.1 p. 69.
	2.2 describing how to manage risks associated with conflicts or dilemmas between an individual's rights and the duty of care See Evidence activity 2.2 p. 69.
	2.3 explaining where to get additional support and advice about conflicts and dilemmas See Evidence activity 2.3 p. 70.
Learning outcome **3**: Know how to respond to complaints by:	**3.1** describing how to respond to complaints See Practice activity 3.1 p. 72.
	3.2 explaining the main points of agreed procedures for handling complaints See Practice activity 3.2 p. 74.

Good luck!

Web links

Skills for Health	www.skillsforhealth.org.uk
Skills for Care and Development	www.skillsforcareanddevelopment.org.uk
Care Quality Commission	www.cqc.org.uk
General Social Care Council	www.gscc.org.uk
Nursing and Midwifery Council	www.nmc-uk.org

Principles of safeguarding and protection in health and social care

For Unit HSC 024

What are you finding out?

Everyone has a responsibility to help keep children and adults safe and free from abuse. Individuals using health and social care services are vulnerable and particularly at risk of neglect, harm or exploitation for a multitude of reasons, such as their age, mental, physical or intellectual ability, or state of health. Providers of health and social care services have a duty to comply with safeguarding legislation set up to protect vulnerable people, and health and social care workers have a responsibility to follow policies and procedures that enable them to recognise and respond promptly and appropriately to suspicions or allegations of abuse.

The reading and activities in this chapter will help you to:

■ Know how to recognise signs of abuse

■ Know how to respond to suspected or alleged abuse

■ Understand the national and local context of safeguarding and protection from abuse

■ Understand ways to reduce the likelihood of abuse

■ Know how to recognise and report unsafe practices.

LO1 Know how to recognise signs of abuse

Abuse is a violation of an individual's human and civil rights by another person. Abuse can occur in any relationship, and abusers or perpetrators may be relatives and family members, professional staff, paid care workers, personal assistants, volunteers, other service users, neighbours, friends, people who deliberately exploit vulnerable people, and strangers. It may consist of a single act or repeated acts. It may be physical, verbal or psychological; it may be neglect; or it may occur when a vulnerable person is persuaded to enter into a financial or sexual transaction to which they have not consented or cannot consent.

No secrets: Guidance on developing and implementing multi-agency policies and procedures to protect vulnerable adults from abuse. **www.dh.gov.uk**

Whatever the abuse, it may result in significant harm to, or exploitation of, the person subjected to it. It can never be condoned.

1.1 Define the different types of abuse

■ **Physical abuse** is defined as any pain, suffering or injury that is **wilfully** inflicted. It includes hitting, slapping, pushing, kicking; rough handling, for example during a moving and handling procedure; forcing people to do things that are inappropriate or against their wishes, such as being sent to their room as punishment; hiding medication in food or giving medication inappropriately, for example to control or subdue; restraint, such as tying down to a chair or toilet; keeping the environment too hot or too cold; and denying food and drink.

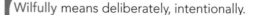

Key term

Wilfully means deliberately, intentionally.

■ **Sexual abuse** is defined as sexual assault or involving someone in sexual activity to which they have not consented or do not fully understand. It includes inappropriate kissing or touching, for example of the breasts and genitals;

vaginal, anal or oral rape, including penetration with objects; and exposure to sexually explicit language and pornography.

■ **Emotional/psychological abuse** is defined as the wilful infliction of mental suffering by someone in a position of trust. It includes threats of harm or abandonment, deprivation of contact, humiliation, blaming, controlling, intimidation, coercion, harassment, verbal abuse, isolation or withdrawal from services and supportive networks. Emotional/psychological abuse is also the wilful failure of someone in a position of trust to prevent mental suffering inflicted by somebody else.

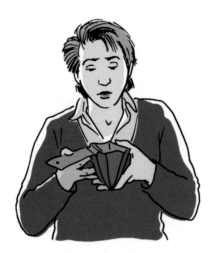

Figure 5.1 Financial abuse

■ **Financial abuse** is defined as the theft or misuse of someone's money, property or resources by someone in a position of trust. Theft and misuse include fraud, exploitation, extortion; pressure, for example in connection with wills, inheritance and financial transactions; and swindling someone out of their savings, investments or benefits.

■ **Institutional abuse** is defined as repression of an individual's needs or choices due to poor professional practice and priority being given to rigid organisational procedures. It takes place, for example, when there is no choice regarding what to eat and drink and when to get up, go to bed, go to the toilet; when clothing and toiletries are shared; when an individual is not allowed to make their own decisions; when medication is not given at the right time; and when someone's personal information is shared without their permission.

■ **Neglect** is defined as the failure of someone who is responsible for a vulnerable person to give them the necessary degree of care. Neglect includes ignoring physical care needs, such as help with personal hygiene and toileting, prevention of pressure sores and protection from health and safety hazards; failure to provide access to, for example, services and social contact; and withholding the necessities of life, such as adequate nutrition, warmth and shelter.

■ **Self-neglect** is defined as the failure, usually of an adult, to care for and protect themselves, for example by living in unsanitary, hazardous conditions; failing to eat and drink properly or maintain personal hygiene; failing to seek help when ill; and failing to take prescribed medication.

Time to reflect

1.1 Self-neglect

Health and social care workers have a hard job. They need to be fit, have a nutritious diet and have sufficient rest and relaxation. If they neglect their health in any way, they can't do their job properly and jeopardise their and other people's safety. Do you look after yourself properly?

 1.2 Identify the signs and/or symptoms associated with each type of abuse

A sign is an indication of health status that can be seen, such as the pallor of the skin; heard, as when blood pressure is measured using a sphygmomanometer; or touched, such as feeling with the fingers for a pulse. Symptoms are the feelings someone has when they are ill, such as pain, confusion, depression.

Table 5.1 Types of abuse and their signs and symptoms

Type of abuse	Signs include:	Symptoms include:
Physical	Cuts, scratches, bite marks; bruises; burns from cigarettes, rough handling, use of restraint; pressure ulcers; scalds and blisters; fractures; withdrawal; abuse of others.	Fear, belittlement, anger; loss of self-confidence and self-esteem; pain due to injuries.
Sexual	Love bites; injuries to the mouth, genitals or anus; blood stained underwear; urinary tract and sexually transmitted infections; pregnancy; withdrawal; inability to develop normal sexual relationships; overtly sexual behaviour.	Fear, shame, guilt; loss of dignity and self-respect; pain due to injuries and infection.
Emotional/ psychological	Rocking, flinching; self-harm; comfort eating; tearfulness; withdrawal; aggression.	Embarrassment, fear, humiliation, resignation; loss of self-confidence, self-esteem and sense of belonging.
Financial	Unexplained loss of money and personal possessions; missing receipts; insufficient money for bills; being bought products that do not match capacity to pay; care workers/ carers benefiting from 'buy-one-get-one-free' offers when doing the shopping; dependency on others; diminishing health status due to reduced quality of life.	Anxiety about financial affairs and fears for the future; loss of independence and control.
Institutional	Loss of interest in the environment and loss of ability to make choices, act independently, communicate; loss of clothing and personal possessions; withdrawal; aggression.	Loss of independence and control over own life; anger; frustration; depression; despair; hopelessness.
Neglect and self-neglect	Dirty, smelly; under/overweight; poor health; poor living conditions; inadequate clothing; loss of interest; withdrawal.	Symptoms associated with poor health status, such as pain due to pressure ulcers, hunger, cold; loneliness.

Evidence activity

 and Types of abuse and associated signs and symptoms

This activity enables you to demonstrate your knowledge of the different types of abuse and associated signs and symptoms.

Produce a set of cards to which everyone at your workplace can refer in order to help them establish if abuse is taking place. There should be a card each for physical, sexual, emotional/ psychological, financial and institutional abuse, and neglect and self-neglect. The cards should:

- state what is meant by each type of neglect

- describe the signs associated with each type of abuse and neglect

- describe the symptoms associated with each type of abuse and neglect.

Describe factors that may contribute to an individual being more vulnerable to abuse

The setting or situation in which people find themselves can have an impact on their vulnerability to abuse. For example, living alone, isolated from social support networks such as family and friends can make people welcoming of company or assistance but unable to assess its trustworthiness. Tales of elderly people being exploited for this reason abound in the media. Social isolation can also mean restricted access to services such as health and social care, transport and the police. As a result, signs of abuse are less likely to be detected, giving free rein to perpetrators.

Poor housing and overcrowding breed aggression, leading to abuse from which, for some, there may be no escape. In addition, shared accommodation increases the risk of having to live with people you wouldn't choose to live with because of their potential to be abusive.

Residential care accommodation is not without risk of abuse. People who have experience of being abused, which includes health and social care workers and people using the services, very often become abusers themselves. Care work gives people power and authority, which, if taken advantage of, can lead to abuse. In addition, work practice that fails to provide the necessary degree of care amounts to neglect. For these reasons, safeguarding legislation is in place that service providers and their employees have a duty to obey.

Shocking as it may seem, living alone or with family or friends and depending on their care is also not without risk. Relying on family and friends to care often puts the **carer** under a huge strain. The needs of vulnerable people often exceed the ability and empathy of their carers, who usually have to change their lifestyle to carry out their caring role and, in doing so, can become socially isolated and develop their own personal difficulties. The consequence is often a soured relationship, which unfortunately may lead to abuse. www.carers.org

Key term

A carer is someone who, without payment, provides help and support to a partner, child, relative, friend or neighbour, who could not manage without their help.

Some people are more vulnerable to abuse than others, for example, because they have:

- limited life experience and sex education, so find it difficult to anticipate abusive situations

- learning, understanding and communication difficulties, so are unaware of their rights and do not know how to complain

- personal, often intimate care needs

- low self-esteem, so lack power in relationships

- a history of violent behaviour, alcoholism, substance misuse or mental illness

- financial problems, such as debt, low income.

In addition, people's age or physical disability can make them victims of discrimination, which is a further form of abuse.

Time to reflect

 Vulnerability to abuse

Think about the people at school who were bullied. Why do you think they were emotionally abused in this way? Was it, for example, because they had learning or physical difficulties, low self-esteem or were poor? How do you think they felt? How would you feel if you were a victim? How do you feel now, if you were a perpetrator?

Evidence activity

Factors that may contribute to vulnerability to abuse

This activity enables you to demonstrate your knowledge of the factors that can make an individual more vulnerable to abuse.

Think about three individuals where you work who you think are especially vulnerable to abuse. What is it about these individuals that makes them more vulnerable? Is it, for example, where they live, the setting in which they are supported, their particular needs? It is important that you are able to identify individuals who are especially vulnerable and why, in order to safeguard them effectively.

LO2 Know how to respond to suspected or alleged abuse

 2.1 Explain the actions to take if there are suspicions that an individual is being abused

If you suspect a colleague or someone in an individual's personal network, for example, their carer or a visitor, of abuse, speak with them politely about your concerns. Never ignore your suspicions of abuse, but never accuse anyone until you understand the reason for their behaviour. For example, it may not seem quite right to you if someone asks a person to walk to the toilet when they have requested a wheelchair, but they may simply be encouraging independence and the ability to walk. On the other hand, they may not be aware that their behaviour is wrong or that they are causing suffering.

If you remain concerned, you have a responsibility to speak out, regardless of any concerns you may have about the consequences of doing so. Your workplace will have a procedure telling you how to deal with suspicions of abuse. However, as a rule of thumb:

■ Discuss your concerns with your supervisor or line manager or, in the case of suspected child abuse, with the Child Protection Officer, in private, without delay. They will decide an appropriate course of action, for example, whether to contact the police, health or social services and family. Do not overstep your responsibilities – dealing with suspected abuse will be someone else's responsibility.

■ Record your concerns on the appropriate report form. Records should be clear, easy to understand, concise and relevant. Only state things as they appeared to you – do not embellish for the sake of 'a good story'.

■ Make every effort to preserve any evidence of abuse. You will read about this later.

■ Request to be kept informed about what is decided and why.

If you suspect your supervisor or line manager of abuse, check to understand the reason for their behaviour. If you remain concerned, talk things over with someone in a more senior position straightaway. If the person you suspect has seniority where you work, talk to the owner or manager of your organisation or to the body that regulates the quality of care in your part of the UK, for example the Care Quality Commission

(CQC) in England, the Commission for the Regulation of Care in Scotland (SCRC) and Ofsted, which regulates services for children and young people. Expect to make a record of your suspicions and request to be kept informed about proceedings.
www.cqc.org.uk; www.carecommission.com; www.ofsted.gov.uk

If you suspect that you have a tendency to be abusive, perhaps verbally because swearing is part of your everyday language, discriminatory because you allow your prejudices to show through, or physically because you are time-poor and liable to rough handling in order to finish a task quickly, share your concerns with a trusted colleague or your line manager. If talking things through doesn't convince you that your suspicions are unfounded, request extra supervision, counselling or training. Ask to be relieved of working with certain people or of tasks that you know you do not perform well. Ultimately, you are responsible for your behaviour so it is up to you to make the necessary changes.

 Evidence activity

2.1 Actions to take regarding suspicions of abuse

This activity enables you to demonstrate your understanding of what to do in the event of suspicions of abuse.

■ Check out your workplace's procedure about how to deal with suspicions of abuse. What are the reasons for following the various actions it describes?

■ What should you do if you suspect that your behaviour is not all it should be?

2.2 Explain the actions to take if an individual alleges that they are being abused

There are a number of ways in which abuse can be alleged, including a victim disclosing that something has happened to them, or an accusation being made by an observer. It takes a great deal of courage for someone to allege abuse, because they may fear that by doing so things will get worse, or that they will be blamed. They might also think that no one will believe them.

Time to reflect

 Alleging abuse

What might stop you alleging an abuse, either of yourself or of someone else? Can you understand why people hesitate to do so?

Your workplace will have a procedure in place that describes how you should deal with allegations of abuse. However, when someone makes a disclosure to you, as a general rule:

■ Accept what they say and reassure them that you take them seriously. Different people have different ideas of what constitutes abuse, for example, you might take no notice of sexually explicit language whereas others become deeply distressed. Do not let your views and emotions prevent you from treating the victim with dignity and taking what they say seriously.

■ Do not 'interview' the person and do not interrupt. Listen calmly to what they say, avoid asking lots of questions and be comfortable with silences. Silences provide thinking time. Try to remember what they say so that you can record it later, before you forget.

■ Do not promise to keep things confidential. Explain that you need to tell another person, but only someone who needs to know so that they can help.

■ Take steps to make them safe.

■ Make every effort to preserve any evidence of abuse.

You will need to make a detailed report of what you are told, including:

■ when the disclosure was made

■ who was involved and the names of any witnesses

■ what happened – what you were told: facts only, no interpretations

■ any other relevant information, such as details of previous incidents that have caused concern.

Use the relevant report form and keep it safe and confidential until you can give it to the appropriate person. Avoid the alleged perpetrator and do not discuss the incident with anyone as this could breach the victim's confidentiality and alert the perpetrator that suspicions have been aroused. It could also complicate any internal or police investigations. Request to be kept informed about what is decided and why.

Evidence activity

 Actions to take regarding allegations of abuse

This activity enables you to demonstrate your understanding of what to do in the event of an individual alleging that they are being abused.

Check out your workplace's procedure about what to do if an individual tells you they are being abused. What are the reasons for following the various actions it describes?

2.3 Identify ways to ensure that evidence of abuse is preserved

Because the police could be involved in a suspected or alleged case of abuse, it is important to preserve any evidence relating to the incident. Failing to preserve evidence is often described as 'decontamination'. If you are in any doubt about how to preserve evidence, including footprints, fingerprints and anything else that may have been left behind by the suspect, consult the police on the telephone prior to their arrival.

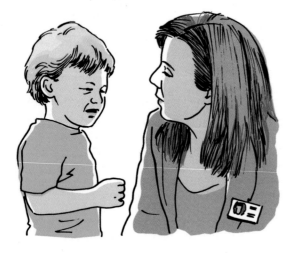

Figure 5.2 Listening to a disclosure

Ten top tips to ensure that evidence of abuse is preserved

1. Do not remove or alter documentation relating to the incident, and preserve video recordings if security cameras are present. You will be held accountable if you destroy or invalidate evidence.

2. Do not allow anyone to enter the scene of the incident until the police arrive, with the exception of medical staff. A medical examination should only take place to decide the extent of injury, provide first aid or arrange for transfer to hospital.

3. Make a note, before you forget, of the state of the alleged victim and perpetrator's clothing, their physical and emotional condition, and of any obvious injuries.

4. Do not let the victim and alleged perpetrator come into contact with each other once the allegation has been made.

5. Do not allow anyone to have physical contact with either the victim or the alleged perpetrator in the event of alleged sexual abuse.

6. Do not move anything.

7. Do not touch anything unless you have to. If anything is handed to you, take care not to destroy fingerprints.

8. Do not clean up and do not wash anything, for example to remove blood or semen.

9. Do not throw anything away. If sexual abuse has been alleged, keep hold of any items that might provide evidence, such as used condoms, objects.

10. Do not assume that it is too late if an allegation is made days after the alleged offence. It may still be possible to collect forensic evidence. Let the police decide.

Evidence activity

 How to preserve evidence of abuse

This activity enables you to demonstrate your knowledge of how to preserve evidence in the event of abuse.

Use a search engine such as Google, or research local and national newspapers, for reports of abuse. If you, as a worker, had been associated with these incidents, how would you have preserved evidence in order not to impair any police investigations?

LO3 Understand the national and local context of safeguarding and protection from abuse

 Identify national policies and local systems that relate to safeguarding and protection from abuse

Following the murders of Jessica Chapman and Holly Wells by Ian Huntley, a school caretaker, the government commissioned the Bichard Inquiry (2002). One of the issues this inquiry looked at was the way employers recruit people to work with children and vulnerable adults.

Research & investigate

3.1 Recruitment where you work

Find out how your organisation goes about recruiting staff to work with vulnerable people.

The Bichard Inquiry's recommendations led to the Safeguarding Vulnerable Groups Act 2006 and the Vetting and Barring Scheme, which is run by the Independent Safeguarding Authority (ISA). The ISA works closely with the **Criminal Records Bureau (CRB)** and uses information in the **PoVA** (Protection of Vulnerable Adults) and **PoCA** (Protection of Children Act) lists and in **List 99** to assess or vet anyone who wants to work or volunteer with children or vulnerable adults. As a result of vetting, the ISA either:

■ gives them ISA registration, which demonstrates that they are able to work with children or vulnerable adults, or

■ puts them on one of the ISA Barred Lists. One records people prevented from working with children and the other people prevented from working with vulnerable adults. **www. isa-gov.org.uk; www.crb.homeoffice.gov.uk**

Key terms

The **Criminal Records Bureau (CRB)** holds information about individuals, such as convictions, cautions, reprimands and warnings.

List 99 is a list of teachers who are considered unsuitable or banned from working with children in school.

The **PoVA** and **PoCA** schemes were replaced by the Vetting and Barring Scheme in October 2009.

A **Green Paper** is a consultation document issued by the government, which contains policy proposals for debate and discussion before a final decision is taken on the best policy option.

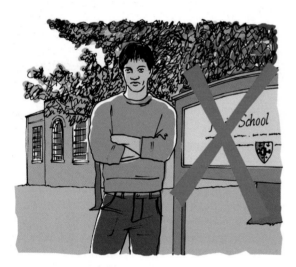

Figure 5.3 You can't work here!

At the time of writing (July 2010), the new coalition government has halted the Vetting and Barring Scheme for review. However, the following safeguarding regulations continue to apply:

■ A person who is barred from working with children or vulnerable adults is breaking the law if they work or volunteer, or try to work or volunteer, with these groups.

■ An organisation that knowingly employs someone who is barred from working with these groups is breaking the law.

■ Organisations that work with vulnerable groups have a legal duty to give ISA information about people who they believe have harmed or may pose a risk of harm to children or vulnerable adults.

Following the report into the death of Victoria Climbié, who was horrifically tortured and eventually killed by her great aunt and her partner, the government published the **Green Paper** 'Every Child Matters' (2003). This paper prompted wide consultation about services for children, young people and families. As a result, the government passed the Children Act in 2004, which provides the legislation for ensuring the safety and protection of children, young people and families.

'Every Child Matters' spells out how professionals must work together to provide children's care. It is based on five outcomes, which Local Authorities use to put together their 'Children and Young People's Plans'. These plans describe how services are to be developed and delivered, and are used to measure success. One of these outcomes is that children 'stay safe', in other words, that they have security, stability, are cared for and that they are safe from:

■ maltreatment, neglect, violence and sexual exploitation

■ accidental injury and death

■ bullying and discrimination

■ crime and antisocial behaviour in and out of school.

In March 2010, the Government published the guidance document 'Working Together to Safeguard Children'. This document describes the roles of the different agencies that are involved in safeguarding and protecting children and young people, including public sector organisations such as health care providers, police, probation services, Youth Offending Teams, schools, Connexions, early years services, Children and Family Court Advisory and Support Service (Cafcass) and the UK Border Agency (UKBA); voluntary sector organisations, such as the NSPCC and Barnardo's; and parents, carers and faith communities.

■ Children's Trusts consist of all the agencies working to safeguard and protect children within a locality.

■ Children's Trust Boards oversee the **inter-agency working** agreements made between the different agencies.

■ Local Safeguarding Children Boards (LSCBs) have a legal responsibility to agree how agencies will work together in implementing the local 'Children and Young People's Plans'.

Key term

Inter-agency working is when two or more agencies or organisations work together. Direct payments are local council payments to people who have been assessed as needing help from social services, and who would like to arrange and pay for their own care and support services instead of receiving them directly from the local council.

The media continues to report tragedies that demonstrate a lack of safety and protection for vulnerable adults. The Human Rights Act 1998 is in place to promote everyone's right to freedom from torture, inhuman and degrading treatment, and public sector health and social care providers have a responsibility to comply with the Act in their work with vulnerable adults. However, unless providing services on behalf of the public sector, private providers do not have any such responsibility. In addition, providers of services to **direct payment** users are, at the time of writing, not liable for human rights abuses, although the government is considering a review of the situation. www.equalityhumanrights.com; communitycare.co.uk

Research & investigate

(3.1) Legislation relating to abuse

The Human Rigts Act is one of a number of pieces of information that aims to protect vulnerable people from abuse. Find out which ones shape your work

In its publication 'No secrets', the government describes its requirement for multi-agency working to ensure that vulnerable adults are protected against abuse. In complying with 'No secrets', and to reflect legal requirements such as the National Minimum Care Standards and professional body standards such as the General Social Care Council Codes of Practice, local agencies have developed Safeguarding Adults Boards and Vulnerable Adults Safeguarding Policies and Procedures.

No Secrets: **Guidance on developing and implementing multi-agency policies and procedures to protect vulnerable adults from abuse. Department of Health. www.dh.gov. uk; www.gscc.org.uk**

Safeguarding Adults Boards bring together local agencies that work with vulnerable adults and monitor their use of safeguarding policies and procedures. Agencies include public sector organisations such as health care providers, learning disability teams, residential, sheltered and supported housing, the police and DSS Benefits Agency; voluntary sector organisations such as MIND, Age UK, the Alzheimer's Society, Mencap and CAB; carer support groups and user groups; private organisations such as lawyers; and multi-agency groups such as Safer Community Partnerships.

www.mind.org.uk; alzheimers.org.uk; www. ageuk.org.uk; www.citizensadvice.org.uk; www.mencap.org.uk; www.carersuk.org

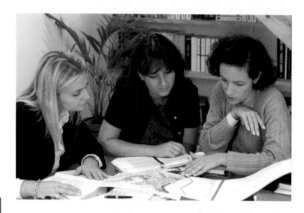

Figure 5.4 Multi-agency working

Evidence activity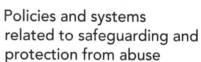

(3.1) Policies and systems related to safeguarding and protection from abuse

This activity enables you to demonstrate your knowledge of national and local safeguarding and protection policies and systems.

Explore a variety of information sources, such as websites (try googling the title of this activity), your local authority, health service providers, the police, and voluntary organisations that work with vulnerable people, to find out what safeguarding and protection policies and systems are at work in your area, and what influence national government has had on shaping their existence.

3.2 Explain the roles of different agencies in safeguarding and protecting individuals from abuse

As you read earlier, Safeguarding Children Boards have a responsibility to agree how agencies will work together in implementing local 'Children and Young People's Plans'. In sum, it is the responsibility of all involved to commit to cooperative working and information sharing, and to:

■ be alert to the potential indicators of abuse or neglect

■ be alert to the risks of harm that abusers or potential abusers may pose to children

■ show respect in their interactions with children, see situations from their perspective, and ensure that their wishes and feelings underpin assessments and any safeguarding activities

■ share and help to analyse information so that an assessment can be made of the child's needs and circumstances and whether they are suffering or likely to suffer harm

■ contribute to whatever actions are needed to safeguard and promote the child's welfare

■ take part in regularly reviewing the outcomes for the child against plans for their welfare

■ work cooperatively with parents, unless this is inconsistent with ensuring the child's safety.

Working Together to Safeguard Children: A guide to inter-agency working to safeguard and promote the welfare of children, Crown copyright 2010

Safeguarding Adults Boards bring together and oversee the agencies that work with vulnerable adults, to ensure effective inter-agency working. It is the responsibility of all involved to commit to cooperative working and information sharing, and to:

■ empower and promote the well-being of vulnerable adults

■ support their rights to be independent and make choices; recognise when they are unable to make decisions and give advice, support and protection as appropriate

■ help them to understand the hazards associated with any risks they want to take and minimise those risks as far as possible

■ ensure their safety by following procedures

■ ensure that they receive the protection of the law and access to the judicial process.

Evidence activity

3.2 Roles of different agencies in safeguarding and protecting against abuse

This activity enables you to demonstrate your understanding of the roles of different agencies in safeguarding and protecting individuals from abuse.

Think about the group of individuals with whom you work. It may be children, elderly people, people with mental health problems, people with learning difficulties. What agencies, apart from the one you work for, are involved in supporting these people? What is their particular role in providing support and why do they have this role?

3.3 Identify reports into serious failures to protect individuals from abuse

Abuse may be perpetrated by carers, such as family and volunteers; care workers, such as professional staff and personal assistants; people who deliberately exploit vulnerable people; friends, neighbours and strangers. And it can take place in any context, for example in the person's own home, in nursing, residential or day care settings, in hospitals, even in public and in places previously assumed safe.

You read above about the shocking deaths of Jessica Chapman, Holly Wells and Victoria Climbié; and you have also heard about Baby Peter. Each died at the hands of either family or people they trusted, and because the potential for abuse had not been properly assessed. According to NSPCC research, during 2009:

■ 15,800 children and young people were the victims of neglect

■ 4,400 of physical abuse

■ 2,000 of sexual abuse

■ 9,100 of emotional abuse

■ 2,900 were the victims of abuse for other, mixed reasons.

In other words, a total of 34,000 children and young people were suffering from some sort of abuse, not counting the cases that went unobserved or unreported.

www.nspcc.org.uk

Failure to protect vulnerable adults is reported on a regular basis in the media. You may have witnessed it yourself. Search engines such as Google list endless reports of, for example, neglect, self-neglect and financial abuse of elderly people; sexual and emotional abuse of people with learning difficulties; self-neglect and institutional abuse of people with mental health problems; and physical and emotional abuse of people with disabilities. But, tragically, many incidents of abuse go unobserved or unreported.

(3.3) **Failures to protect individuals from abuse**

This activity enables you to demonstrate your knowledge of reports into serious failures to protect individuals from abuse.

The reports of Lord Laming and Sir Michael Bichard have been catalysts for the reform of safeguarding and protection. Check out their reports (try googling the title of this activity), as well as those published by the CQC (Care Quality Commission); private, charitable and voluntary organisations; specialist health and social care journals; and health and social care providers in your locality/region.

What do you think? How much progress have we made when it comes to protecting individuals from abuse? Why does it still happen?

(3.4) **Identify sources of information and advice about own role in safeguarding and protecting individuals from abuse**

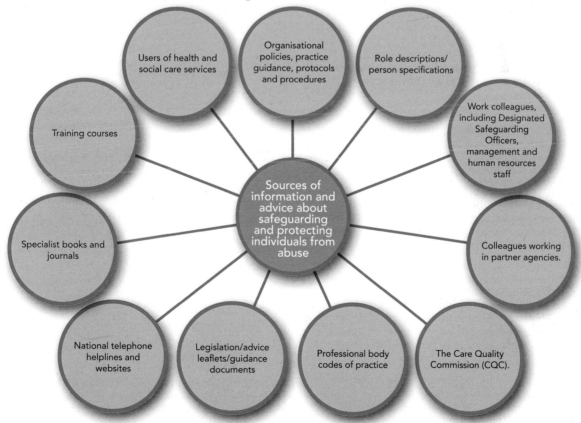

Figure 5.5 Where can you find information and advice about safeguarding and protecting individuals from abuse?

Evidence activity

 Sources of information and advice on safeguarding and protecting

This activity enables you to demonstrate your knowledge of where you can find information and advice about your role in safeguarding and protecting individuals from abuse.

Make a list of five people and five places that you can use to find out what you should be doing to help protect people from abuse.

LO4 Understand ways to reduce the likelihood of abuse

4.1 Explain how the likelihood of abuse may be reduced

Abuse occurs as the result of deliberate intent or negligence, and usually stems from the fact that perpetrators have little or no regard for their victims. They do not value them as people. Best practice in health and social care settings requires workers to use person-centred values in their work. By doing so, they demonstrate respect for:

■ Personal values, beliefs, preferences and life experiences – a lack of respect for, for example, the value someone puts on family and treasured possessions, their religious and political beliefs, their likes and dislikes and their life history can be emotional abuse.

■ Choices – denying a choice of food can be physical abuse, and preventing someone from getting up and going to bed when they decide can be a form of institutional abuse.

■ Rights – for example, a failure to protect from danger and denying medication amount to physical abuse; unfair treatment and discrimination is emotional abuse; denying someone their pocket money or benefit payments is financial abuse; denying personal privacy could amount to sexual abuse; and not promoting dignity could be seen as neglect.

■ Active participation and independence – we all need to be involved in everyday life and to develop and maintain independence. Failure to encourage an individual to take part in activities and relationships on a day-to-day basis and to live their life independently may be both emotionally and institutionally abusive. In addition, preventing someone from being an active partner in their care can be emotional abuse.

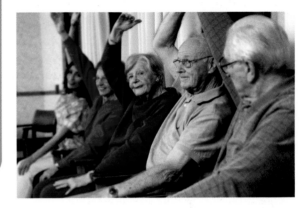

Figure 5.6 Active participation and independence

The likelihood of abuse is reduced by working with person-centred values, promoting choice and rights and encouraging active participation. Anything else is bad practice and synonymous with abuse.

Evidence activity

 How to reduce the likelihood of abuse

This activity enables you to demonstrate your understanding of how to reduce the likelihood of abuse by working with person-centred values, encouraging active participation and promoting choice and rights.

Why does:

■ having respect for someone's personal values, beliefs, preferences and life experiences reduce the likelihood of their being abused?

■ showing respect for someone's right to choice, safety, medical care, fair treatment, financial support, privacy and dignity reduce the likelihood of their being abused?

■ being actively involved in day-to-day life reduce the likelihood of an individual being abused?

4.2 Explain the importance of an accessible complaints procedure for reducing the likelihood of abuse

Because abuse is a violation of an individual's human and civil rights and very often illegal, it cannot be condoned. A complaint must be made.

All health and social care providers are legally required to have a complaints procedure.

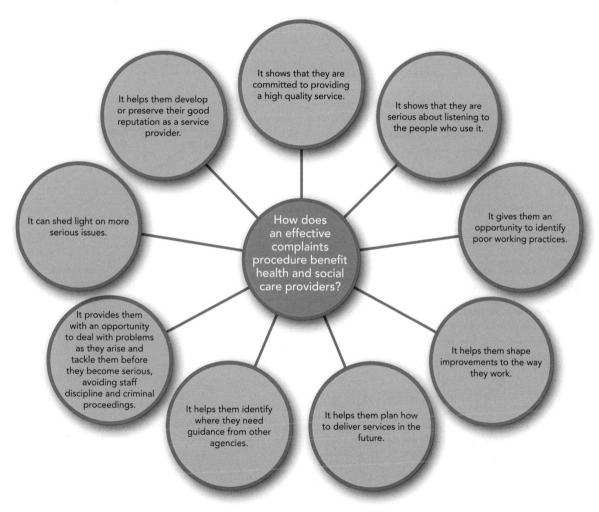

Figure 5.7 The benefits of complaints procedures

Complaints procedures need to be accessible. This is particularly important given the vulnerability of people using health and social care services. Accessibility of complaints means that they must:

■ be publicised and easy to get hold of, to advertise that people have a right to complain and to encourage them to do so. This includes everyone who suspects, has witnessed or is a victim of abuse.

■ be clear and understandable. Style and language are very important. For example,

children, people with learning difficulties and speakers of foreign languages would have difficulty understanding a complaints procedure written for English adults, as would someone who uses Braille or has a sight impairment. Complaints procedures must be published in a variety of formats to reflect the age, understanding, ability and communication needs of the different people involved.

■ ensure confidentiality. Information leaks can have a serious impact on both the complainant and the person it was about, and therefore discourage complaints being made.

■ ensure that complainants will be listened to and taken seriously. Anything less would be neglect.

■ ensure that complainants will be treated fairly, honestly and with respect. Anything less would be in breach of their human and civil rights.

■ reassure complainants that they will receive support that meets their needs while their complaint is being investigated and a response when the investigation is complete.

Evidence activity

 Importance of an accessible complaints procedure

This activity enables you to demonstrate your understanding of the need for an accessible complaints procedure.

Check out your organisation's complaints procedure.

■ Does everyone who might want to use it know it exists?

■ Is it easy to get hold of? Think in terms of its location – is it accessible by a wheelchair user? And is anxiety when asking for the procedure anticipated and dealt with?

■ Is it clear and understandable – does it meet everyone's communication needs?

■ Does it reassure people that their complaint will be taken seriously and that confidentiality will be maintained?

■ Does it describe what will happen once the complaint has been made and promise a response within a given time?

Hopefully your answers will all be positive. If not, talk the procedure over with your manager. It might not have occurred to them that the procedure is not fit for purpose.

LO5 Know how to recognise and report unsafe practices

 Describe unsafe practices that may affect the well-being of individuals

Unsafe, abusive work practices that can affect an individual's well-being include:

■ rough handling, for example pushing, pulling and dragging

■ misuse of medication, for example hiding medication in food or giving medication to control or subdue

■ ignoring health needs, such as pressure ulcers, and social needs, such as clean clothing and personal hygiene

■ keeping the environment too hot, too cold, drafty, stuffy

■ not providing food and drink when requested

■ not taking someone to the toilet when they need to go; leaving them in soiled, wet clothing or bedding

■ inappropriate restraint, such as tying down to a bed, chair or toilet

■ dismissing dignity needs, such as invading privacy and helping someone to wash or use the toilet in a less than private situation

■ making people do things they do not want to do, for example eat or go to bed when they are not ready

■ controlling people, making decisions for them, not allowing them to do as they wish

■ abandoning people and isolating them, for example to punish

■ belittling people

■ using crude or sexually explicit language

■ shopping for someone and taking advantage of buy-one-get-one-free offers; collecting points for their purchases onto your club card; not giving them their receipts

■ coercing someone to buy from your personal shopping catalogue.

Resource and operational difficulties can also impact on well-being. Resources are the things you need in order to do your job safely and avoid abuse. They include health and safety training and supervision to ensure you work safely;

access to policies, procedures and guidance documents, including safeguarding procedures that guide you in safe practice and enable you to report concerns; safe, well-maintained equipment; personal protective equipment and hand-washing facilities; safe disposal facilities; time. A lack of resources leads to unsafe practice and a threat to well-being.

Time to reflect

 Time to own up …

Are you guilty of any of these abusive work practices? It could be that you have been unaware of your behaviour, that no-one pointed it out to you, that nothing more was expected of you. Now you know what constitites abuse, there is no going back. How can you ensure that you will work more safely in the future?

Resource and operational difficulties can also impact on well-being. Resources are the things you need in order to do your job and avoid abuse. They include health and safety training and supervision to ensure you work safely; access to policies, procedures and guidance documents, including safeguarding procedures that guide you in safe practice and enable you to report concerns; safe, well maintained equipment; personal protective equipment and hand washing facilities; safe disposal facilities; and time. A lack of resources leads to unsafe practice and a threat to well-being.

Operational difficulties result from the way an organisation is managed. They, too, nurture unsafe practice and are a threat to well-being. For example, understaffing means a stressed, time-poor workforce with low morale, leading to neglect and accidents; a poorly trained and uncommitted workforce results in high staff turnover, poor continuity of care and the possibility of abuse and neglect due to inexperience; security issues, such as intruders and missing people, create untold worry and concern.

 Evidence activity

 Unsafe practices

This activity enables you to demonstrate your knowledge of unsafe practices that can affect people's well-being.

Evaluate how you and your colleagues carry out work activities and any resource and operational difficulties. Make a note of anything that you feel could impact on safety and well-being.

5.2 Explain the actions to take if unsafe practices have been identified

Health and social care providers are obliged to ensure that their staff use safe practice and help them improve their performance. They must also have systems in place to enable staff to report inadequate resources or operational difficulties that could affect the delivery of safe care.

What should you do if you identify unsafe work practice? Initially, discuss your concerns with the person concerned.

Be discrete and sensitive – they may be unaware that their work is unsafe, and pointing this out in public could be embarrassing and humiliating. If you feel that your intervention has been in vain, or perhaps that your work practice is not all it should be, follow your workplace's procedure for reporting unsafe practice. Usually this involves discussing concerns with your manager and recording them on a specific report form.

What should you do if you experience resource or operational difficulties? Follow your workplace's procedure for reporting and recording your concerns. If, for example, an activity requires you to:

- use unsafe, ill-maintained equipment
- cut corners, because of time
- handle body fluids and contaminated waste without wearing protective clothing
- carry out an activity alone, the procedure for which requires a team

carry out an activity in which you haven't been trained, or work with a colleague who also lacks training, report and record your concerns as required and do not carry on with the activity until your concerns have been resolved. Not only would you be putting your own safety at risk, you would also be compromising that of the people you work with.

 Evidence activity

5.2 Actions to take if unsafe practices have been identified

This activity enables you to demonstrate your understanding of what to do should you identify unsafe practices.

Look back at your response to Evidence activity 5.1, where you identified work practice that could impact on safety and well-being. What should you do?

5.3 Describe the action to take if suspected abuse or unsafe practices have been reported but nothing has been done in response

If you are concerned that any report you make of suspected abuse or unsafe practice is not acted upon, tell your manager. She or he will then be responsible for taking the matter forward, and you should ensure that they report back to you within an agreed timescale.

If you are concerned that management is involved in abuse or unsafe practice, speak to someone in authority on who you can rely to deal with the situation, for example your Trade Union Representative, someone in a more senior position than the manager concerned, or the organisation that regulates health and social care services where you work.

Reporting or disclosing abusive or negligent behaviour in the interest of the people you work with is described as 'whistle blowing'. The Public Interest Disclosure Act 1998 protects workers who 'blow the whistle' from victimisation by their manager or employer, providing they follow the correct procedure. You are protected as a whistle blower if you:

are a 'worker'

believe that malpractice is happening at work, has happened in the past or will happen in the future

disclose information of the right type (a 'qualifying disclosure')

disclose to the right person, and in the right way (making it a 'protected disclosure')

www.direct.gov.uk; www.hse.gov.uk

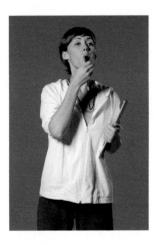

Figure 5.8 Whistle blowing!

 Evidence activity

5.3 Action to take if a report has not been acted on

This activity enables you to demonstrate your knowledge of what to do should a report of suspected abuse or unsafe practice not be acted on.

Check out what to do in the event that your employer fails to deal with a report of suspected abuse or unsafe practice. If there is no such procedure, check online for a whistle blowing procedure and produce a poster or information leaflet for everyone at work that describes what to do in the event that suspected abuse or malpractice is swept under the carpet.

Assessment summary

Your reading of this chapter and completion of the activities will have prepared you to demonstrate your learning and understanding of the principles of safeguarding and protection in health and social care.

To achieve the unit, your assessor will require you to:

Learning outcomes	Assessment Criteria
Learning outcome 1: Show you know how to recognise signs of abuse by:	**1.1** defining the following types of abuse: • Physical abuse • Sexual abuse • Emotional/psychological abuse • Financial abuse • Institutional abuse • Self neglect • Neglect by others See Evidence activity 1.1 and 1.2 p. 79.
	1.2 identifying the signs and/or symptoms associated with each type of abuse See Evidence activity 1.1 and 1.2 p. 79.
	1.3 describing the factors that may contribute to an individual being more vulnerable to abuse See Evidence activity 1.3 p. 80.
Learning outcome 2: Know how to respond to suspected or alleged abuse by:	**2.1** explaining the actions to take if there are suspicions that an individual is being abused See Evidence activity 2.1 p. 81.
	2.2 explaining the actions to take if an individual alleges that they are being abused See Evidence activity 2.2 p. 82.
	2.3 identifying ways to ensure that evidence of abuse is preserved See Evidence activity 2.3 p. 83.

Learning outcomes	Assessment Criteria
Learning outcome **3**: Understand the national and local context of safeguarding and protection from abuse by:	**3.1** identifying national policies and local systems that relate to safeguarding and protection from abuse See Evidence activity 3.1 p. 85.
	3.2 explaining the roles of different agencies in safeguarding and protecting individuals from abuse See Evidence activity 3.2 p. 86.
	3.3 identifying reports into serious failures to protect individuals from abuse See Evidence activity 3.3 p. 87.
	3.4 identifying sources of information and advice about own role in safeguarding and protecting individuals from abuse See Evidence activity 3.4 p. 88.
Learning outcome **4**: Understand ways to reduce the likelihood of abuse by:	**4.1** explaining how the likelihood of abuse may be reduced by: • working with person-centred values • encouraging active participation • promoting choice and rights See Evidence activity 4.1 p. 88.
	4.2 explaining the importance of an accessible complaints procedure for reducing the likelihood of abuse See Evidence activity 4.2 p. 90.
Learning outcome **5**: Know how to recognise and report unsafe practices by:	**5.1** describing unsafe practices that may affect the well-being of individuals See Evidence activity 5.1 p. 91.
	5.2 explaining the actions to take if unsafe practices have been identified See Evidence activity 5.2 p. 92.

Learning outcomes	Assessment Criteria
Learning outcome 5: Know how to recognise and report unsafe practices by:	(5.3) describing the action to take if suspected abuse or unsafe practices have been reported but nothing has been done in response See Evidence activity 5.3 p. 92.

Good luck!

Web links

Department of Health	www.dh.gov.uk
Princess Royal Trust for Carers	www.carers.org
Care Quality Commission (CQC)	www.cqc.org.uk
Commission for the Regulation of Care (SCRC)	www.carecommission.com
Independent Safeguarding Authority (ISA)	www.isa-gov.org.uk
Criminal Records Bureau	www.crb.homeoffice.gov.uk
Equality & Human Rights Commission	www.equalityhumanrights.com
Community Care website	www.Communitycare.co.uk
General Social Care Council	www.gscc.org.uk
Mind (mental health)	www.mind.org.uk
Alzheimer's Society	www.alzheimers.org.uk
AGE UK (Age Concern/Help the Aged)	www.ageuk.org.uk
Citizen's Advice Bureau	www.citizensadvice.org.uk
Mencap (learning disability)	www.mencap.org.uk
Carers UK	www.carersuk.org
National Society for the Prevention of Cruelty to Children	www.nspcc.org.uk
Office for Standards in Education, Children's Services and Skills	www.ofsted.gov.uk
Government website for public services	www.direct.gov.uk
Health & Safety Executive	www.hse.gov.uk

The role of the health and social care worker

For Unit HSC 025

What are you finding out?

Best practice in any work setting is underpinned by effective working relationships, an ability to follow agreed ways of working and an ability to work in partnership with others.

In health and social care settings, effective work relationships are based on professionalism and principles of care, which require workers to have respect for and promote the rights of everyone with whom they work. This includes team members, colleagues, other professionals, the individuals who need care and support and everyone who is important to them, such as their families, friends and advocates.

Ways of working in health and social care settings are described in an organisation's formal written policies and procedures, and more informally in records that have been agreed by all concerned and that allow needs to be met more flexibly. They are based on legislation, government reports and guidance documents, and professional body codes of practice. Workers are

required to follow these ways of working to promote and maintain the health, safety and well-being of everyone in the workplace.

Collaborative or partnership working in health and social care settings requires input from all the relevant **stakeholders**. Team members, colleagues, other professionals and people working in voluntary agencies are all stakeholders in meeting the care and support needs of individuals, but equally important is the input of the individuals themselves, their families, friends and advocates. Partnership working through 'joined up' care ensures a best practice **holistic approach** to care needs.

The reading and activities in this chapter will help you to:

■ Understand working relationships in health and social care

■ Be able to work in ways that are agreed with the employer

■ Be able to work in partnership with others

Key terms

A holistic approach is one that meets all aspects of an individual's care needs, including physical, intellectual, emotional, social and spiritual.

A stakeholder is a person or group having an interest in the success of an activity, enterprise etc.

LO1 Understand working relationships in health and social care

1.1 The difference between working and personal relationships

Relationships are probably the most involved and emotionally charged area of our lives. From the moment we are born we form relationships, each one requiring something different from us and giving us something different in return. We learn to identify people we like and don't like. We learn that we need to relate differently to different people; that some relationships are satisfying and rewarding while others are almost impossible to navigate. However, relationships are a basic human need and something which the majority of us strive to develop and maintain throughout our lives.

All relationships involve some level of **interdependence**. People in personal relationships, for example family members, friends, sexual and business partners, tend to influence each other, share personal and sometimes intimate thoughts and feelings, engage in activities together and give and take emotional, physical and financial support. Because of this interdependence, things that impact on one member of the relationship will also impact on the other.

Key terms

Interdependence means dependence between two or more people.
Integrity is the quality of being morally upright, credible, trusting.

According to the psychologist George Levinger, the natural development of a personal relationship follows four or five stages:

■ **Acquaintance** – This begins a relationship and can continue indefinitely, without any build-up.

■ **Build-up** – This is when people begin to trust and care about each other.

■ **Continuation** – This is when people commit to a long-term friendship or romantic relationship, perhaps marriage. Mutual trust is important for sustaining the relationship.

■ **Deterioration** – Not all relationships deteriorate, but in those that do, people become bored, resentful, dissatisfied and uncommunicative. There is betrayal and a loss of trust.

■ **Termination** – This marks the end of the relationship, either by death in the case of a healthy relationship, or by separation.

Time to reflect

 Personal relationships

Think about the personal relationships you have experienced during your life.

- Why did they develop from just an acquaintance?

- What sort of personal relationship did they become? Friendship? Romantic? Marriage? Business? Something else?

- Which of them have survived?

- Of those that haven't survived, what was the reason for the termination?

When a personal relationship terminates because one or other of the people in it have become bored, resentful, dissatisfied or uncommunicative, we say it has lost its **integrity**. Because it is absolutely inconceivable that users of health and social care services should lose their trust in and feel betrayed by workers on whom they depend, best practice in a health and social care setting is built on the integrity of work relationships.

An integral, morally upright work relationship in a health and social care setting is built on professionalism. Professionalism is a set of values, attitudes and behaviours that underpin best practice and help shape positive outcomes for the individuals you work with.

While it is not appropriate to make personal disclosures in a professional working relationship, some individuals you support may need to relax in your company, especially if you help them with personal care needs. Letting work relationships become more personal does not mean you need to disclose personal things about yourself or ask personal questions. However, mentioning holiday plans, remembering birthdays and asking after grandchildren, for example, can create a deeper relationship, which helps you get to know each other better, making working together easier and more efficient. It also shows that you are approachable and that you are human!

Case Study

(1.1) Betrayal of trust

The following is a synopsis of a report published in the *Telegraph* online in 2007 (www.telegraph.co.uk).

A teacher who had sex with one of his female pupils has been jailed for five years.

Mr X, a teacher for 21 years at the time of the offences – when the girl was 14 – was involved in after-school sports clubs at the school. The girl was a member of an after-school running club, and Mr X would go into the changing room to talk to her. The girl, who had never had sexual intercourse before, but who had been emotionally involved and had not resisted, said they had sex four times in the store room and at his home, when contraception was not used.

Mr X told the court that he bitterly regretted his actions and had betrayed his professional principles and his position of responsibility, and for that there was no excuse. He said he was unable to comprehend his actions, had lost his self-respect and dignity, and had shattered the lives of all the people he loved.

1. According to the paper, the girl was willing. Does this excuse Mr X's behaviour? If not, why not?

2. Mr X told the court that he had betrayed his professional principles. What do you think he meant by this?

3. What impact do you think this event will have on both people's lives?

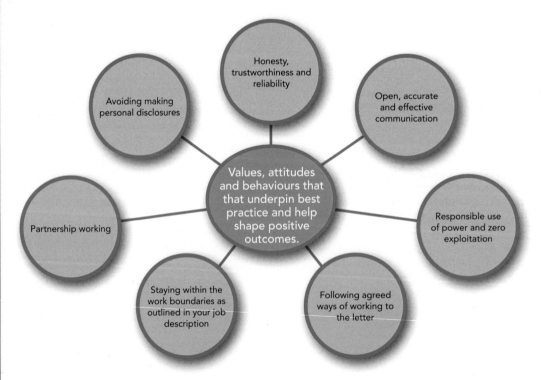

Figure 6.1 Professional practice

Finally, and as you read earlier, effective work relationships are based on principles of care. This means that, whatever your job role, when you support individuals with health and care needs, you must:

■ show respect for their beliefs, opinions, life experiences and social, cultural and ethnic backgrounds

■ shape the way you work around their wishes, expectations and preferences

■ support their rights to dignity, choice, privacy, independence, equality and fair treatment, risk taking, protection from harm, confidentiality, communicate using a method of their choice, and care that meets their specific needs.

Evidence activity

 How a working relationship differs from a personal relationship

This activity enables you to demonstrate your understanding of the differences between a working relationship and a personal relationship.

Use the following table to compare aspects of the relationships you have with a friend and someone you support and care for at work.

Behaviours	My friend	The person I support at work	Reasons for the differences in my behaviour.
How I communicate:			
How I show respect:			
What I tell them about me:			
What I ask them about:			
What we do together:			

1.2 Different working relationships in health and social care settings

Everything you do as a health and social care worker involves joint working, with individuals at your workplace and with people from other agencies (inter-agency working). As a result, you are required to develop working relationships with:

■ the individuals you support

■ their carers, family, friends and advocates

■ everyone at your workplace, including your colleagues, members of work teams, your manager

■ professionals from other agencies

■ voluntary organisations including faith groups, and voluntary workers including members of support groups

■ people with whom you liaise about your work, for example inspection agencies, manufacturers and suppliers of equipment, and maintenance and repair staff.

See *Working Together to Safeguard Children: A guide to inter-agency working to safeguard and promote the welfare of children* (www. dcsf.gov.uk) and your Local Authority's Inter-Agency Policies and Procedures for, for example, working with vulnerable adults.

Each of these relationships will have different requirements of you, but in general you will need to be:

■ a clear verbal and written communicator

■ courteous, reliable, trustworthy, responsible, cooperative, well organised and a good time-keeper

■ able to get on with others, use your initiative and work under pressure

■ able to take, follow and give instructions

■ willing to learn new skills and develop your understanding.

It is worth mentioning here that the general public is very much dependent on professional working relationships for their own and their loved ones' support and care. Health and social care workers are therefore perceived to be in a working relationship with the public. Unfortunately, events continue to undermine public trust in health and social care services. You therefore have a responsibility to behave, both at work and outside, in such a way as to develop and maintain public trust and confidence in the profession.

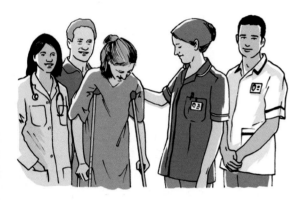

Figure 6.2 Working relationships

Research & investigate

(1.2) A loss of public trust

You will be familiar with the video footage of Ian Tomlinson, showing him to have been struck on the leg and pushed to the ground by a police officer during G20 protests in London in 2009. At the time of writing (July 2010), prosecutors have been unable to prove beyond reasonable doubt that there was any link between his death and the alleged abuse. As a result, an intense debate is taking place about the deteriorating trust and confidence that the public have in the police force.

Research the internet, local and national **media** and ask family, friends and colleagues for information about other events that have rocked public trust and confidence in different sectors and professions. What impact do you think a decline in trust and confidence in the health and social care sector has in the short and long term on everyone concerned?

Key term

Media are the means of communication, such as radio and television, newspapers and magazines, that reach or influence people widely.

Evidence activity

(1.2) Different working relationship in health and social care settings

This activity enables you to demonstrate your knowledge of the range of working relationships in which you are involved.

Make a list of all the working relationships in which you are involved, identify the people you work with and describe the personal qualities and skills expected of you in your role as a partner.

LO2 Be able to work in ways that are agreed with the employer

2.1 The importance of adhering to the agreed scope of your job role

The scope of your job role comprises the different tasks or activities that need to be carried out to get your job done. It is in effect a 'contract' in that it defines what you have to do, how you should do it, with whom, where, in what circumstances and by when. Because it also includes details about what you are aiming to achieve, it is used to judge your performance. So the more well defined it is, the better your chance of success.

The scope of your job role should also clarify what you must not do. This could include activities for which you have yet to be trained; activities that you are not capable of doing, for example, because of your health status or lack in seniority or of experience; activities that your age, sex or understanding prevents you from carrying out, such as helping someone of the opposite sex with intimate care needs; and your criminal record. Working in ways that are clearly defined as 'no go' puts the health, safety and emotional well-being of all concerned at risk.

Given that the scope of your job role is used to measure your performance, it is important that you are consulted about what is expected of you. Informal supervision, such as observation, enables your supervisor to identify your strengths and limitations and chat with you about your performance. Formal supervision, such as appraisals, gives you an opportunity to resolve your limitations by discussing concerns and suggestions you have regarding:

■ your understanding and performance

■ improving your learning and performance

■ adapting activities to make them more successful

■ situations you find difficult to handle

■ personal, resource and operational difficulties that impact on your performance.

The aim of supervision is to reach a mutual agreement about the scope of your job role. You should come away with a clear remit of what you can and cannot do, an improved understanding of your work activities and how you can improve your performance, and an updated Continuous Personal Development (CPD) plan that describes your learning and performance needs and how and when they will be met.

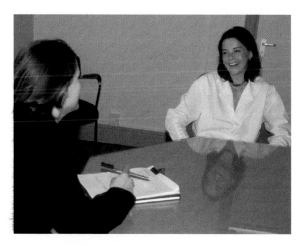

Figure 6.3 Agreeing your job scope

 Evidence activity

2.1 **The importance of adhering to the agreed job scope**

This activity enables you to demonstrate your knowledge of the importance of adhering to the agreed scope of your job role.

■ Make a list of all the activities for which you have a responsibility. What is the purpose of each? What could happen if you failed to carry them out as required?

■ What activities aren't you allowed to undertake? Why not? What could happen if you carried them out?

2.2 **Access full and up-to-date details of agreed ways of working**

Workplace policies set out the arrangements that a workplace has for complying with legislation. For example, in order to comply with the Health and Safety (First Aid) Regulations, every workplace should have a policy that describes how it manages first aid.

Procedures describe the ways of working that need to be followed for policies to be implemented. They record who does what, when and how in order to maintain health, safety and well-being at all times. For example, first aid procedures describe the roles of first aiders, the people responsible for maintaining first-aid equipment and facilities, when and how to call the emergency services and when and how to complete an accident report form.

Most workplace procedures are extremely rigid and prescriptive. However, because individual needs and capabilities and the environments in which needs are met are so diverse, some procedures have to be more flexible. For example, fire evacuation procedures will differ according to where people live – a purpose-built residential care home will be equipped with fire doors and fire-fighting equipment, but not so the family home in which your grandmother wants to live out her remaining days. Similarly, a purpose-built residential care home will be equipped with hoists and stair lifts, whereas your grandmother's house may not have room for moving and handling equipment. In such situations, ways of working have to be devised and agreed by all concerned.

Case Study

 Meeting needs flexibly

Dorrie, aged 9, has spastic cerebral palsy, which means she has stiffness, movement difficulties and visual and hearing problems. During the week she lives in a residential care home, where she has therapy to help with movement, balance and coordination, eating, drinking and swallowing. At weekends she lives at home with her mother, father and baby sister. Dorrie has a care plan that describes her needs, but obviously the care home is equipped to meet them in a different way from her family home.

Identify four of Dorrie's needs, including a physical, an intellectual, an emotional and a social need, and compare how they might be met differently in the care home and at home with her family.

All workplaces have procedures and agreed ways of working in place to ensure that work practice conforms to a vast array of legislation. Because health and social care settings vary in the type of work they do, their procedures and agreed ways of working will also vary. However, in general, health and social care settings have procedures and agreed ways of working that address:

- safeguarding and protection
- equal opportunities
- confidentiality
- record keeping
- medicines administration
- first aid
- concerns and complaints
- missing persons
- emergency evacuation.

It is a legal requirement that you follow procedures and agreed ways of working to the letter. They promote and maintain safe work practice and failure to follow them jeopardises the health, safety and well-being of everyone concerned. It could also mean the loss of your employer's reputation as a well-regarded service provider and the end of your career in health and social care.

Workplace procedures and agreed ways of working are usually stored centrally, where they are accessible to everyone who might need to know their content. They must be updated regularly in response to, for example:

- Changes in legislation – failing to amend a procedure or agreed way of working to allow for a change in legislation results in illegal practice.

- Government and **Sector Skills Council (SSC)** initiatives, such as the changes in work practice recommended in the government guidance document 'Working Together to Safeguard Children'. Failure to work according to such initiatives means failure to use best practice.

- Technological advances that translate into more effective and efficient ways of working, for example day surgery and medicines administration.

Key term

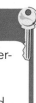

Sector Skills Councils (SSCs) are employer-led organisations in the UK that cover specific economic sectors, such as the social care, health care and child care and development sectors.

Updates to agreed ways of working are also made in response to changes in the condition and needs of the individuals you support. This ensures that care needs continue to be met appropriately.

Practice activity

 Access full and up-to-date details of agreed ways of working

This activity gives you an opportunity to practice accessing full and up-to-date details of agreed ways of working.

- Where does your organisation store procedures and agreed ways of working? Why is it important that you know this?

- Identify 3 activities that you carry out on a regular basis and, for each, check the procedure or agreed way of working to make sure you work as required. What is likely to happen if you don't fulfil your duties?

contd.

Practice activity

■ How do you know that the procedure or agreed way of working is up-to-date? What can you do to check that it is? Why is it important to ensure that agreed ways of working are up-to-date?

 2.3 Implement agreed ways of working

Ten top tips for implementing procedures and agreed ways of working.

1. Only carry out a procedure or agreed way of working if it is included in the scope of your job role and you have had the relevant training.

2. Make sure you know and understand what you have to do before you start working. If there is anything you don't understand, ask for help.

3. If you identify operational problems, such as short staffing, or problems with resources, such as faulty equipment, tell the appropriate person and do not proceed until you are confident that the problem has been solved.

4. Constantly monitor the activity for hazards. If anything happens that could put health, safety and well-being at risk, stop working and get help.

5. If the activity provides care and support to an individual, give them clear and accurate information about what you have to do and encourage them to work with you.

6. If the activity involves teamwork, accept and follow the team leader's instructions. If you are the team leader, give clear, authoritative instructions.

7. Take responsibility for your own actions and those of the people to whom you give directions.

8. Accept responsibility for and learn from your mistakes so that you don't repeat them.

9. Accept and use feedback from others to enable you to improve your understanding and performance.

10. Report and record any problems with the activity and be prepared to suggest how the activity could be improved.

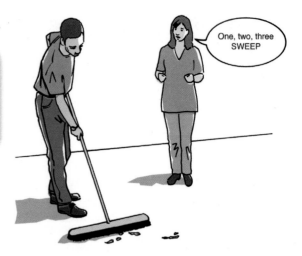

Figure 6.4 Give clear, authoritative instructions

Time to reflect

2.3 Working as required?

Look at the 'Ten top tips for implementing procedures and agreed ways of working'. Can you honestly say you bear each of them in mind when carrying out your activities? Are there any top tips you would add to the list?

Practice activity

 2.3 Implement agreed ways of working

This activity gives you an opportunity to practise putting agreed ways of working into action.

Ask for supervision as you carry out your activities and for feedback regarding how well you perform. Keep a diary to show how you are developing professionally. The entries you make will be useful for appraisals and for completing your CPD plan, the document in which you record your learning and performance needs and how and when they will be met.

LO3 Be able to work in partnership with others

3.1 The importance of working in partnership with others

Partnership working in health and social care is the coming together of agencies that have a shared interest in supporting people who have care needs. The key principles of partnership working are shared values, agreed goals or outcomes for the individuals they support, and regular communication.

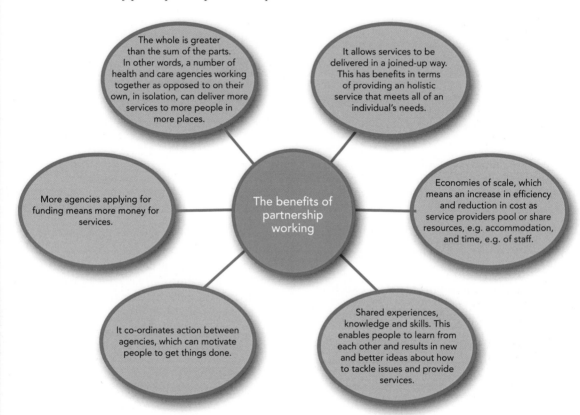

The whole is greater than the sum of the parts. In other words, a number of health and care agencies working together as opposed to on their own, in isolation, can deliver more services to more people in more places.

It allows services to be delivered in a joined-up way. This has benefits in terms of providing an holistic service that meets all of an individual's needs.

More agencies applying for funding means more money for services.

The benefits of partnership working

Economies of scale, which means an increase in efficiency and reduction in cost as service providers pool or share resources, e.g. accommodation, and time, e.g. of staff.

It co-ordinates action between agencies, which can motivate people to get things done.

Shared experiences, knowledge and skills. This enables people to learn from each other and results in new and better ideas about how to tackle issues and provide services.

Figure 6.5 The benefits of partnership working

Evidence activity

3.1 Explain why it is important to work in partnership with others.

This activity gives you an opportunity to demonstrate your understanding of the importance of working in partnership with others.

Make a list of all the people you work with, both individually and in a team. Why is it important to work with each of these people? What are the benefits to all concerned? What might be the outcome if you failed to work with them?

3.2 Ways of working that can help improve partnership working

Partnership working is spread right across the public, private and voluntary sectors. The partners or 'stakeholders' that you work with will include the individuals you support, their carers, family and friends; your colleagues and team members; other professionals; and people who are important to the individuals you support, such as advocates and members of faith and support groups.

You can help encourage and improve partnership working by promoting the three key principles: shared values, agreed goals or outcomes for the individuals you support, and regular communication.

Shared values

■ Have a genuine desire, commitment and enthusiasm for working with other people.

■ Be open, trustworthy, honest and professional in order to gain the confidence of everyone concerned.

■ Always have the interests of the individuals you support at the heart of your work.

■ Be prepared to learn new things and adapt the way you work.

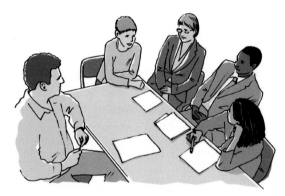

Figure 6.6 Partnership working

Agreed goals or outcomes

■ Understand what goals or outcomes the partnership is trying to achieve, and by when. If you don't understand, ask.

■ Understand exactly what is expected of you in achieving goals or outcomes, but remember not to act beyond your job scope or competence. If you have any concerns about what is expected of you, talk to your manager.

■ Understand exactly what is expected of everyone else. If you're not sure, ask.

■ Keep people informed about what you have been doing. The more you inform, the more satisfied people will be.

Regular communication

■ Make sure you attend all meetings and appointments; be punctual and well presented.

■ Use **jargon**-free communication. The individuals you support, their carers, family and friends, volunteers and people working in other agencies may not understand the language of your workplace, so using it would put them at a disadvantage.

Key term

Jargon is the specialist or technical language of a trade or profession.

■ Listen actively to others and show that you value their contribution.

■ Be sensitive to and supportive of each other's well-being, and acknowledge and respect their perceptions and points of view.

■ Ensure confidentiality.

■ Remain positive if communication becomes tense and conflicts develop.

Practice activity

(3.2) Improving partnership working

This activity gives you an opportunity to practise demonstrating that you can help improve partnership working.

■ The most important people in any partnerships in which you are involved are the individuals you support and the people that are important to them. Ask them how they feel about your efforts to secure and deliver care that meets wishes and needs. Do they have any suggestions as to how you could improve their situation?

■ Working partnerships are usually led or chaired by someone who has the ability and authority to ensure that the partnership's objectives are met. Talk to the leader or chair of the partnerships in which you are involved. Find out how they think you perform within the partnership, whether you demonstrate shared values and goals and whether your communication skills promote partnership working. Do they have any suggestions as to how you could improve your ways of working?

(3.3) Skills and approaches needed for resolving conflicts

Because partnership working requires individual people and agencies to set aside their own agendas and work towards a common goal, there is always a risk of conflict. Conflict is not necessarily a bad thing. If it is dealt with effectively, we can learn from it and develop personally and professionally. However, if it is not resolved effectively, the results can be damaging. Conflicting goals can rapidly turn into personal dislike; teamwork breaks down; talent is wasted as people remove themselves from the partnership; and in a health and social care scenario, individuals fail to receive appropriate care and support.

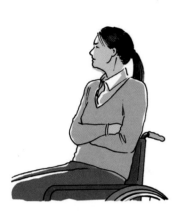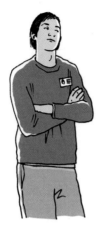

Figure 6.7 Conflict!

The guiding principles behind successful conflict resolution are mutual respect, effective communication, an open mind and a desire to understand different points of view, an enthusiasm to work cooperatively with others, and a willingness to consult, negotiate and compromise.

Time to reflect

(3.3) Rocky relationships ...

Think about a meeting you recently attended. How did it go? Was it obvious that everyone had shared goals and values? Was communication positive? Was there agreement about the way forward? Or was there disagreement? Did people go away from the meeting unconvinced and irritated? If so, why?

Because partnership working requires individual people and agencies to set aside their own agendas and work towards a common goal, there is always a risk of conflict. Conflict is not necessarily a bad thing. If it is dealt with effectively, we can learn from it and develop personally

contd.

Time to reflect

contd.

and professionally. However, if it is not resolved effectively, the results can be damaging. Conflicting goals can rapidly turn into personal dislike; teamwork breaks down; talent is wasted as people remove themselves from the partnership; and in a health and social care scenario, individuals fail to receive appropriate care and support.

Five steps to conflict resolution

Step 1: Effective communication

Effective communication is far more successful at resolving conflict than aggression. People who are involved in a conflict must be given an opportunity to express their perception of the problem, and active listening ensures that they are heard and understood.

■ Show that you are interested in what the other person is saying, for example by maintaining eye contact.

■ Show that you are trying to understand their point of view, for example by mirroring their facial expressions and tone of voice; by using appropriate body movements, such as head nods; and by making affirmative noises such as 'mmm' and 'yes'.

■ Check your understanding by asking questions, **paraphrasing** what they tell you and summarising what you understand them to have said.

Key term

Paraphrasing is rephrasing in your own words what someone else has said.

And make sure that when you talk, you are calm, courteous and assertive rather than confrontational and aggressive.

Step 2: Research

Everyone has their own interests, needs and concerns. Conflict arises when someone feels that theirs are being ignored or not taken into account. Try to understand how the partnership's way of doing things is impacting on an individual, for example, is it affecting their work performance, disrupting teamwork, hampering decision-making? Or is it affecting the way an individual feels cared for or supported? Be objective – focus on work issues and leave personalities out of the discussion.

Step 3: Identify the problem

Everyone needs to have a clear understanding of the problem. As you read above, different people have different needs, interests and concerns, and as a result they perceive problems differently. You need to reach an agreement about what the problem is before you can find a mutually acceptable solution.

Step 4: Negotiate a win–win solution

If everyone is to feel comfortable with the way a problem is solved, they need to be involved in identifying possible solutions. Involvement means being open to all ideas, including the ones they hadn't thought of. If agreement cannot be reached, consider making a compromise.

Step 5: Problem-solving

Action the agreed or compromise solution, and monitor it to ensure that it does resolve the problem. Be prepared to try out any of the other proposed solutions to see whether they might prove more effective.

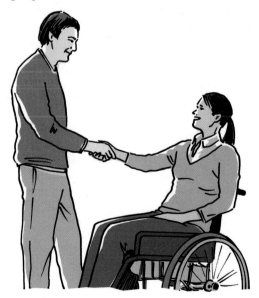

Figure 6.8 Problem solved!

Evidence activity

(3.3) Identify skills and approaches needed for resolving conflicts

This activity gives you an opportunity to demonstrate your knowledge of how to behave in order to resolve a conflict.

Produce a poster for display in the staff room, entitled 'Conflict Resolution', which describes the skills and approaches needed to get to the bottom of and settle a conflict.

 (3.4) How and when to access support and advice about partnership working and resolving conflicts

Working with other people can present hazards. For example, there may be a personality clash or you may be asked to carry out an activity that:

■ is outside the scope of your job role

■ is within the scope of your job role but for which you have yet to be trained or, because of inexperience, you are not confident to do with competence

■ is not written into an individual's care plan

■ would compromise your integrity, for example if you were asked to disclose confidential information

■ would compromise the professional boundaries between you and an individual you support, for example if you were asked to use your position to exploit them in some way.

Where can you go for advice and support in the event that you have concerns about partnership working or conflict is rearing its ugly head? First of all, talk to the person concerned as soon as possible and before things get any worse. Be assertive but not confrontational. Tell them how you feel and why, and do not make accusations.

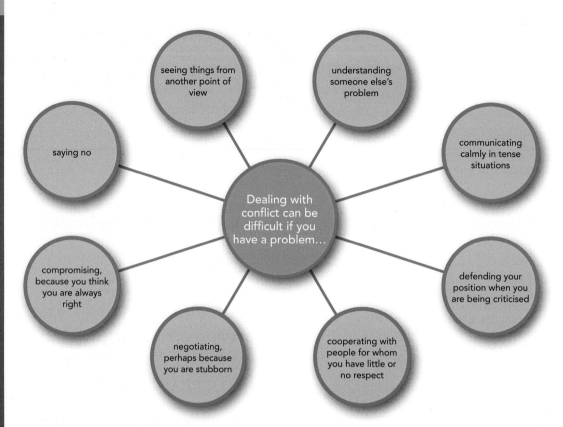

Figure 6.9 Difficulties in dealing with conflicts

If talking doesn't resolve the problem, or if the person you find it difficult to work with or with whom you have a dispute is your manager, get advice or support from a higher level. Most organisations have procedures in place to deal with disputes and conflicts. They may require you to speak with someone in human resources, a union representative or an outside source, such as a **mediator** or the **Advisory, Conciliation and Arbitration Service (ACAS)**.

www.acas.org.uk

Key terms

The Advisory, Conciliation and Arbitration Service (ACAS) provides confidential and impartial advice to assist workers in resolving issues in the workplace.

A mediator is an intermediary third party, who is neutral and helps negotiate agreed outcomes.

Practice activity

(3.4) **Demonstrate how and when to access support and advice about partnership working and resolving conflicts**

This activity gives you an opportunity to practice demonstrating how and when to access support and advice about partnership working and resolving conflicts.

■ Talk to your manager about what you should do and when in the event of a conflict or when you experience difficulties in working within a partnership.

■ Check out your workplace procedures and agreed ways of working in the event that talking doesn't resolve a problem.

contd.

Practice activity

- Research Acas and mediators in your locality. Find out how they can help in the event of a dispute.

- Produce an information sheet for circulation within your workplace that details your findings.

If you want to complain about being a victim of a dispute or conflict, keep a record of what happened, when and where as well as anything else you think might be relevant, such as emails, texts, notes and letters. If it gets as far as a hearing, you will need these as evidence.

Disputes and unresolved conflicts affect people professionally and personally, so should never be ignored.

Assessment summary

Your reading of this chapter and completion of the activities will have prepared you to demonstrate your learning and understanding of the principles of safeguarding and protection in health and social care. To achieve the unit, your assessor will require you to:

Learning outcomes	Assessment Criteria
Learning outcome **1**: Understand working relationships in health and social care by:	**1.1** explaining how a working relationship is different from a personal relationship See Evidence activity 1.1, p. 99.
	1.2 describing different working relationships in health and social care settings See Evidence activity 1.2, p. 100.
Learning outcome **2**: Be able to work in ways that are agreed with the employer by:	**2.1** describing why it is important to adhere to the agreed scope of the job role See Evidence activity 2.1, p. 101.
	2.2 accessing full and up-to-date details of agreed ways of working See Practice activity 2.2, p. 102.
	2.3 implementing agreed ways of working See Practice activity 2.3, p. 103.
Learning outcome **3**: Be able to work in partnership with others by:	**3.1** explaining why it is important to work in partnership with others See Evidence activity 3.1, p. 104.
	3.2 demonstrating ways of working that can help improve partnership working See Practice activity 3.2, p. 105.

Learning outcomes	Assessment Criteria
Learning outcome **3**: Be able to work in partnership with others by:	(3.3) identifying skills and approaches needed for resolving conflicts See Evidence activity 3.3, p. 107.
	(3.4) demonstrating how and when to access support and advice about: • partnership working • resolving conflicts See Practice activity 3.4, p. 108.

Good luck!

Web links

The Department for Education, previously the Department for Children, Schools and Families and Schools	www.dcsf.gov.uk
Care Quality Commission (CQC)	www.cqc.org.uk
Commission for the Regulation of Care (SCRC)	www.carecommission.com
Advisory, Conciliation and Arbitration Service	www.acas.org.uk

Promote person-centred approaches in health and social care

For Unit HSC 036

What are you finding out?

The essence of a person-centred approach is that it is individual to, and owned by, the person being supported. But how can we ensure that this happens and how can we support others to work in a person-centred way?

The reading and activities in this chapter will help you to:

■ Understand what person-centred approaches are

■ Understand how to work in a person-centred way

■ Understand the role risk assessment plays in enabling a person-centred approach.

LO1 Understand the application of person-centred approaches in health and social care

1.1 Explain how and why person-centred values must influence all aspects of health and social care work

Person-centred care is a way of providing care that is centred around the person, and not just their health or care needs. To explain this in simple terms, we are all individual – no two people are the same, so it is not appropriate to say that because two people have dementia they both have the same care and support needs. Person-centred values ensure a comprehensive understanding of individual needs and the development of appropriate individual care plans for all.

Person-centred values cover the total care of the person. The person is the centre of the plan, so they must be consulted and their views must always come first. The approach should include all aspects of their care: social services, health, family and the voluntary sector.

Person-centred planning is central to the White Paper 'Valuing People' (Department of Health, 2001). One of the challenges this presents is how we can fully involve people with high support needs, who may not use words to speak, in person-centred planning. Traditionally, when we have considered how we can involve people in planning we have concentrated on the planning meeting. The **personalisation agenda** is leading some of the changes happening in social care today.

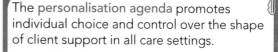

Key term

The personalisation agenda promotes individual choice and control over the shape of client support in all care settings.

The White Paper 'Our health, our care, our say' confirms the vision of high-quality support meeting people's hopes for independence and greater control over their lives, making services flexible and responsive to individual needs. A useful guide to receiving direct payments is available from the Department of Health.

The Mental Capacity Act (MCA) 2005

It may be that the individual cannot always make decisions for themselves. The Mental Capacity Act 2005 is intended to support such times. It came into effect from 1 April 2007 and covers England and Wales. The Act provides a statutory framework for people who may not be able to make their own decisions because of mental disability. It promotes fair treatment for people who may be affected, and protects the rights of some of the most vulnerable people in society.

More than two million people in England and Wales may lack the capacity to make decisions by themselves. They may be people with:

- dementia
- learning disabilities
- mental health problems
- people who have suffered stroke and head injuries.

The Mental Capacity Act 2005 will help people to make their own decisions. It will also protect people who cannot make their own decisions about some things. This is called lacking capacity.

The Act tells people:

- what to do to help someone make their own decisions about something
- how to work out if someone can make their own decisions about something
- what to do if someone cannot make decisions about something sometimes.

A lack of mental capacity could be due to:

- a stroke or brain injury
- a mental health problem
- dementia
- a learning disability
- confusion, drowsiness or unconsciousness because of an illness or the treatment for it
- substance misuse.

The type of decisions that are covered by the MCA range from day-to-day decisions such as what to wear or eat, through to more serious decisions about where to live, having an operation or what to do with a person's finances and property. Some types of decisions (such as marriage or civil partnership, divorce, sexual relationships, adoption and voting) can never be made by another person on behalf of someone who lacks capacity. This is because these decisions or actions are either so personal to the individual concerned or because other laws govern them and the Mental Capacity Act does not change this. The MCA applies to situations where a person may be unable to make a particular decision at a particular time because their mind or brain is affected, for instance by illness or disability, or the effects of drugs or alcohol.

 Evidence activity

1.1 **The impact of the Mental Capacity Act 2005**

What impact would the Mental Capacity Act 2005 have on individuals in your care?

Who could you ask for help and guidance?

1.2 **Evaluate the use of care plans in applying person-centred values**

A care plan sets out in some detail the daily care and support that it has been agreed should be provided to an individual. If you are employed as a carer, it acts as a guide to you in terms of what sorts of activities are expected of you. It does not stand still, of course. There will be regular reviews, and the individual and you should be involved in discussion about how it is working and whether parts need changing.

Person-centred planning is much more than a meeting. It is a process of continually listening and learning, focused on what is important to the person now and in the future, and acting upon this in alliance with their family and friends. It is vital that we think about how the person can be central throughout the process, from gathering information about their life, preparing for meetings, monitoring actions and on-going learning, to reflection and further action. There is a danger that efforts to develop person-centred planning simply focus on having better meetings. Any planning without implementation leaves people feeling frustrated and cynical, which is often worse than not planning at all.

Very often you will only be caring for and supporting people when they are in a vulnerable position. The quality of care that you can provide will be improved if you have knowledge of the whole person, not just the current circumstances: for example, knowledge can help us to understand better why people behave in the way they do. A care plan, based on a person-centred approach, will help in understanding some of this, but what else might help? Person-centred planning, then, demands that you see the person whom you are supporting as the central concern. You need to find ways to make care and support individual, not 'one size fits all'. The relationship should move from being one of carer and cared for towards one based on a partnership: you become a resource to the person who needs support.

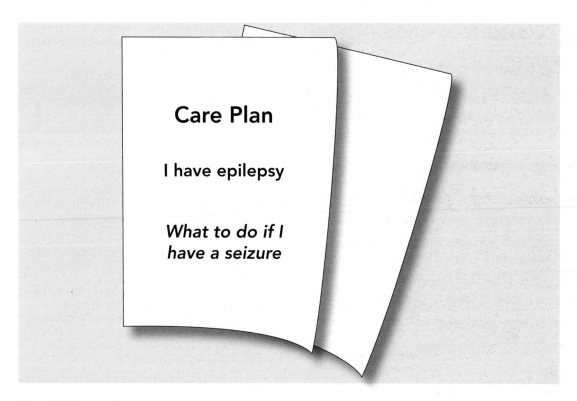

Care Plan

I have epilepsy

What to do if I have a seizure

Figure 7.1 A care plan

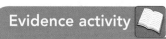
Evidence activity

1.2 Care plans

What do you think a care plan should contain? Write a list of what you think should be in it and state why.

LO2 Be able to work in a person-centred way

Person-centred planning is a way of helping people to think about what they want now and in the future. It is about supporting people to plan their lives, work towards their goals and get the right support. It is a collection of tools and approaches based upon a set of shared values that can be used to plan *with* a person, not *for* them. Planning should build the person's circle of support and involve all the people who are important in that person's life.

Person-centred planning is built on the values of inclusion and looks at what support a person needs to be included and involved in their community. Person-centred approaches offer an alternative to traditional types of planning,

which are based upon the **medical model of disability** and which are set up to assess need, allocate services and make decisions for people.

Key term

The medical model of disability views disability as a 'problem' that belongs to the disabled individual.

Person-centred working

Person-centred working involves a number of approaches which people who provide support can use to help them work in a more person-centred way, such as:

■ how to sort what is important to a person from what is important for them

■ how to address issues of health, safety and risk while supporting choice

■ how to identify what the core responsibilities are for those who provide paid support

■ how to consider what makes sense and what does not make sense about a person's life

■ how to ensure effective support by matching characteristics of support staff to the person's needs.

Research & investigate

 Comparing care plans

Look for copies of care plans and compare them. What are the differences and which do you think offers more choices for individuals?

Person-centred teams

Person-centred approaches are not only for people who use services, they can also be very useful tools for enabling teams to work together effectively. Person-centred team plans help teams to be clear about their purpose, to understand what is important to each member and what support they need to do a good job.

Evidence activity

 Teamworking

Draw a spider diagram to show the people you think would be part of a care team. What are their roles?

 Work with an individual and others to find out the individual's history, preferences, wishes and needs

Person-centred planning can work for anyone. It is especially useful for people who may need help planning their future, or who find that services often do the planning for them. Lots of people feel like this, so person-centred planning suits lots of different people.

There are key features of person-centred planning that will help anyone reviewing plans to ensure the person is at the centre and has their say.

Key features are:

1. The person is at the centre. This means that the person has had genuine choice and involvement in the process, and in deciding who is involved, where, when and how the planning takes place.

2. Family members and friends are full partners. People will come together to work

flexibly and creatively to ensure that the person is getting the supports they need to have a better life.

3. Person-centred planning reflects the person's capacities, what is important to the person (now and for the future) and specifies the support they require to make a valued contribution to their community. The plan identifies choices about how the person wants to live, and then demonstrates how the proper supports are provided.

4. Person-centred planning builds a shared commitment to action that will uphold the person's rights and encourages their participation in community life.

5. Person-centred planning leads to continual listening, learning and action, and helps the person to work towards getting what they want/need out of life. The plan is not focused only on services provided, but on what might be possible in the future. The person-centred plans include negotiation so that resources and supports reflect what the individual wants and needs.

The essence of a person-centred plan is that it is individual to, and owned by, the person being supported.

There is no single approach that can be applied to working with someone in a person-centred way, and no approach that exclusively covers all of the processes that may be needed in developing a person-centred plan.

Research & investigate

 New ways of working

Carry out some research into new ways of working and how this can improve individual's lives

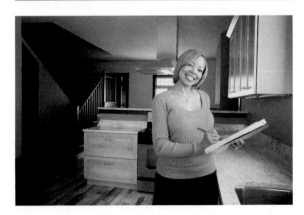

Figure 7.2 The inspection process

2.2 Demonstrate ways to put person-centred values into practice in a complex or sensitive situation

Person-centred planning is a process of life planning with individuals, using the principles of inclusion and a social model rather than a medical model. With a medical model, a person is seen as the passive receiver of services and their impairment is seen as a problem; this often leads to segregation and to them living and working away from the community. A social model sees a person as being disabled by society. In this model, a person is proactive in the fight for equality and inclusion.

The concept of person-centred planning is not new. One of the first people to develop the model was John O'Brien. His 'five accomplishments' (respect, choice, participation, relationships and ordinary places) were the foundation for person-centred planning in the USA.

Person-centred planning has five key features:

1. The person is at the centre of the planning process.

2. Family and friends are partners in planning.

3. The plan shows what is important to a person now and for the future and what support they need.

4. The plan helps the person to be part of a community of their choosing and helps the community to welcome them.

5. The plan puts into action what a person wants for their life and keeps on listening – the plan remains 'live'.

Evidence activity

2.2 Responsibility for care plans

Who is responsible for reviewing care plans and service delivery in your setting?

2.3 Adapt actions and approaches in response to an individual's changing needs or preferences

An important first step in person-centred approaches is to understand each person's

unique way of getting their message across. This can vary from person to person, and can depend on the person's level of spoken language, their eye contact and their body language. It is important, when getting person-centred planning started, that each individual is recognised as having their own particular way of communicating. Without an understanding of this we will struggle to achieve a person-centred approach, to hear about people's hopes and needs, and to achieve a better life for each person.

The person at the centre

Good communication depends on:

■ how well you can hear

■ how well you can see

■ how comfortable you are feeling

■ how alert and attentive you are

■ how well you can understand what is happening

■ how well you can express yourself to someone else

■ how interested and motivated you are to communicate.

Case Study

2.3 Signing

The manager of a day centre does not approve of using sign language as he feels it makes people with learning disabilities stand out and look funny. Service users are not encouraged to use signing, and staff are not taught or supported in learning it.

Janet came to the centre from school, with poor speech and good signing skills. After two weeks, she was no longer using her signs in the centre, although she continued to do so at home. Staff found her difficult to understand, and she became increasingly withdrawn.

What could be done to make communication more effective?

What you need to do:

■ Make sure that the person can hear, see and is comfortable.

■ Check when the person last had a hearing or vision test; get an up-to-date assessment.

■ Make sure that hearing aids or glasses are used if necessary, and that they work properly!

■ Make sure you speak clearly and allow the person to read your lips if necessary.

■ Use signs/gestures and pictures to back up your speech.

■ Make sure you present information clearly for people to see.

■ Make sure people are positioned for good communication – seating is key.

■ Make sure that the environment is quiet and there are not too many distractions.

■ Check out the person's general health and comfort – pain, physical difficulties, effects of medication.

■ Get a person's attention before starting to speak.

■ Show that you respect a person's way of communicating by using it with them.

■ Make sure communication books/aids are available to the person when they need them – not stuck in a cupboard!

■ Be a good observer and respond to all communicative signals.

■ Make sure the person can see your hands and face if you are signing and talking.

■ Give enough time for the person to listen to you and respond.

■ Check that you have understood by talking to others and helping the person to tell you when you have got it wrong. Don't pretend you can understand if you really can't!

LO3 Be able to establish consent when providing care or support

3.1 Analyse factors that influence the capacity of an individual to express consent

Every adult must be presumed to have the mental capacity to consent or refuse treatment, unless they are

■ unable to take in or retain information provided about their treatment or care

■ unable to understand the information provided

■ unable to weigh up the information as part of the decision-making process.

It is primarily the responsibility of the clinician providing the treatment or care to assess whether or not an adult lacks the capacity to consent, but nurses and midwives have a responsibility to participate in discussions about this assessment.

Nurses and midwives have three overriding professional responsibilities with regard to obtaining consent:

■ to make the care of people their first concern and ensure they gain consent before they begin any treatment or care

■ to ensure that the process of establishing consent is rigorous, transparent and demonstrates a clear level of professional accountability

■ accurately to record all discussions and decisions relating to obtaining consent.

Valid consent must be given by a competent person (who may be a person lawfully appointed on behalf of the person) and must be given voluntarily. Another person cannot give consent for an adult who has the capacity to consent.

In exceptional cases, for example, where consent was obtained by deception or where not enough information was given, this could result in an allegation of battery (or civil assault in Scotland). However, only in the most extreme cases is criminal law likely to be involved.

Usually the individual performing a procedure should be the person to obtain consent. In certain circumstances, you may seek consent on behalf of colleagues if you have been specially trained for that specific area of practice.

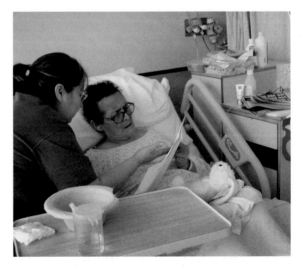

Figure 7.3 The consent process

Forms of consent

A person may demonstrate their consent in a number of ways. If they agree to treatment and care, they may do so verbally, in writing or by implying (by cooperating) that they agree. Equally, they may withdraw or refuse consent in the same way. Verbal consent, or consent by implication, will be enough evidence in most cases. Written consent should be obtained if the treatment or care is risky, lengthy or complex. This written consent stands as a record that discussions have taken place and of the person's choice. If a person refuses treatment, making a written record of this is just as important. A record of the discussions and decisions should be made.

When consent is refused

Legally, a competent adult can either give or refuse consent to treatment, even if that refusal may result in harm or death to him or her. Nurses and midwives must respect their refusal just as much as they would their consent. It is important that the person is fully informed and that, when necessary, other members of the health care team are involved. A record of refusal to consent, as with consent itself, must be made.

Evidence activity

3.1 Refusing consent

Why do you think someone might refuse to give consent? What action should you take if this happens?

Consent of people under 16

If the person is under the age of 16 (a minor), carers must be aware of local protocols and legislation that affect their care or treatment. Consent of people under 16 is very complex, so local, legal or membership organisation advice may need to be sought. Children under the age of 16 are generally considered to lack the capacity to consent or to refuse treatment. The right to do so remains with the parents, or those with parental responsibility, unless the child is considered to have significant understanding and intelligence to make up his or her own mind about it.

Children of 16 or 17 are presumed to be able to consent for themselves, although it is considered good practice to involve the parents. Parents, or those with parental responsibility, may override the refusal of a child of any age up to 18 years. In exceptional circumstances, it may be necessary

to seek an order from the court. Child minders, teachers and other adults caring for the child cannot normally give consent.

Consent of people who are mentally incapacitated

It is important that the principles governing consent are applied just as vigorously to people who are mentally incapacitated.

A person may be described as mentally incapacitated for a number of reasons. There may be temporary reasons, such as sedatory medicines, or longer-term reasons, such as mental illness, coma or unconsciousness.

The courts have identified certain circumstances when referral should be made to them for a ruling on lawfulness before a procedure is undertaken. These are:

- sterilisation for contraceptive purposes

- donation of regenerative tissue such as bone marrow

- withdrawal of nutrition and hydration from a patient in a persistent vegetative state

- where there is doubt as to the person's capacity or best interests.

3.2 Establish consent for an activity or action

If your work involves treating or caring for people (anything from helping people with dressing to carrying out major surgery), you need to make sure you have the person's consent for what you propose to do, if they are able to give it. This respect for people's rights to determine what happens to their own bodies is a fundamental part of good practice. For a person's consent to be valid, the person must be:

- capable of taking that particular decision

- acting voluntarily (not under pressure or duress from anyone)

- provided with enough information to enable them to make the decision.

Seeking consent is part of a respectful relationship and should usually be seen as a process, not a one-off event. When you are seeking a person's consent to treatment or care, you should make sure that they have the time and support they need to make their decision. People who have given consent for a particular intervention are entitled to change their minds and withdraw their consent at any point if they have the capacity (are 'competent') to do so.

Similarly, they can change their minds and consent to an intervention which they have earlier refused. It is important to let the person know this, so that they feel able to tell you if they change their mind.

Adults with the capacity to take a particular decision are entitled to refuse the treatment or care being offered, even if this will clearly be detrimental to their health. Mental health legislation does provide the possibility of treatment for a person's mental disorder without their consent (in which case more specialist guidance should be consulted). Detention under mental health legislation does not give a power to treat unrelated physical disorders without consent.

Consent is a process. Legally, it makes no difference if people give their consent verbally, non-verbally (for example, by holding out an arm for blood pressure to be taken) or by signing a consent form. A consent form is only a record, not proof that genuine consent has been given. It is good practice to seek written consent if treatment or care is complex, or involves significant risks or side effects. If the person has the capacity to consent to treatment or care for which written consent is usual, but cannot write or is physically unable to sign a form, a record that the person has given verbal or non-verbal consent should be made in their notes or on the consent form.

Some people may therefore have capacity to consent to some treatment or care provisions but not to others. People suffering from the early stages of dementia, for example, would probably still have the capacity to make many straightforward decisions about their own treatment or care but might lack the capacity to take very complex decisions. It should never be assumed that people can take no decisions for themselves, just because they have been unable to take a particular decision in the past. A person's capacity may also fluctuate: they may, for example, be able to take a particular decision one day even if they had not been able to take it the day before. Where a person's capacity is fluctuating you should, if possible, delay treatment or care decisions until a point when the individual has the capacity to make their own decision. People close to the person may sometimes be able to assist you in choosing an appropriate time to discuss his or her health or social care wishes and options.

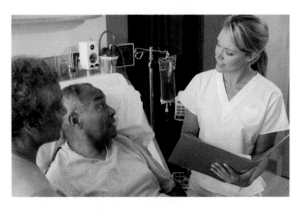

Figure 7.4 Seeking agreement

 3.3 Explain what steps to take if consent cannot be readily established

When adults lack capacity

Even where information is presented as simply and clearly as possible, some people will not be capable of taking some decisions. This will obviously apply when a person is in a coma, for example. It may also apply to people with severe dementia, although you should never automatically assume that a person lacks capacity simply because they have dementia. A person's capacity should always be assumed until proved otherwise.

If a person is not capable of giving or refusing consent, it is still possible for you lawfully to provide treatment and care, unless such care has been validly refused in advance. However, this treatment or care must be in the person's 'best interests'. No one (not even a spouse, or others close to the person) can give consent on behalf of adults who are not capable of giving consent for themselves. However, those close to the incapacitated person should always be involved in decision-making, unless the older person has earlier made it clear that they don't want such involvement. Although, legally, the health and social care professionals responsible for the person's care are responsible for deciding whether or not particular treatment or care is in that person's best interests, ideally decisions will reflect an agreement between professional carers and those close to the person.

 Research & investigate

3.3 When consent cannot be given
Find out what action you should take if consent cannot be given.

Evidence activity

3.2 Seeking consent

You are seeking consent from an individual. What information do they need? How can you help them get this?

LO4 Be able to implement and promote active participation

 Describe different ways of applying active participation to meet individual needs

A crucial aspect of relationship building in your job role is making sure that people are able to make choices and take control over as much of their lives as possible. This is known as empowerment and simply means doing everything you can to enable people to make their own decisions. Many people who receive care services are often unable to make choices about what happens in their lives. This might be due to many factors, for example their physical ability, where they live, who provides care and the way services are provided.

Individuals who are unable to make choices and exercise control may also suffer from low self-esteem and lose confidence in their own abilities. There are other factors which may impact on self-esteem, including the degree of encouragement and praise a person is given from important people in their lives; the amount of satisfaction someone gets from their job and whether a person has positive and happy relationships with friends and family.

Self-esteem has a major effect on people's health and well-being. Individuals who have a positive and more confident outlook are far more likely to be interested and active in the world around them than those lacking confidence and belief in their own abilities. It is therefore easy to see how this can affect an individual's quality of life and their overall health and well-being.

If self-esteem is about how we value ourselves, then self-image is how we see ourselves – both are equally important. As part of empowering individuals, you need to consider how you can promote individuals' sense of their own identity. This involves making sure you recognise the values, beliefs, likes and preferences individuals have and not ignoring or discounting them if they do not fit in with the care system.

A little thought and consideration can ensure that people feel they are valued and respected as individuals. For example, finding out how an individual likes to be addressed is important. Some older people, for example, like to be addressed as Mr or Mrs as this indicates respect.

You will also need to make sure that people have been asked about their religious or cultural beliefs, particularly in relation to food,
acceptable forms of dress and the provision of personal care.

Evidence activity

 Beliefs

Think of the things that might irritate you or annoy you. Are they your beliefs or just a passing dislike? How do you stop these things impacting on your job role?

 Work with an individual and others to agree how active participation will be implemented

Individuals should be enabled to have control over their lives. How are you going to support them to do this? Person-centred approaches are about the service user being the centre of any care plan. Person-centred approaches are quite simply getting people a life and not just a service. What is important to that person? What support do they need? What are their dreams and ideas for their future?

The General Social Care Council (GSCC) Codes of Practice for Social Care Workers and Employers directs social care workers to:

■ treat each person as an individual

■ respect and, where appropriate, promote their individual views and wishes

■ and support their right to control their lives and make informed choices.

The Nursing and Midwifery Council (NMC) Standards of conduct, performance and ethics for nurses and midwives reflect this thinking by stating that health care workers should listen to the people in their care and respond to their concerns and preferences. Reflect on the diversity of the people you are supporting, and enable them to communicate their needs and choices so that they have quality of life.

Evidence activity

 GSCC Code of Practice

Look for the GSCC Code of Practice and make note on the key points it addresses in relation to person-centred care.

4.3 & 4.4 Demonstrate how active participation can address the holistic needs of an individual & Demonstrate ways to promote understanding and use of active participation

First you must be sure that you give information in a way that can be understood by the individuals concerned. You must ensure that any specific communication needs are met. For example, people may require information in Braille, or to be communicated with using signing. You will need to find out how to change the format of the information, or how to access it in a suitable format. Promoting choice and empowerment is about identifying the practical steps you can take in daily working activities to give individuals more choice and more opportunities to make decisions about their own lives and the activities they wish to become involved in.

You will also need to consider the circumstances when you pass on information about a particular service or facility. You should take into account the situation of the individual at that particular time. An obvious example is that you would not pass on information about social clubs and outings to someone whose partner had just died. You also need to take into account an individual's state of health and any medical treatment that may affect the relevance or usefulness of the information.

Make sure that the information is accessible by:

- presenting it in the most useful format
- making it available at the right time
- taking all the circumstances into account.

Evidence activity

4.3 Providing information

You need to provide some information to an individual you provide care for. How can you make sure they can understand this information?

When individuals want to make choices about their lives, you must ensure that you are doing your best to help them identify any barriers they may meet and help them overcome them. When working with individuals in their own home, it is generally easier for them to make day-to-day choices for themselves.

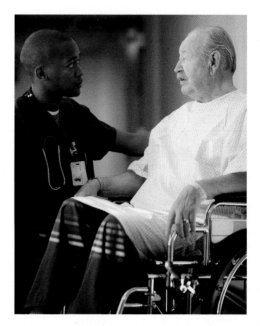

Figure 7.5 Multicultural needs

Everyone is different, but we can tend to make sweeping generalisations which we think apply to everyone in a particular group. So, in order to provide quality, empowering care, we must take the time to find out about personal beliefs and values and consider all aspects of individuals' lives. Although you may hold a different set of values or beliefs from the individual you provide care for, you must not impose your beliefs on them. You may need to act as an advocate for their beliefs even if you do not personally agree with them. Value each person as an individual and be sure to be open to what others have to say.

The range of services and facilities that individuals may want to use is large and varied. Once people have the information on what is available, the next stage is to support them to make use of it. This may involve completing application forms or other paperwork, and you may need to support individuals to fill in any forms that are required to access their selected networks or services.

Overcoming barriers

There are many barriers that can restrict access or prevent people from using networks, participating in or developing relationships. Information is one of the keys to overcoming barriers. An individual with plenty of accurate and current information is far more likely to be able to challenge or overcome difficulties than someone who feels anxious or uncertain because of lack of information and support. Barriers to access tend to fall into three key categories: environmental, communication and psychological.

Environmental barriers include:

- lack of disabled facilities
- narrow doorways
- no ramps
- no lifts
- no interpretation of signage for those with a sensory impairment
- lack of transport
- lack of ease of access.

Communication barriers include:

- lack of loop systems
- poor-quality communication skills
- lack of translators or interpreters
- lack of information about the network or facility
- lack of information in an appropriate format.

Psychological barriers include:

- unfamiliarity
- lack of confidence
- fear or anxiety
- unwillingness to accept help in order to access resources or networks.

Evidence activity

 Identifying barriers

Look around your work setting and identify any barriers you think there may be. How do you think these barriers can be overcome?

LO5 Be able to support the individual's right to make choices

5.1 Support an individual to make informed choices

People need information about the options available to them if they are to be able to make choices about their lives. There are many ways of making information accessible to people. These include the different ways of communicating that we have mentioned above, but also ways of presenting information so that people can become more engaged in the planning process. At the moment there are many barriers that prevent the person at the centre of the planning process from being in control.

Action for person-centred planning

You need to consider:

- what method or combination of methods will be most useful to the person
- how to give the person ownership and control over information about themselves
- allowing enough time to produce information and resources
- linking with other services to make sure that everyone is consistent in what they are doing
- how to store and catalogue resources so that they are not mislaid
- your own training needs. Do you need to go on a signing or ICT course?

There are lots of ways in which the physical space affects communication.

- Noise makes it hard to hear, and makes us tense and jumpy.
- Furniture arranged in a formal way, in lines or round a table, can make us feel inhibited.
- Big spaces make it hard to hear and see people.
- If people are coming in and out of the room it makes us feel our communication is not private.
- Uncomfortable chairs mean we don't feel at ease.
- Bare rooms mean there are fewer topics of conversation.
- Unpainted dirty rooms make us feel devalued and worthless.

Big decisions are the outcome of small decisions. Seeing things from the perspective of the person at the centre means being aware of the importance of small changes. Choosing what to wear, where to sit or what music to listen to may not seem very significant from our point of view, but these small decisions can make someone feel effective and in control of a manageable part of their lives.

Case Study

(5.1) How can you help someone make decisions?

Terry is a service user with profound learning disabilities. He and his advocate have tried out two different activities – shopping in a supermarket and shopping at the local grocery shop. Terry seems more comfortable in the grocery shop, which is smaller and where the shopkeeper says hello and helps him choose fruit. His advocate took photos of the supermarket and the grocers, and after each visit he and Terry sat down together and talked about the experience. Now when Terry leaves the centre to go shopping, he turns in the direction of the grocers, indicating that this is where he would prefer to go.

Learning to make choices also involves learning how to make choices. This means that we need to make the procedures of planning clear and accessible. Having predictable routines that are used consistently will help the person to participate actively. The more consistent experiences we have of making effective choices, the better we get at it.

(5.2) Use own role and authority to support the individual's right to make choices

Making choices is part of everyday life for most of us. It is an essential part of us being recognised and respected as an individual. Such choices contribute to us having control over our lives, and individuals we support also have the right to participate in decisions that affect their lives.

Our practice should recognise the right of individuals to make their own choices. Alongside this, services also need to provide capacity to give their users options. Choosing to 'take it or leave it' is not a real choice. Choice for individuals is now rightly promoted as a quality standard when care organisations advertise their services, and it forms part of how they are judged. The vast majority of decisions – and virtually all choices – can ultimately be tackled by most adults if the right information and options are made accessible to them in terms they can understand. These efforts can involve advocates and other measures to safeguard the choice or decision-making and may, for some parties, require considerable time and expertise in communication. Choice is one of the major core elements of person-centred approaches.

A person's rights can range from everyday human rights to civil and legal rights. Legal and civil rights help to eradicate discrimination in our society. There are also other rights which we might consider to be important, e.g. the right to be treated with dignity and respect, the right to complain. We could refer to these as moral rights. Generally these rights may not have the same legal force behind them as civil and legal rights; they depend more on the goodwill and nature of people to recognise and support them.

Exercising choice is, for most people, part of everyday life. It is also a fundamental part of being recognised as individual and being respected as a person. Whether these choices are minor or major they all contribute to having control over our lives. Minor choices are typically taken for granted. Major choices or decisions are those such as where to live and work, whether to have a particular type of medical treatment or even who to be intimate with. These are the decisions that can have a big impact and long-term effect on people's lives.

Choice for consumers is routinely promoted as a quality standard when care providers advertise their services. For politicians and policymakers alike, choice has become something of a buzzword. For people receiving care and support services there is often a very real gap between the rhetoric and the experience. Consideration should be given to the difference between making a 'choice' and a 'decision'.

Generally speaking, 'choice' is referred to when the options are not too important. A 'decision' is seen to relate to a more fundamental choice that can have a greater impact on an individual's life.

In order to make a major decision a person should have:

■ access to appropriate and sufficient information

■ the capacity to understand the information, the options and the consequences of the various outcomes

■ the opportunity to make their decision freely and without any duress or biased encouragement.

Sometimes, presenting the same information in different ways, or presenting small pieces of information and continually checking understanding, can help with progression to an overall understanding and therefore to a decision. It may become apparent that the person cannot make a decision completely on their own. In this case, every effort should be made to ensure that they have participated in the decision-making process to the fullest degree. Depending on the situation, it may be important to involve a person who knows the individual well. Those close to an individual can teach us a lot about their communication. On other occasions, it may be appropriate to use a person who is completely independent to work with a client, if there are concerns that there may be external pressures from another person, for example a relative or another carer.

 Evidence activity

5.2 Inability to make decisions

Imagine that you can't make decisions; they are all made for you. How would you feel?

5.3 Manage risk in a way that maintains the individual's right to make choices

Risk is usually seen as the possibility that an event will occur, with harmful outcomes for an individual or for others. Such an event may be more likely because of risks associated with:

- disability or impairment
- health conditions or mental health problems
- activities while out in the community, or in a social care setting
- everyday activities, which may be increased by a disability
- delivery of care and support
- use of medication
- misuse of drugs or alcohol
- behaviours resulting in injury, neglect, abuse or exploitation by self or others
- self-harm, neglect or thoughts of suicide
- aggression or violence of self or others.

A pure health and safety approach to risk identifies five key steps:

1. Identify the hazard.
2. Identify the risk (who may be harmed and how).
3. Evaluate the risks and decide on precautions.
4. Record findings and implement them.
5. Review the risk assessment and update if necessary.

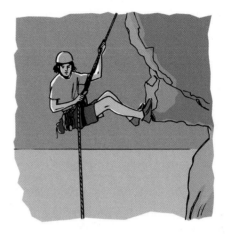

Figure 7.6 Should I? Shouldn't I?

Exploring choice can also expose people to potential risk. Professionals and staff can feel a clear tension between choice and empowerment and risk for the individual. While being aware of their duty of care and wishing to empower individuals to take reasonable risks on the one hand, on the other they are acutely aware of being accountable for their actions and can fear a blame culture. Here is where appropriate risk policies have a role to play, and organisations should develop a clear definition of risk that looks at probability and consequences.

Evidence activity

5.3 Risk vs choice

What do you think would cause tension between risk and choice in the setting you work in? How could a safe compromise be reached?

In certain circumstances it may not be possible to comply with the wishes of the person in this regard, for example, where there are child protection risks or safeguarding risks. Taking risks can help people to learn and gain experience and confidence in leading their lives. Not taking risks can mean that people are not able to develop and grow, and may be prevented from doing things which make them happy. Therefore people should be supported to make real choices, even when these choices may sometimes be unwise or could lead to harm: provided that the assessment and support planning has been undertaken in partnership with the person, has taken all the relevant factors into account and enabled the person to weigh up the advantages and disadvantages of a proposed course of action, and they are able to make an informed choice. It is important when doing this to find out why the person wishes to make a particular choice, what this will bring to their life, and how their life may be adversely affected if they are prevented from making this choice.

 5.4 Describe how to support an individual to question or challenge decisions concerning them that are made by others

In social care, the relationship between the individual and the people involved in assessing their needs or helping them to arrange their support is a relationship which gives rise to a duty of care. Therefore it is essential that risk assessments are carried out in a transparent way, in partnership with people and their carers, and that agreement is reached about the risks, how they will be managed, and who will be responsible for them.

When carrying out risk assessments and risk management, the following factors should be considered:

■ The identification, assessment and management of risk should promote independence and social inclusion.

■ Risks may be minimised, but not eliminated.

■ It may not be possible to manage all risks.

■ Identification of risk carries a duty to do something about it, i.e. to manage the risk.

■ Risks may change as circumstances change, and should be reviewed – an assessment is a snapshot, whereas risk assessment is an ongoing process.

Advocacy

Advocacy is the process of speaking up about an issue that is important to the individual. This can be either self-advocacy, where the individual speaks on their own behalf, or citizen advocacy, where a volunteer from a local advocacy group speaks on the individual's behalf. From time to time, an issues advocate is required to address a specific issue. The process of advocating is to address a specific problem, and once this is resolved it will come to an end. Because of the level

of complexity or expertise required, the advocate could be a paid official or professional, e.g. solicitor or welfare rights consultant. This form of advocacy does not replace the likes of citizen advocacy or self-advocacy but works alongside it.

Research & investigate

5.4 Advocates

Find out when an advocate would be used and what they can do to help someone. Make notes on your findings.

Professionals, organisations and even family carers need to recognise the role and work of advocates in independently supporting people. An individual may be living in a care or supported setting, or with their family, and can still avail themselves of an advocate. In all cases the relationship is confidential to the person and their advocate partner. Such partnerships can grow into long-term friendships which give much to supporting and safeguarding people and their interests, particularly if they live in a long-term care setting.

LO6 Be able to promote individuals' well-being

 6.1 Explain the links between identity, self-image and self-esteem

Evidence activity

6.1 Identity

Ask an older friend or relative how they think their needs and abilities have changed over the years. Do they need any more or less support or help?

What is our personal identity?

Our personal identity is the way we see ourselves and is closely related to our self-image. It is very important to us because it will affect the way we feel about ourselves and how we behave in challenging situations. Our personal identity includes:

- Who we are.
- What makes us unique.
- What our values are.
- Our physical identity (what we think we look like to others), also known as body image.
- Our internal identity (who we think we are in terms of our personality and character, values etc.).
- How we see ourselves in relation to others.
- How we identify ourselves in terms of our job.
- Our personal goals.

The most important thing to realise about our personal identity is that it can be close to how other people see us, in which case we will be at harmony with the world and others around, or it can be very different from how others see us and so we may feel we are misunderstood and that life is a battle to make others appreciate who we are.

One of the biggest problems people have with their personal identity is that they may not accept or may be blind to who they are and what they believe. Most of us today suffer from this to a certain extent because society seems to want us to behave and live in ways which may not be exactly what we want.

The first step towards higher self-esteem is to be clear about who you are and what you believe. This is the goal of self-awareness. Before you can improve your self-esteem or indeed make any positive changes to your life you need to devote time to this form of self-improvement. Therefore, understanding your personal identity is a necessary first step and only after this step can you think about how to change your life positively.

How can our personal identity help improve our self-esteem?

1. Who are you? What makes you tick? Knowing this can lead you closer towards decisions which help you live as you want to, not as others want or how you feel you should.

2. What makes you unique? Nobody else among the billions of people living on this planet now or the billions of people who lived before is or was ever exactly like you.

3. What are your values? If you want to feel good about yourself then you need to understand what your values are and start living them. Many people compromise their

values and believe they must live a certain way, but this is the road to unhappiness and low self-esteem.

4. What is your internal identity? Your personality and character make you unique and you should value them. Focus on what positives you have in these two areas.

5. How do you see yourself in relation to others? This is related to your status as you see it. If you believe you have very low status you will suffer low self-esteem, but if you feel you have a high status this will help you have higher self-esteem.

6. Do you identify yourself in terms of your job? Don't make the mistake of thinking that a job defines who you are – it is only what you do and nothing more.

7. What are your personal goals? These say a lot about who you are and the values you hold, but if you want to improve your self-esteem you should have goals that move you closer to being who you really are.

 ## Analyse factors that contribute to the well-being of individuals

Many factors combine together to affect the health and well-being of individuals and communities. Whether people are healthy or not is determined by their circumstances and environment. To a large extent, factors such as where we live, the state of our environment, genetics, our income and education level, and our relationships with friends and family all have considerable impacts on health and well-being, whereas the more commonly considered factors, such as access and use of health care services, often have less of an impact. The context of people's lives determines their health, so blaming individuals for having poor health or crediting them for good health is inappropriate. Individuals are unlikely to be able directly to control many of the determinants of health.

Evidence activity

6.2 Well-being

What do you understand by well-being? What can affect our well-being?

6.3 **Support an individual in a way that promotes their sense of identity, self-image and self-esteem**

Developing and monitoring service delivery

You may be involved in a care planning meeting organised to develop or review an individual's care plan or to review service delivery. The responsibility for arranging the meeting may also lie with you, but it is important that you provide the necessary information and materials as soon as possible prior to the meeting.

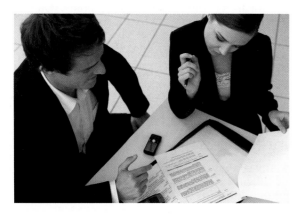

Figure 7.7 It is important to monitor and review care plans

Encouraging participation

Individuals and/or their relatives and friends should have a full part to play in the care planning process. This could mean becoming involved in meetings – either at the actual meeting or in the preparations for it.

Part of your role is to encourage individuals and those close to them to play an active part. A first step may be to give them basic information about things such as:

■ Why your organisation is having the meeting.

■ Where and when the meeting will take place.

■ Whether transport will be needed for the individual to get to the meeting.

■ Who will attend the meeting.

■ Why the different people are there.

■ How the individual should present their views.

■ What will happen when the individual and relative/or friend arrive.

■ What they will be asked to say or do.

■ What happens if they decide to say nothing.

The aim of a person-centred approach is to ensure that the individual is an equal partner with health and social care professionals in assessing, identifying options for and delivering the most appropriate package of care for that individual across organisational boundaries. It involves the provision of full information on all aspects of the individual's needs and available services, and requires the individual to be treated with respect, courtesy and dignity at all times.

To begin with the person must be the centre of the plan, i.e. must be consulted and their views always come first. The plan should include all aspects of care – social services, health services, family and the voluntary sector.

A proactive care setting will follow the principles of person-centred care. Person-centred care aims to see the person as an individual, rather than focusing on their illness and on abilities they may have lost. Instead of treating the person as a collection of symptoms and behaviours to be controlled, person-centred care takes into account each individual's unique qualities, abilities, interests, preferences and needs.

Personal dignity and privacy should be respected at all times. Individual cultural or religious beliefs should also be taken into account. For example, staff should address the person in whichever way the person prefers, whether by their first name or more formally. Individuals, for example those with dementia, have the right to expect those caring for them to try to understand how they feel and to make time to offer support rather than ignoring or humouring them. Staff should sit and chat to residents while they are helping them with physical tasks such as washing and dressing. One member of staff should have particular responsibility for the care of each person. This staff member should have a clear idea of that person's life history, habits and interests.

Evidence activity

6.3 **Recording and storing care plan information**

You have completed a care plan. What do you need to think about in relation to recording and storing the information included on the plan?

6.4 Demonstrate ways to contribute to an environment that promotes well-being

Supporting care plan activities

When a care plan is in place, as well as carrying out your own duties under the plan you will need to support and supervise colleagues to carry out their specified activities.

Monitoring is essential to ensure that any plan of care is continuing to meet the needs it was designed to meet. A care plan will have originally been assessed, planned and put in place to meet a particular set of circumstances. The original plan should include provision for monitoring and review, because plans put in place with even the most thorough assessment and careful planning will not necessarily be appropriate in six months or a year's time, and may not continue to provide services of the quality or at the level originally expected.

Monitoring may seem a complex process but its principles are very simple. Monitoring of care services needs to pick up and address changes in the circumstances of those receiving the services, their carers and service providers. For example, someone recently discharged from hospital following treatment for mental health problems may receive quite extensive support under the care programme approach. However, feedback on their progress may show that their mental health has improved to the point that day care is no longer needed on the previous level and that a lower level of care input can be planned for.

Checking resources

Checking on resources can also be important if changes in the availability of those resources means that a care package will have to be altered in some way. A reduction in the availability or an increase in demand for a particular service may mean that adjustments in the level of service provision will have to be made. Regular monitoring makes it easier to be aware of where resources are being used and where changes can be made.

Ways of monitoring

Whatever approach is taken to monitoring, how a particular plan of care will be monitored and the methods used will be agreed with the individual and their carers at the outset. Your feedback will be an essential part of the process.

This may involve the following key people:

- the individual concerned
- their carers and/or family
- other health care professionals
- the service provider.

The most important person in the monitoring process is the individual receiving the service, so they must be clear about how to record and feed back information on the way the care package is working. This can be achieved by completing a checklist on a regular basis, maintaining regular contact with the care manager or coordinator, or recording and reporting any changes in the needs or in the care provision.

> **Evidence activity**
>
> **6.4 Monitoring and review of care plans**
>
> Why is monitoring and review of care plans important? How do you do this in your setting?

LO7 Understand the role of risk assessment in enabling a person-centred approach

7.1 Compare different uses of risk assessment in health and social care

The emphasis in thinking about providing support and care has moved over the past decade or so towards promoting independence. An important part of this must be the recognition that the people we support have the same rights as any other citizens. This in turn means the right to take risks.

> **Evidence activity**
>
> **7.1 Risks**
>
> We know quite a lot nowadays about what is and is not good for us. Think about yourself, your friends and family. List below some of the things that you and those you know do that are a risk.

The assessment of risk is something that can leave us feeling very anxious. Questions such as, 'What if I get it wrong?' are normal. It makes sense, therefore, to talk about worries with your manager or mentor, because talking things through helps us to get things in better perspective. As a result we learn to feel more confident in our judgements. Policies and procedures can also help, and this part of the standards requires you to look at the risk assessment policy in your organisation. You also need to know what to do with the policy.

Most services are provided on the basis that the service user wishes to follow a plan of treatment/support and that carers are involved wherever possible. Other services also depend on good-quality assessments of need and risk. Local authorities have rules about how much money and resources should be allocated to people with additional needs. Such rules are called 'eligibility criteria' and increase the entitlement of an individual to resources, according to the level of need they have.

The general public take risks every day of their lives. These may be day-to-day risks, such as playing sport, drinking or driving a car, or occasional risks, like going on an aeroplane. Some of us take great pleasure in pushing the boundaries to the limit in what is called extreme sport. Of all the activities that we do, the only ones that require us to be risk assessed or to be tested are those in which others may get hurt, for example driving a car. Taking risks is part of living a full life. For service users to have choice and to live as full a life as possible they must be supported to take risks. Service users must be allowed make bad and good choices, and be supported in the risk and consequences that these bring. For people to learn things about their environment and themselves they must be supported while they make mistakes.

Employers have responsibilities for the health and safety of their employees. They are also responsible for any visitors to their premises, such as relatives, suppliers and the general public.

The Health and Safety at Work Act

The Health and Safety at Work etc Act 1974 is the primary piece of legislation covering work-related health and safety in the United Kingdom. It sets out a lot of your employer's responsibilities for your health and safety at work. The Health and Safety Executive is responsible for enforcing health and safety at work.

Risk assessments

Your employer has a 'duty of care' to look after, as far as possible, your health, safety and welfare while you are at work. They should start with a risk assessment to spot possible health and safety hazards.

They have to appoint a 'competent person' to take on health and safety responsibilities. This is usually one of the owners in smaller firms, or a member of staff trained in health and safety in larger businesses.

You also have responsibilities for your own health and safety at work. You can refuse to do something that isn't safe without being threatened with disciplinary action. If you think your employer isn't meeting their responsibilities, talk to them. Your safety representative or a trade union official may be able to help you with this. As a last resort, you may need to report your employer to the Health and Safety Executive or to the environmental health department of your local authority. If you are dismissed for refusing to undertake an unsafe working practice, you may have a right to claim unfair dismissal at an employment tribunal.

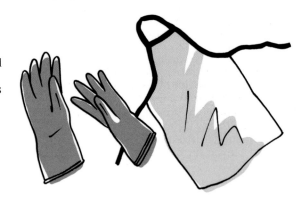

Figure 7.8 Take precautions to protect your health and safety

7.2 Explain how risk-taking and risk assessment relate to rights and responsibilities

Addressing the issue of positive risk-taking is key to the implementation of person-centred planning and approaches, which are aimed at increasing inclusion and promoting people's participation in their communities as valued and contributing citizens. Responsible and responsive organisations (and services) are striving to find ways of balancing their responsibilities as employers with supporting people to live lives which work for them.

Our starting point is the principle that 'everyone in society has a positive contribution to make to that society and that they should have a right to control their own lives.' *Independence, Well-being and Choice* (Social Care Green Paper, March 2005). Positive risk-taking is about people taking control of their own lives by weighing up the potential benefits and harms of exercising one choice of action over another. Positive risk-taking is not negligent ignorance of the potential risks. Risk is a part of everyone's everyday life. Everyone, including people with learning disabilities, has the right to take risks.

Practice outcomes

People will be given the support they need to take the risks they want and to make informed choices. New experiences and greater community involvement potentially involve people taking risks that offer opportunities for the development of independence, confidence and autonomy.

Organisations must be able to demonstrate that a risk-assessing process (i.e. a process of thinking things through properly, involving the focus person and others who know them) has taken place. This may or may not result in a formal written risk assessment. This policy is intended to complement the organisation's health and safety policy.

Everyone is assumed to have capacity unless proven otherwise (Mental Capacity Act, April 2005). Everyone is able to be involved in decision-making, whether they are deemed to have capacity or not.

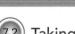

Evidence activity

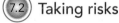

7.2 Taking risks

How can risk-taking be a positive thing? Think of some examples to illustrate this.

 7.3 Explain why risk assessments need to be regularly revised

The following list gives an overview of the types of occasions when a risk assessment needs to be completed:

- when planning activities
- when planning and purchasing new facilities
- when new work practices are introduced
- when an individual develops a special need, or where there is a significant change to their existing needs.

In addition there should be a system for regularly reviewing the risk assessments. No risk assessment should be written without a review date, monthly, quarterly, six monthly or annually, depending upon the need.

The risk assessment form allows risks to be recorded and the actions required to manage the risk easily communicated. This should be cross-referenced to other plans for the individual, especially the care plans. All plans need to be reviewed regularly. However, an additional review needs to take place whenever a significant risk occurs. Forms need to be dated and numbered.

Evidence activity

7.3 Carrying out a risk assessment

What are the steps involved in carrying out a risk assessment? Carry out a short risk assessment of a hazard you identify in your workplace, or out in the community. Record your findings.

Assessment summary

Your reading of this chapter and completion of the activities will have prepared you to be able to engage in personal development in health, social care or children's and young people's settings.

To achieve the unit, your assessor will require you to:

Learning outcomes	Assessment Criteria
Learning outcome **1**: Show that you understand the application of person-centred approaches in health and social care role by:	**1.1** explaining how and why person-centred values must influence all aspects of health and social care work See Evidence activity 1.1, p. 112
	1.2 evaluating the use of care plans in applying person-centred values See Evidence activity 1.2, p. 113
Learning outcome **2**: Be able to work in a person-centred way by:	**2.1** working with an individual and others to find out the individual's history, preferences, wishes and needs See Evidence activity 2.1, p. 114
	2.2 demonstrating ways to put person-centred values into practice in a complex or sensitive situation See Evidence activity 2.2, p. 115
	2.3 adapting actions and approaches in response to an individual's changing needs or preferences See Case study 2.3, p. 115
Learning outcome **3**: Be able to establish consent when providing care or support by:	**3.1** analysing factors that influence the capacity of an individual to express consent See Evidence activity 3.1, p. 117
	3.2 establishing consent for an activity or action See Evidence activity 3.2, p. 118
	3.3 explaining what steps to take if consent cannot be readily established See Research and investigate 3.3, p. 118

Learning outcomes	Assessment Criteria
Learning outcome **4**: Be able to implement and promote active participation by:	**4.1** describing different ways of applying active participation to meet individual needs See Evidence activity 4.1, p. 119
	4.2 working with an individual and others to agree how active participation will be implemented See Evidence activity 4.2, p. 119
	4.3 demonstrating how active participation can address the holistic needs of an individual See Evidence activity 4.3, p. 120
	4.4 demonstrating ways to promote understanding and use of active participation See Evidence activity 4.4, p. 121
Learning outcome **5**: Be able to support the individual's right to make choices by:	**5.1** supporting an individual to make informed choices See Case study 5.1, p. 122
	5.2 using own role and authority to support the individual's right to make choices See Evidence activity 5.2, p. 123
	5.3 managing risk in a way that maintains the individual's right to make choices See Evidence activity 5.3, p. 123
	5.4 describing how to support an individual to question or challenge decisions concerning them that are made by others See Research and investigate 5.4, p. 124
Learning outcome **6**: Be able to promote individuals' well-being by:	**6.1** explaining the links between identity, self-image and self-esteem See Evidence activity 6.1, p. 124

Learning outcomes	Assessment Criteria
Learning outcome **6**: Be able to promote individuals' well-being by:	(6.2) analysing factors that contribute to the well-being of individuals See Evidence activity 6.2, p. 125
	(6.3) supporting an individual in a way that promotes their sense of identity, self-image and self-esteem See Evidence activity 6.3, p. 126
	(6.4) demonstrating ways to contribute to an environment that promotes well-being See Evidence activity 6.4, p. 127
Learning outcome **7**: Show that you understand the role of risk assessment in enabling a person-centred approach by:	(7.1) comparing different uses of risk assessment in health and social care See Evidence activity 7.1, p. 127
	(7.2) explaining how risk taking and risk assessment relate to rights and responsibilities See Evidence activity 7.2, p. 129
	(7.3) explaining why risk assessments need to be regularly revised See Evidence activity 7.3, p. 129

Good luck!

Web links

The Department for Education, previously the Department for Children, Schools and Families and Schools	www.dcsf.gov.uk
Care Quality Commission (CQC)	www.cqc.org.uk
Commission for the Regulation of Care (SCRC)	www.carecommission.com
The place to go for Essential Lifestyle Plans	www.elpnet.net
Valuing People Support Team	http://valuingpeople.gov.uk
Department of Health	www.dh.gov.uk
Families Leading Planning UK	www.familiesleadingplanning.co.uk
In Control	www.in-control.org.uk
Office of Public Sector Information	www.opsi.gov.uk
Support planning	www.supportplanning.org

8 Promote and implement health and safety in health and social care

For Unit HSC 037

What are you finding out?

According to the **Health and Safety Executive (HSE)**, statistics for 2008/9 showed that:

1.2 million people were suffering from an illness they believed was work-related

180 workers were killed at work

131,895 injuries to employees were reported under **RIDDOR**

246,000 **reportable injuries** occurred

29.3 million days were lost overall, 24.6 million due to work-related ill health and 4.7 million due to workplace injury.

www.hse.gov.uk

The reading and activities in this chapter will help you to:

■ Understand your own responsibilities, and the responsibilities of others, relating to health and safety

■ Be able to carry out your own responsibilities for health and safety

■ Understand procedures for responding to accidents and sudden illness

■ Be able to reduce the spread of infection

■ Be able to move and handle equipment and other objects safely

■ Be able to handle hazardous substances and materials

■ Be able to promote fire safety in the work setting

■ Be able to implement security measures in the work setting

■ Know how to manage stress.

Key terms

The Health and Safety Executive (HSE) is the national independent watchdog for work-related health, safety and illness, working to reduce workplace death and serious injury. Reportable injuries are injuries that keep someone away from work or unable to do their normal duties for more than three days. RIDDOR stands for Reporting of Injuries, Diseases and Dangerous Occurrences Regulations.
A work sector is a division of the national economy, for example the manufacturing sector, the private sector.

The type of work carried out within the health and social care **work sector** is closely associated with a high risk of accident, injury and ill health caused, for example, by slips and trips, unsafe moving and handling, contact with hazardous materials, spread of infection and stress. Accidents, injuries and ill health in staff also have a knock-on effect on their delivery of health and social care services.

LO1 Understand own responsibilities, and the responsibilities of others, relating to health and safety

1.1 Legislation relating to health and safety in a health or social care work setting

There are a number of important pieces of health and safety legislation that affect health and social care settings.

Table 8.1 Health and safety legislation

Legislation	Purpose of the legislation
Health and Safety at Work etc Act (HASWA) 1974	Ensures the health and safety of everyone who may be affected by work activities.
Management of Health and Safety at Work Regulations (MHSWR) 1999	Require employers and managers to carry out risk assessments to eliminate or minimise risks to health and safety.
Workplace (Health, Safety and Welfare) Regulations 1992	Minimise the risks to health and safety associated with working conditions.
Manual Handling Operations Regulations (MHOR) 1992	Minimise the risks to health and safety associated with moving and handling activities.
Personal Protective Equipment at Work Regulations (PPE) 1992	Minimise the risks to health and safety associated with cross infection.
Reporting of Injuries, Diseases and Dangerous Occurrences Regulations (RIDDOR) 1995	Require that certain work-related injuries, diseases and dangerous occurrences are reported to the HSE or local authority.
Control of Substances Hazardous to Health Regulations (COSHH) 2002	Minimise the risks to health and safety from the use of hazardous substances.
Provision and Use of Work Equipment Regulations (PUWER) 1998	Minimise the risks to health and safety associated with the use of equipment.
Electricity at Work Regulations 1989	Minimise the risks to health and safety associated with electricity.
Regulatory Reform (Fire Safety) Order 2005.	Minimises the risks to health and safety of fire.
Health and Safety (First Aid) Regulations 1981	Ensure that everyone can receive immediate attention if they are injured or taken ill in the workplace.
Disability Discrimination Act (DDA) 1995	Ensures that people with a disability have safe access to the workplace and a safe way out in the event of needing to evacuate the premises.
Food Safety Act 1990 and the Food Hygiene Regulations 2006	Minimise the risks to health and safety associated with food handling.
Data Protection Act 1998	Ensures everyone's right to privacy of their personal information.
Corporate Manslaughter and Homicide Act 2007	Allows an organisation to be convicted when, due to negligence, the death occurs of someone to whom it owes a duty of care, such as a worker or person using the service.

Evidence activity

Legislation relating to health and safety

Bearing in mind the needs of the people you support and the type of service that your workplace provides, make a list of the Acts and Regulations in Table 8.1 that you think apply to your work setting. Talk your answer through with your manager or employer.

Health and safety policies and procedures

Health and safety policies set out the arrangements that a workplace has for complying with legislation. For example, in order to comply with the Health and Safety (First Aid) Regulations, every workplace should have a policy that describes how it manages first aid.

Health and safety procedures describe the activities that need to be carried out for policies to be implemented. They record who does what, when and how in order to maintain health and safety at all times. For example, first aid procedures will describe the roles of first aiders and the people responsible for maintaining first-aid equipment and facilities. They will also describe when and how to call the emergency services and when and how to complete a record of an accident.

It is a legal requirement that you follow workplace health and safety procedures to the letter. Failure to do so could mean the end of your career in care.

Research & investigate

Failing to follow health and safety procedures

Check out the consequences of you failing to follow health and safety procedures at work. What could happen to you, the people you work with, your colleagues and your workplace?

Evidence activity

Health and safety policies and procedures agreed with the employer

This activity enables you to demonstrate your understanding of the reasons why policies and procedures shape the way you do your work.

1. Make a note of three policies that govern practice at your workplace. Why is it necessary for these policies to be in place?

2. Make a note of three procedures you must follow as you carry out your activities. Why is it necessary for you to follow these procedures?

Main health and safety responsibilities

Your responsibilities

The Health and Safety at Work etc Act 1974 states that it is your duty, while at work, to:

- take reasonable care of yourself and anyone else who may be affected by your actions, including colleagues, the individuals you work with, their families, carers and **advocates**

- cooperate with your employer or manager in relation to health and safety issues

- not interfere with or misuse anything provided in the interest of health and safety, for example first aid and fire fighting equipment, health and safety notices.

Key term

Advocates are people who support or speak on behalf of someone else.

In addition, you have a responsibility to follow health and safety policies and procedures to the letter, participate in and stay up-to-date with health and safety training, and not carry out any task in which you have not been trained.

Table 8.2 The responsibilities of your employer or manager

Legislation	Responsibilities of your employer or manager
Health and Safety at Work etc Act 1974	• Write health and safety policies and procedures and make you aware of them. • Ensure everyone's health, safety and welfare, including visitors and the people using the service, as far as is reasonably practicable.
Management of Health and Safety at Work Regulations 1999	• Carry out risk assessments to eliminate or reduce risks to health and safety. • Set up emergency procedures and inform everyone about them. • Provide you with clear information, supervision and training to ensure that you are competent to carry out your work.
Workplace (Health, Safety and Welfare) Regulations 1992	Meet minimum standards with regard to buildings and equipment, lighting, temperature, and the provision of first aid, drinking water and rest and toilet facilities.
Manual Handling Operations Regulations 1992	• Train you in safe moving and handling. • Eliminate or reduce all risks associated with moving and handling activities.
Personal Protective Equipment at Work Regulations (PPE) 1992	Provide you with appropriate protective clothing and equipment.
Reporting of Injuries, Diseases and Dangerous Occurrences Regulations (RIDDOR) 1995	Train you in how to report injuries, diseases and dangerous occurrences.
Control of Substances Hazardous to Health Regulations (COSHH) 2002	Carry out risk assessments on all activities that involve using hazardous substances and write procedures for their correct and safe use.
Provision and Use of Work Equipment Regulations (PUWER) 1998	• Train you in the use of equipment and supervise you to make sure you use it safely and correctly. • Ensure that the equipment you use is safe, well maintained and appropriate for the job.
Electricity at Work Regulations 1989	• Carry out risk assessments on all activities that involve electricity. • Ensure safe systems of working and that all electrical equipment is well maintained.
Regulatory Reform (Fire Safety) Order 2005	• Assess the risk of fire, paying particular attention to the needs of vulnerable people. • Equip the workplace with fire detection and fire-fighting equipment. • Train you in fire prevention and what to do in the event of a fire.

Legislation	Responsibilities of your employer or manager
Health and Safety (First Aid) Regulations 1981	• Provide adequate and appropriate first-aid equipment and facilities. • Provide an adequate number of qualified first aiders and appointed persons to take charge of first-aid arrangements.
Disability Discrimination Act 1995	Ensure that people with a disability have safe access to your workplace and a safe way out in the event of needing to evacuate the building.
Food Safety Act 1990 and the Food Hygiene Regulations 2006.	• Ensure that you have good personal hygiene and that the workplace meets hygiene standards. • Ensure that food safety hazards are identified and controlled.
Data Protection Act 1998.	Train you in maintaining the security of personal information.
Corporate Manslaughter and Homicide Act 2007.	Have in place adequate risk management systems.

The responsibilities of others in the work setting

Like you, your colleagues have a responsibility to follow procedures in their work. Visiting family, carers and advocates also have a responsibility to consider health and safety, especially with respect to helping maintain security, hand washing, complying with no smoking rules, and their general conduct.

The health and safety of the people you work with depends to a large extent on your ability to work together, in partnership. For example, the risks associated with moving and handling activities are greatly reduced when they fulfil their responsibility to assist with a move as much as they can. Other responsibilities they have include:

■ helping to maintain their personal hygiene, in order to reduce the spread of infection

■ remaining aware of what to do in the event of a fire

■ using any equipment assigned to them, such as glasses and mobility aids, appropriately and safely.

Evidence activity

1.3 Analyse health and safety responsibilities

Think of one work activity that you carry out on a regular basis. What responsibilities do the following people have in ensuring that it is carried out safely?

■ you

■ your colleagues

■ your employer or manager

■ the people you work with

1.4 Specific tasks in the work setting that should not be carried out without special training

You read earlier that one of your main responsibilities is to not undertake any task in which you have not been trained. Some of these tasks are described below.

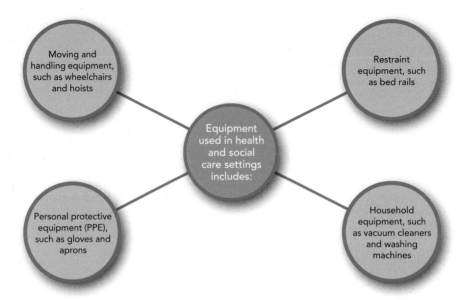

Figure 8.1 Equipment used in health and social care settings

Inappropriate use or misuse of equipment can result in alleged abuse, spread of infection, injury or death, as can using equipment that hasn't been maintained or is in a state of disrepair. Only use equipment that you have been trained to use, and use it according to written procedures. If you have any concerns about equipment, report and record your worries and don't use it again until your concerns have been resolved.

While an untrained person who gives first aid in an emergency in good faith won't be running the risk of being sued, they could be charged with negligence or incompetence, especially if they make an incorrect diagnosis and give the wrong treatment. First aid training improves competence and can make the difference between a life lost and a life saved.

Try out the interactive quiz on the Test Your Skills pages of www.bbc.co.uk/health/treatments/first_aid to find out how much you know about first aid.

Medication should only be given by staff who are trained and can demonstrate competence. The effects of a missed administration, an incorrect dose, a dose given at the wrong time or given incorrectly, such as by mouth instead of anally, or as a tablet instead of a fluid, can be devastating, even fatal for the person concerned. Training in the handling of medicines prevents accidents happening and demonstrates **duty of care**.

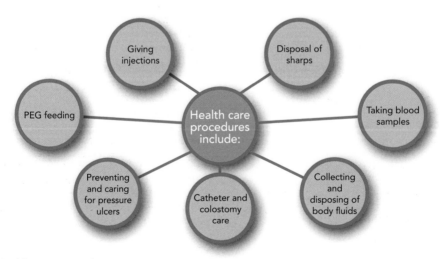

Figure 8.2 Health care procedures

Key term

Duty of care is acting in the very best interests of the people you work with.

Cross-infection is the transfer of harmful bacteria, viruses, fungi or parasites from one person, object, place or part of the body to another.

PEG feeding is feeding via a tube inserted through the skin and into the stomach.

Sharps are items of equipment that can cause cuts or puncture injuries.

Health care procedures are specialist activities and should never be carried out without training. In addition, they carry a high risk of **cross-infection** and therefore should never be carried out without training in infection control.

Food safety legislation requires that everyone who handles food, including storing, preparing, cooking and serving, supporting people to eat and drink, and disposing of waste, should be trained in food hygiene. Training helps reduce the risk of cross-infection and the debilitating, sometimes fatal, effects of food poisoning.

Evidence activity

(1.4) **Tasks that should not be carried out without special training**

Make a list of all the activities you are able to do now because you have had training and those you are not permitted to do until you have had the appropriate training.

LO2 Be able to carry out own responsibilities for health and safety

(2.1) **Use policies and procedures or other agreed ways of working that relate to health and safety**

Most health and safety procedures are extremely prescriptive. They describe the who, what, when and how of activities in very narrow, rigid terms, for example the correct way to dispose of sharps. This is because any other method of working could jeopardise the health and safety of everyone concerned. Imagine the consequences of a child coming across a used syringe in the kitchen bin. However, because individual needs and capabilities, and the environments in which needs are met, are so diverse, some procedures have to be more flexible. For example, fire evacuation procedures will differ according to where people live – a purpose-built residential care home will be equipped with fire doors and fire-fighting equipment, but not so the family home in which your grandmother wants to live out her remaining days. Similarly, the purpose-built residential care home will be equipped with hoists and stair lifts, whereas your grandmother's house may not have room for moving and handling equipment. In such situations, safe ways of working have to be devised and agreed by all concerned.

Time to reflect

(2.1) Health and safety at home

Think about three or four emergencies that could happen in the home of someone with health or social care needs. How would you deal with these emergencies? What might happen if you didn't deal with them?

You are now familiar with a range of legislation relating to health and safety in a health or social care work setting. Some of the policies that ensure legislation is put into practice include Health and Safety, Moving and Handling, Personal Protective Equipment, Use of Hazardous Substances, Use of Equipment, Fire Safety and Infection Control. Each policy will have a number of procedures for carrying out activities and, as you read earlier, it is your responsibility to follow those procedures to the letter. You also have a responsibility to keep up to date with changes in the way you are required to perform activities – methods of working are constantly in flux due to changes in legislation and advances in technology.

Practice activity

2.1 Policies and procedures related to health and safety

This activity gives you an opportunity to practise using policies and procedures or other agreed ways of working that relate to health and safety.

Keep a log to show when you have referred to policies, procedures or other agreed ways of working in order to carry out a task. Ask a colleague or your manager or employer to observe how well you carry out the task, and use their feedback to improve your way of working so that you become fully competent.

2.2 Support others to understand and follow safe practices

By following safe working practices, you are fulfilling your responsibility for the health and safety of yourself and anyone else who may be affected by your actions. You also have a responsibility to promote health and safety in your workplace by supporting others to understand and follow safe practice.

We all have role models, people who possess the qualities we would like to have and who inspire us to be better people. Role models in the workplace inspire us to become more competent. By demonstrating consistent use of safe work practices and approved methods, you will inspire others to take your lead.

A good role model is also a mentor. Mentoring is a way for people to learn from each other. It involves teaching, advising and guiding. By becoming a role model you have an opportunity to improve your mentees' understanding of why you work as you do, and the consequences of failing to follow safe practice. You also have the opportunity to advise and guide them in making improvements. And because mentoring is a two-way process, you too have an opportunity to learn!

Practice activity

2.2 Support others to understand and follow safe practices

This activity gives you an opportunity to practice showing how you support others to understand and follow safe practices.

Ask your manager or employer to set up a buddy-system that will enable you to mentor a member of staff who is newer than you to the work setting. Monitor your mentee's work practice on an informal basis and get together as frequently as possible to:

- help them improve their understanding of safe working practice
- advise on methods that will enable them to work more safely.

Keep a record of how you support your mentee, along with their evaluation of how you have helped them.

2.3 Monitor and report potential health and safety risks

A health and safety risk is the likelihood that a hazard will cause harm. Hazards include chemicals and medication, faulty equipment, obstructions in passageways and on stairs, challenging behaviour, lack of security and unsafe food handling. The harm they cause ranges from burns, fractures, infection, illness, stress, asphyxiation, through to death. While it is not always possible to fully eliminate risks to health and safety, legislation requires employers and managers to minimise them as far as possible.

Health and social care workers are best placed to identify health and safety hazards. However, even when following tried and tested safe working practices, they have to be on the ball to deal with, for example, unexpected threatening behaviour, and moving and handling equipment that up until yesterday was in good working condition. But identifying hazards is not enough on its own – they need to be reported in order that the associated risk can be either eliminated (i.e. removed), or minimised, which involves amending work practices to take account of the hazard.

How should you report a hazard? Practices for making reports vary between workplaces, but in general, report the hazard verbally to your line manager or health and safety coordinator, then record it in writing using the appropriate form. Finally, take steps to isolate the person, equipment or work area in question and warn others of the hazard by posting warning notices.

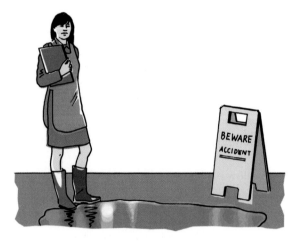

Figure 8.3 Potential health and safety risks

Practice activity

2.3 Monitor and report potential health and safety risks

This activity gives you an opportunity to practise monitoring and reporting potential health and safety risks.

Identify three potential health and safety risks in your work setting and, using your workplace's procedure, report and record the hazard posing the risk, what harm you think each may cause and the degree of risk involved.

Identifying and reporting health and safety hazards is the first stage of a risk assessment.

2.4 Use risk assessment in relation to health and safety

Under the Management of Health and Safety at Work Regulations, your manager or employer has a responsibility to carry out risk assessments to eliminate or reduce risks associated with particular hazards.

According to the HSE, there are five steps to a risk assessment:

Step 1: Identify hazards by visually inspecting the workplace, talking with colleagues and anyone else who visits, and looking at records relating to accidents, near misses and ill health.

Step 2: Decide who might be harmed and how. Think about everyone where you work, not just colleagues and the individuals you work with.

Step 3: Evaluate the risks arising from the hazards and decide whether the existing precautions are adequate or if more should be done. If something needs to be done, take steps to eliminate or control the risks.

Step 4: Record the findings and say how the risks can be controlled to prevent harm. Inform everyone about the outcome of the risk assessment as everyone will be involved in controlling the risk.

Step 5: Review the assessment from time to time and revise it if necessary, for example if work activities change.

Because you have a responsibility to cooperate with your employer's or manager's efforts to improve health and safety, you should be thinking 'risk assessment' as you carry out your activities.

Practice activity

2.4 Use risk assessment in relation to health and safety

This activity gives you an opportunity to practise showing that you can use risk assessment in relation to health and safety.

Identify three caring activities that you carry out on a day-to-day basis and discuss your answers to the following questions with your manager or employer:

■ What hazards are associated with each task?

■ Who might be harmed and how?

■ How great – or small – is the risk of harm, and are existing precautions sufficient or does more need to be done? If the latter, what further precautions do you think could be put in place?

2.5 Demonstrate ways to minimise potential risks and hazards

The working environment is fraught with potential risks and hazards. Slips and trips are the most common cause of major injuries at work, and the main risk is of broken bones. They are caused by, for example, ill-fitting, poorly maintained floor coverings; wet floors due to spills, cleaning, condensation; poorly maintained external walkways; obstructions such as equipment and furniture, trailing flexes and articles left on stairs; inappropriate footwear; lighting that is too dim or too bright; physical conditions such as visual impairment, restricted mobility and poor balance; and the side effects of medication, which can cause people to fall.

Six top tips for minimising the risk of slip and trip hazards

1. Use your initiative – if you identify a hazard, either clean it up or remove it yourself. If that isn't possible, report the situation without delay and erect a sign to warn others.

2. Check that lighting is adequate.

3. Make sure that equipment is stored properly and furniture arranged such that it doesn't cause an obstruction.

4. Wear sensible footwear and try to persuade others at work to do likewise.

5. Ensure that people who are at risk of falling have their needs catered for. For example, check that the prescription for their glasses is current and that they use appropriate walking aids.

6. Follow procedures for reporting accidents.

The health and social care services report over 5000 moving and handling injuries every year, approximately half of which happen during the handling of people. They affect the **musculoskeletal system**.

Key term

The musculoskeletal system is the system of muscles and tendons, bones, joints and ligaments that move the body and maintain its form.

Six top tips for minimising risks when moving and handling a person

1. Follow moving and handling safe working procedures to the letter.

2. Don't carry out moving and handling activities or use moving and handling equipment in which you haven't been trained.

3. Remain on the alert for incidents that could complicate or endanger a move, such as unpredictable behaviour and unexpected problems with equipment.

4. Think about how an activity could be done more safely and make your ideas known to your manager.

5. Remind the person you are working with to assist in the activity.

6. Follow procedures for reporting accidents.

Users of health and social care services are vulnerable, so they need special protection from the spread of infection, and health and social care workers need to be protected from infectious diseases. Infection spreads through physical contact with, for example, an infected person, their blood, clothing and **waste products**, and through the use of instruments that have been contaminated with their **body fluids**. It can also be spread by eating contaminated food and drink, by insects, and can be dust-, air- and water-borne.

Key terms

Body fluids include blood, plasma and cerebrospinal fluid.
Waste products include urine, faeces, tears and mucous.

Six top tips for minimising spread of infection

1. Follow infection control and food hygiene procedures to the letter.

2. Seek training in how to reduce the spread of infection.

3. Maintain a high standard of personal hygiene; keep your hands scrupulously clean at all times; and stay away from work if there is any chance you might have an infectious condition.

4. Always wear appropriate personal protective equipment (PPE), put on clean PPE for every person you work with, and dispose of soiled PPE and laundry, sharps and **clinical waste** correctly.

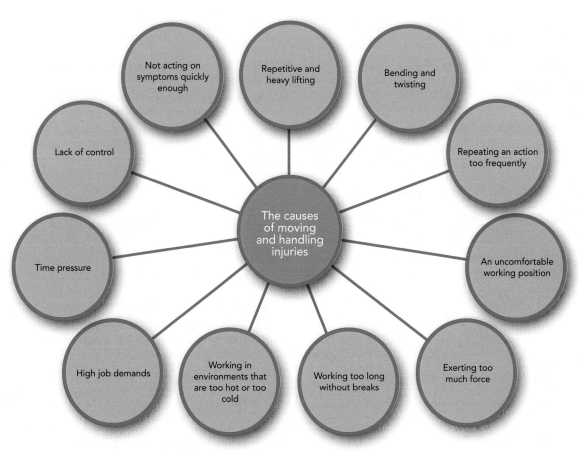

Figure 8.4 Moving and handling injuries

5. Decontaminate equipment according to the manufacturer's instructions.

6. Follow procedures for reporting illness.

Key term

Clinical waste is any material that has the potential to put health at risk, e.g. soiled dressings, incontinence pads and colostomy bags.

Every year, thousands of workers are made ill by hazardous substances, which include cleaning materials, detergents, beauty and hairdressing products, body fluids and waste, medication and gases contained in gas cylinders. The risks to health include skin disease such as dermatitis, lung disease such as asthma, and cancer. Some hazardous substances are flammable. Others are a source of infection.

Six top tips for minimising risks from hazardous substances

1. Follow COSHH procedures to the letter.

2. Don't work with hazardous materials until you have been appropriately trained.

3. Always wear appropriate PPE when working with hazardous material.

4. Store, handle and dispose of hazardous materials according to the manufacturer's instructions.

5. Know what to do in the event of an accident involving hazardous material.

6. Follow procedures for reporting accidents.

Fire in the workplace leads to death or serious injury but, in the main, is easily avoided.

Six top tips for minimising risks from fire

1. Report any tampering with fire safety notices and fire fighting equipment.

2. Know how to prevent a fire from starting.

3. Know how to prevent fire from spreading.

4. In the event of a fire, follow procedures to the letter.

5. Know how to protect people, such as vulnerable people and those who are not familiar with the workplace, from fire.

6. Follow procedures for reporting accidents.

Work-related stress is widespread in the working population. It has widespread effects on health and can result in poor performance, an increase in accidents and lengthy periods of sick leave. Stress can also occur because of ill health, disability, having to live in residential care with people you don't particularly like, and so on. In such situations, stress can cause aggressive behaviour and social withdrawal.

Six top tips for minimising risks from stress

1. Know the signs and symptoms of stress in yourself and in the people you work with.

2. Know what can trigger your stress and stress in the people you work with.

3. Know how to manage your own stress.

4. Know how to support others who are stressed.

4. Know where to get help.

6. Follow procedures for reporting accidents.

Reports of tragic incidents relating to a lack of security in health and social care settings appear in the media all too often. They include rape, kidnap, theft and murder and could all have been avoided if security measures had been tightened up.

Six top tips for minimising risks due to security issues

1. Follow security procedures to the letter, including missing persons procedure in the event that someone goes missing.

2. Always check the identity of visitors, report any concerns to your manager without delay and follow procedures for reporting incidents in the event of a breach of security.

3. Never give out information about anyone at work unless you have been given permission to do so.

4. Know your responsibilities in dealing with security emergencies and don't overstep them.

5. If your workplace has provided you with a key pad code number, don't share that number with anyone else. Similarly, if it has provided you with a swipe card, don't lend your card to anyone else.

6. Always let colleagues know where you are, particularly if you are working alone.

Case Study

 2.5 A security issue

A teenager who was out on bail for a series of burglaries dragged an 86-year-old woman from her Bradford care home and raped her. The young man was high on drink and drugs when he entered the care home and kidnapped the victim. The pensioner, who was bed-bound and suffered from dementia and incontinence, was left bruised and bloodied after the attack last September.

This story was published in the *Yorkshire Post* on 3 February 2010.

1. What lapses in security do you think took place?

2. How do you think this event will have impacted on everyone at the home?

3. How do you think events like this could be avoided in future?

Practice activity

 2.5 Minimising potential risks and hazards

This activity gives you an opportunity to practise showing that you can minimise potential risks and hazards.

Look back at your response to practice activity 2.3, in which you assessed the degree of risk to health and safety from three hazards. For this activity, suggest ways that would minimise those risks. Talk with your employer or manager about your ideas, and if they give permission, put your suggestions into practice.

2.6 Access additional support or information relating to health and safety

Health and safety is a hot topic! Many people think its abundance of rules and regulations are rather excessive. However, there is no doubt that workplace health and safety legislation protects the health, safety and welfare of everyone at work – and that means you!

This chapter has pointed you in the direction of legislation, policies and procedures that identify your responsibilities for promoting health and safety. Where can you look for further information? The internet is awash with useful sites – try googling 'health and safety' and you will be presented with a huge list of websites, including:

- official government websites, such as HSE (an excellent source of information with numerous free leaflets to download)
- websites belonging to Sector Skills Councils and trades unions
- websites promoting training courses and advertising books and journals
- websites of organisations that provide support in resolving health and safety issues.

There may be a trades union representative and a health and safety officer in your workplace. Either will be able to provide you with health and safety information. They will also be able to support you with any concerns you may have, as will your manager or employer and the staff in your human resources department.

Libraries and community centres can provide information on a range of health and safety issues, as can fire stations, GP practices, hospitals, manufacturers of materials and equipment used in health and social care settings, and so on. Finally, check out your local FE College for face-to-face courses, **e-learning** programmes or **distance learning** programmes and organisations like St John's Ambulance for a wide range of health and safety training courses.

Key terms

Distance learning allows you to learn in your own time while being supported by a tutor by telephone, email etc.
E-learning is learning that takes place electronically, over the internet.

Practice activity

2.6 Access additional support or information relating to health and safety

This activity gives you an opportunity to practice showing that you can access additional support or information relating to health and safety.

Choose an aspect of health and safety that interests you and using as many sources of information as you can find, put together a portfolio of fliers, posters, computer print outs, course leaflets, etc to show your developing skills in accessing information and support.

LO3 Understand procedures for responding to accidents and sudden illness

3.1 Different types of accidents and sudden illness that may occur in your work setting

Workplace accidents can happen at any time to anybody, but some types of accidents are more common than others, depending on the work sector.

Accidents leading to musculoskeletal disorders such as strains, sprains, slipped discs and fractures are the biggest cause of sickness absence in the health and social care sector. Indeed, according to the results of a Labour Force Survey (LFS), the **prevalence rate** in 2007/08 and 2008/09 of musculoskeletal disorders was higher in the health and social care sector than in any other sector. In addition, health and social care workers can be as much as four times more likely to experience accidents caused by violence and aggression than other workers. The main causes of violence are frustration, anxiety, resentment, and drink, drugs and mental instability.

Key term

Prevalence rate means frequency.

Needle-stick injuries are particular to health and social care workers. A needle-stick injury is a stab wound from a needle or other sharp object, a bite or a scratch, that can result in exposure to the blood or body fluids of a person carrying a blood-borne virus, for example hepatitis B (HBV), hepatitis C (HCV) and human immunodeficiency virus (HIV).

Sudden illness, such as a heart attack and stroke, is a medical emergency that requires professional help. If professional help is not immediately available, it needs emergency first aid straightaway to prevent the condition worsening, aid recovery and preserve life. The signs and symptoms of sudden illness include chest pain or pressure with sweating and shortness of breath, vomiting, loss of consciousness, severe bleeding, seizures or convulsions, sudden numbness or paralysis, loss of vision, a very bad headache, and a change in mental ability, such as confusion and memory loss.

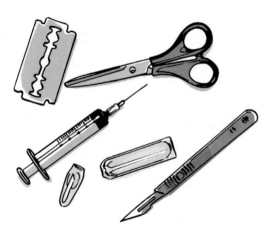

Figure 8.5 Causes of needle-stick injuries

Evidence activity

(3.1) Different types of accidents and sudden illness

Talk with you colleagues, manager or employer, and look through your workplace Accident Record Book and any care plans that are accessible to you, to find out what accidents and sudden illnesses are particular to where you work. Familiarise yourself with what can cause the accidents and with the signs and symptoms of each sudden illness. Use what you have learnt to make an awareness-raising presentation to your colleagues.

(3.2) Procedures to be followed if an accident or sudden illness should occur

The following is basic advice on first aid for use in an emergency and is not a substitute for effective training.

DR ABC

D: Check for Danger

Don't put yourself in danger, make the area safe, assess all casualties and get someone to call 999 for an ambulance. They should be prepared to describe what happened and where, the number of people affected and their condition.

R: Response

Gently shake the casualty's shoulders and ask loudly, 'Are you all right?' If there is a response, reassure them that help is on its way. If there is no response:

- Check that help is on its way.
- Open their airway.
- Check for normal breathing.
- Take appropriate action – cardiopulmonary resuscitation (CPR) if necessary.

A: Airway

To open the airway, place your hand on the casualty's forehead, gently tilt the head back and lift the chin with two fingertips. Remove any visible obstructions from the mouth and nose. Check that help is on its way.

B: Breathing

Look for chest movements that indicate breathing, listen at the casualty's mouth for breath sounds and feel for air on your cheek. If the casualty *is* breathing normally, place them in the recovery position to keep the airway open. If the casualty is not breathing normally, check that help is on its way and start and cardiopulmonary resuscitation (CPR).

C: Circulation

If breathing is not normal, circulation is not normal, so you need to start CPR. CPR is a series of chest compressions and rescue breaths that maintain circulation. Do not carry out CPR unless you have been trained and shown yourself to be competent. Check that help is on its way.

Severe bleeding

Apply direct pressure to the wound and raise and support the injured part (unless broken) to promote the flow of blood back to the heart. Firmly apply a dressing and, if bleeding seeps through, put an extra dressing on top. Get help.

Needle-stick injury

Encourage bleeding and wash with soap and running water. If blood or body fluids have splashed into the eyes or mouth, wash with large amounts of cold water. Get help.

Broken bones and spinal injuries

If you suspect a broken bone or spinal injury, get help. Do not move the casualty unless they are in immediate danger.

Sprains and strains

Rest the injured area to promote healing, and elevate if possible. Apply ice to reduce swelling, and use a compression bandage and sling, if appropriate, to give support. Get help.

Burns

Cool with cold water to relieve the pain, and continue cooling while taking the casualty to hospital. Hazardous chemicals can seriously irritate or damage the skin. Flood the affected area with cold water for at least 20 minutes and continue cooling on the way to hospital. Remove any contaminated clothing that is not stuck to the skin.

Dealing with violence

The risk of violence to someone working in health and social care depends on the kind of work they do, the setting in which they work and the type of people they work with. Workers who may be at risk should be trained in how to defuse violence before there is a need for first aid. In the event of exposure to violence, they should receive post-incident counselling and first aid as appropriate.

Record keeping

It is good practice to record all incidents involving injury or illness that you have attended. Include the following information in your entry:

- The date, time and place of the incident.

- The name of the injured or ill person.

- Details of the injury/illness and any first aid given.

- What happened to the casualty immediately afterwards (e.g. went back to work, went to hospital).

- Your name and signature.

This information can help identify accident trends and areas for improvement in the control of health and safety risks.

Basic advice on first aid at work, HSE 2006, www.hse.gov.uk; www.nhs.uk

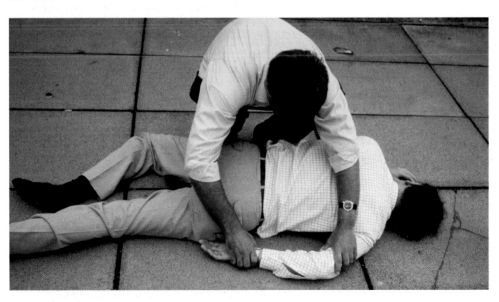

Figure 8.6 The recovery position

Time to reflect

 Dealing with accidents and emergencies

Think about two or three occasions in the past when you have witnessed or helped out at an accident or emergency. Are you confident that the situation was dealt with effectively? Or were you concerned with what you were asked to do or with the way the situation was handled? If you had an accident or became suddenly ill, how would you like to be dealt with?

Evidence activity

 Procedures to be followed

This activity enables you to demonstrate your understanding of the procedures to be followed if an accident or sudden illness should occur where you work.

Using your own words, produce a series of memory cards that describe first aid procedures for the accidents and sudden illnesses that most frequently occur in your workplace. Your memory cards should include explanations for why these procedures should be followed.

LO4 Be able to reduce the spread of infection

4.1 Your role in supporting others to follow practices that reduce the spread of infection

You have a responsibility to promote health and safety by supporting others to understand and follow practices that reduce the spread of infection. By demonstrating your understanding and application of best practice you will inspire others to take your lead.

Ten top tips for supporting others to follow practices that reduce the spread of infection

1. Always follow procedures. Remind others to do the same and report any concerns you have that procedures aren't being followed.

2. Never undertake any activity in which you haven't been trained, and don't ask your colleagues to carry out activities in which they haven't been trained.

3. Find opportunities to check that everyone is aware of infection control procedures, for example, request 10 minutes of meeting times to review knowledge and assess whether procedures need updating. Involve everyone in the review so they can take ownership of the way they work. People are more effective in their jobs if they are listened to and have some control over what they do.

4. Request training opportunities so that everyone can keep up to date with new infection control methods. Find out what's on offer, for example, there may be distance learning courses and classes at your local FE college. People are more likely to learn and develop if they can do it in a way that best suits them.

5. Demonstrate a high standard of personal hygiene and be kind and discrete when telling others if they fall short of the required standard.

6. Wash your hands as recommended, and remind others to do the same. Check that decent soap, alcohol rub, good-quality paper towels and hand cream are always available.

7. Don't let standards slip with regard to the use and disposal of PPE, soiled laundry, sharps and clinical waste. Set an example and be courteous but firm in reminding others of the correct procedures.

8. Make sure everyone understands the manufacturer's instructions for decontaminating equipment, and let them know that you are willing to help whenever necessary.

9. Make sure that everyone is immunised appropriately.

10. Make sure everyone understands the need to report and record unexpected illness.

Evidence activity

4.1 Supporting others to follow practices

This activity enables you to show your understanding of your role in supporting others to reduce the spread of infection.

Write a procedure entitled 'Support others to reduce the spread of infection' that explains to colleagues how they should work in order to promote best practice.

4.2 Demonstrate the recommended method for hand washing

Hand hygiene is the single most important method of preventing and controlling infection. Our hands normally have a resident population of **micro-organisms** that do us no harm, but transient micro-organisms picked up during everyday activities can cause infectious disease. Hand washing with soap and warm water should remove transient organisms before they are spread, for example, to another person or a piece of equipment.

Key term

Micro-organisms are organisms of microscopic or sub-microscopic size, for example bacteria and viruses.
Aseptic means free of disease-causing micro-organisms.
A care episode is one of a series of care tasks in the course of a continuous care activity.

Always wash your hands:

- when they are visibly soiled
- before and after handling food
- after using the toilet, smoking, touching your body or hair, or coughing or sneezing into your hands
- before an **aseptic** procedure, such as changing dressings and giving injections
- after a dirty procedure, such as disposing of body waste or soiled linen, even if you wore gloves

- between different patients and between **care episodes** for one patient.

Wash your hands effectively using soap and water:

- palm to palm
- right palm over the back of the left hand, left palm over the back of the right hand
- palm to palm fingers interlocked
- backs of fingers to opposing palms with fingers interlocked
- rotational rubbing of right thumb clasped in left palm and vice versa
- rotational rubbing backwards and forwards with clasped fingers of right hand in left palm and vice versa.

Don't forget to wash your wrists, dry your hands thoroughly with a disposable paper towel and apply hand cream to help keep your skin in good condition.

Washing with an alcohol rub is a useful alternative when your hands are not visibly dirty or when adequate hand washing facilities are not available. It also increases the removal of transient bacteria and should always be used prior to aseptic procedures. When using an alcohol rub, use enough to rub into all areas of the hands, paying attention to the thumbs, fingertips, between the fingers and the backs of the hands, until the hands feel dry.

www.hpa.org.uk, *Hand Hygiene for Health Care* and *Social Care Staff Stop! Have You Washed Your Hands?* HPA 2009

Practice activity

4.2 Demonstrate the recommended method for handwashing

This activity enables you to demonstrate that you wash your hands effectively. Practice washing your hands using the technique described above.

4.3 Demonstrate ways to ensure that your own health and hygiene do not pose a risk to an individual or to others at work

If you don't look after your health, you won't be able to do your job properly, which will jeopardise health and safety. If you have poor personal hygiene, you will carry and spread infectious micro-organisms. Good practice dictates that you:

■ have scrupulously clean hands at all times

■ are 'bare below the elbow'

■ keep your skin, teeth, hair, feet, fingernails and clothes clean and your hair tied out of the way

■ are smart, well presented and don't smell, for example of body odour, food or cigarettes

■ don't wear false nails, nail polish or jewellery

■ cover skin breaks with a waterproof dressing; get medical advice if your skin is damaged by conditions such as eczema or psoriasis

■ wear suitable shoes that are comfortable and provide good support

■ eat a nutritious diet and get enough non-work related exercise

■ watch your alcohol intake, don't use drugs and if you smoke, try to give up

■ get enough sleep and relaxation and know how to manage your stress

■ make sure you are appropriately immunised.

Practice activity

 Your own health and hygiene

This activity gives you an opportunity to show that your health and hygiene don't pose a risk to the health and safety of others.

Keep a diary for a couple of weeks to show what you eat and drink, how much sleep and relaxation you have, and how much exercise you take outside of work. Record any poor health behaviours, such as smoking, and vaccinations you have had and when any boosters are due. Note down your personal hygiene routine and how you present yourself for work.

Are you confident that your health and hygiene do not pose a risk to others? Can you make any improvements?

LO5 Be able to move and handle equipment and other objects safely

 The main points of legislation that relate to moving and handling activities

The Manual Handling Operations Regulations (MHOR) 1992 (amended 2002, revised 2007), apply to a wide range of moving and handling activities, including lifting, lowering, pushing, pulling or carrying. The load may be inanimate, for example a box or a trolley, or animate, such as a person.

MHOR require your employer or manager to minimise any risk of injury from moving and handling, so far as is reasonably practicable, and to train you in safe moving and handling techniques. As an employee you have a duty to:

■ follow safe moving and handling procedures

■ only carry out moving and handling activities in which you have been trained

■ use moving and handling equipment properly and appropriately

■ inform your employer or manager if you identify hazardous moving and handling activities

■ ensure that your activities do not put others at risk.

Getting to grips with manual handling, HSE 2004

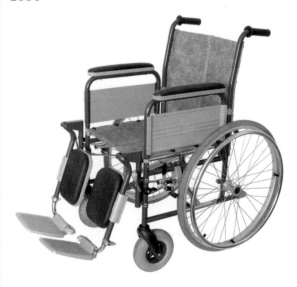

Figure 8.7 Moving and handling equipment

The Provision and Use of Work Equipment Regulations 1998 (PUWER) are in place to prevent or control risks to health and safety from equipment used at work. Your employer or manager is required to ensure that work equipment is suitable for the intended use, is maintained in a safe condition, has protective devices, such as guards, markings and warnings, and that you are trained to use it.

Simple guide to the Provision and Use of Work Equipment Regulations 1998, HSE 1999

The Lifting Operations and Lifting Equipment Regulations (LOLER) aim to reduce risks to health and safety from lifting equipment such as slings and hoists. Your employer or manager is required to ensure that lifting equipment is suitable for the intended use, maintained in a safe condition, positioned and installed to minimise any risks (e.g. from the load falling), used safely, and that you are trained to use it.

Simple guide to the Lifting Operations and Lifting Equipment Regulations 1998, HSE 1999

Research & investigate

5.1 Complying with safe moving and handling legislation

Carry out a health and safety survey on the moving and handling equipment you use at work, for example check for evidence of safety inspections, that protective devices are in place, and that it is well maintained and appropriately positioned. While doing your inspection, check whether colleagues have been trained in its use, are confident that they know how to use it safely, and know what to do should they have any concerns about its safety.

Evidence activity

5.1 Legislation that relates to moving and handling

Select three moving and handling activities that you carry out on a day-to-day basis. For each one, identify the legislation that governs the activity, and your and your employer's or manager's legal responsibilities with regard to ensuring that the activity is safe. Explain why it is important that you comply with legislation and meet your responsibilities.

As an employee, you don't have responsibilities under PUWER and LOLER but you do have a duty under HASWA and the MHSWR to take reasonable care of yourself and of others who may be affected by your work activities.

5.2 Basic principles for safe moving and handling

1. Always follow procedures and never carry out an activity in which you haven't been trained.
2. Wear appropriate clothing and footwear.
3. If the load is a person, explain what you are going to do, reassure them throughout the move and remind them to assist in the move as much as they can. Be prepared for unexpected movements and have a plan for how you would cope.
4. Use the recommended equipment. Before you start, make sure that all equipment is

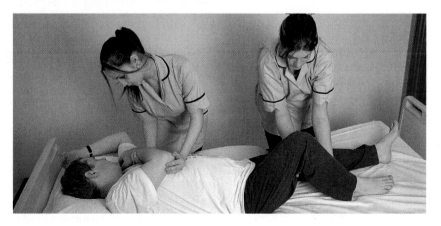

Figure 8.8 Safe moving and handling

safe to use and, if you are using equipment with wheels (e.g. a hoist or a wheelchair), that the brakes are on. But be prepared – accidents can happen, so have a plan for how you would cope.

5. Make sure there is enough room to carry out the activity safely.

6. Maintain a natural 'S'-shaped spinal posture and create a stable base with your legs slightly apart, one foot in front of the other, your knees slightly bent. Avoid stooping, squatting and twisting.

7. Ensure help is at hand. If you are working with colleagues, identify a team leader to give clear instructions, such as 'One, two, three, move!'

8. Use your large thigh and buttock muscles to power the activity, keep the load as close to you as possible, and make sure you have a good handgrip. In the case of a person, check that the movement and your grip do not cause any discomfort.

9. Take your time and if, for any reason, you are not happy with the activity, get advice and report your concerns.

10. Know your own personal limitations and do not exceed them.

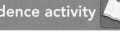 Evidence activity

 5.2 **Explain the principles for safe moving and handling**

Think about a couple of moving and handling activities that you carry out regularly and break them down into stages. Write down exactly how and why you carry out each stage of the activity in order to maintain the health and safety of everyone concerned.

5.3 Move and handle equipment and other objects safely

More than a third of injuries reported each year are caused by handling loads or by pushing and pulling using bodily force. The following sections describe basic safe procedures – they are not a substitute for training. Also, your workplace will have its own procedures to follow for different moving and handling activities. It is your responsibility to follow these procedures to the letter.

Safe lifting, holding, carrying, and lowering

■ Plan the activity. Are you dressed appropriately? Will you need help? Have you got enough room to move? Where will you set the load down? If it will be a long manoeuvre, where can you rest the load, for example to change grip?

■ Should you be using equipment? If so, what equipment should you use? Are you confident that you know how to use it properly and that you are physically able to use it? Is there evidence to show that it is in good repair and safe to use?

■ If it isn't appropriate to use equipment, adopt a good posture and stable position (see 5.2) and be prepared to move your feet to maintain stability.

■ Bend at your hips and knees and slightly at your waist. Avoid stooping or squatting and don't twist or lean sideways when picking up the load.

■ Get a good hold. Hugging a load close to the body is safer than gripping it tightly with your hands.

■ Maintain the natural shape of your back and use your thigh and buttock muscles to power you into an upright position. Never lift above shoulder height.

■ Turn by moving your feet. Keep your shoulders level and facing in the same direction as your hips, and keep your head up. Look ahead, not down at the load.

■ Carry the load slowly and smoothly.

■ Lower the load by bending at the hips and knees and slightly at the waist. Slide it into the desired position.

■ Don't handle more than you can easily manage. If in doubt, seek advice or get help. And don't forget, if the load is a person, remind them to assist in the move as much as they are able.

Safe pushing and pulling

■ Push rather than pull when moving a load.

■ Keep your feet well away from the load and walk, don't run.

■ The handles of wheeled equipment, such as trolleys and wheelchairs, should be comfortable to hold and at a height between your shoulder and waist. Wheels should run smoothly and brakes should be reliable!

■ Get help if you find it difficult to negotiate a slope or ramp, and to move a load over soft or uneven surfaces.

Case Study

5.3 The importance of training in safe moving and handling

Following an investigation in early 2010, the Scottish Commission for the Regulation of Care has stated that manual handling training needs to be delivered to care home workers on a systematic basis and that refresher training should always be available. The investigation was conducted after the Care Commission received a complaint that one care provider was not supplying proper training to its staff, particularly at the induction stage. The complainant was especially concerned about the staff's lack of proper knowledge about safe moving and handling procedures. The investigation found that although there was a clear moving and handling policy in place, nineteen members of staff had not received any moving and handling training despite the fact that they were involved in carrying out moving and handling tasks.

1. Why might staff not have been trained?

2. How might their lack of training in moving and handling affect them and the people they work with?

3. How should this situation impact on the employer?

LO6 Be able to handle hazardous substances and materials

6.1 Describe types of hazardous substances that may be found in the work setting

A hazardous substance or material is one that poses a risk to health. Hazardous substances or materials in health and social care settings include the following:

■ Chemicals, for example in cleaning materials, paint, ink, glue and cosmetics. Inhalation of chemicals can cause conditions

such as asthma; contact with chemicals can burn and trigger skin conditions such as dermatitis; and **ingestion** of chemicals can cause damage to the internal organs. Some chemicals are **carcinogenic**. The labelling of a product shows its potential for harm.

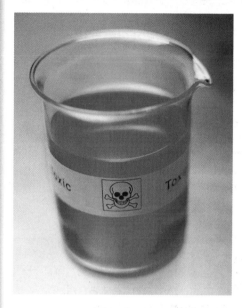

Figure 8.9 Read the label!

Key terms

Carcinogenic means capable of causing cancer.
Ingestion is taking something into the body through eating or drinking.
Maladministration means incompetent management.
Pathogenic means able to cause disease.

■ Medication. You read earlier, in section 1.4, about the potential for **maladministration** of medicines and how it can have tragic results.

■ Food contaminants, for example, **pathogenic** micro-organisms, pest droppings and substances accidentally introduced into food, such as chemicals and metals can all cause food poisoning.

■ Body fluids and waste, such as mucous, blood, vomit, urine and faeces; clinical waste, such as used dressings; and soiled linen, such as clothing and bed linen all have the potential to carry pathogenic organisms and spread disease.

■ Contaminated sharps, for example, needles, scalpels, stitch cutters, razor blades and glass ampoules all have the potential, through cuts and puncture injuries, to spread infection.

■ Dust and dirt within the environment may contain pathogenic micro-organisms and can, if inhaled, trigger conditions such as asthma.

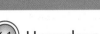

Evidence activity

6.1 Hazardous substances

This activity gives you an opportunity to show that you know which of the substances you use at work are hazardous.

Produce a poster for display in the staff room that identifies all the hazardous substances that you are exposed to at work. Briefly describe how each affects health and safety.

6.2 Safe practices for storing, using and disposing of hazardous substances and materials

COSHH Regulations require that your employer or manager has procedures in place for the correct and safe storage, use and disposal of hazardous substances and materials. Manufacturers' instructions also describe safe storage, use and disposal. It is your responsibility to follow these procedures to the letter, as well as procedures for use of PPE, cleaning up spills and dealing with accidents. In addition, only work with hazardous substances if you have had the relevant training.

Note that what follows does not provide a substitute for effective training in safe storage and disposal of hazardous substances and materials!

Storing hazardous substances

■ Keep hazardous substances in a locked cupboard, to which only named people have access.

■ Keep the storage area clean and well organised, and store containers with their labels facing forward and lids securely in place to prevent leaks and spills.

■ Keep hazardous substances in their original containers. Never transfer anything into an unlabelled storage container and never re-use an empty container for something else.

■ Report any dangerous storage situations to your manager.

Using hazardous substances

Follow procedures and report any concerns you have to your employer or manager.

Disposal of hazardous substances and materials

■ Return unused medication to the pharmacy.

■ Dispose of body waste and fluids down the sluice.

■ Dispose of used sharps in approved lidded containers, for example sharps bins, and send containers for incineration when three quarters full. Never resheath used needles.

■ Report any dangerous storage situations to your manager.

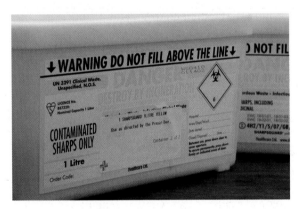

Figure 8.10 Safe disposal of sharps

■ Bag waste as follows:

■ yellow bag – clinical or infected waste, to be incinerated

■ clear alginate bag inside a red plastic bag – soiled and infected linen, to be laundered

■ black bag – domestic waste that is not infected or contaminated

■ pink and blue bag – food waste.

■ Report any dangerous waste disposal situations to your manager.

www.infectioncontrolservices.co.uk

Practice activity

(6.2) **Safe practices for hazardous substances and materials**

This activity gives you an opportunity to show that you know how to safely store, use and dispose of hazardous substances and materials.

Ask a colleague, your manager or employer to supervise your use and disposal of hazardous substances and materials, and your management of the storage area. Act on their feedback until everyone concerned is confident in your competence.

LO7 Be able to promote fire safety in the work setting

(7.1) **Describe practices that prevent fires from starting and spreading**

There is no better way of dealing with a fire than preventing it from starting in the first place.

Forty per cent of deaths caused by fires in the home are caused by smoking. If smoking is allowed in the setting where you work, make sure that cigarettes are never left unattended and are put out properly, that no one smokes in bed, that proper ashtrays are used and frequently emptied, and that matches and lighters are kept out of the reach of children and people whose use of them could put others at risk.

How to help prevent fires in the kitchen

■ Keep anything flammable away from a source of heat.

■ keep electrical leads and appliances away from water and don't overload sockets.

■ Use appropriate containers for cooking.

■ Never fill a deep fat fryer more than a third full, dry food before putting in the fryer and don't allow fat or oil to get so hot that it smokes.

Fires can be caused by faulty wiring in plugs and electrical appliances and by electrical equipment not being used safely.

■ Get wiring checked if plugs and sockets become hot or have brown scorch marks, fuses blow for no reason, lights flicker or wires become loose. Replace damaged cables and don't run them under carpets or rugs – you won't be able to see them if they become damaged.

■ Unplug electrical appliances when not being used; use the correct fuse for the appliance; avoid using multi-way adapters and overloading electric sockets; and have appliances serviced regularly.

■ Use electric blankets according to the manufacturer's instructions; have them serviced every three years, replaced at least every 10 years and replaced if they are damaged in any way or don't carry the British Standard Kitemark (BSK) and the British Electrotechnical Approvals Board (BEAB) symbols.

At bedtime, unplug electrical equipment; put a guard in front of an open fire; extinguish candles, cigarettes etc.; check that fire escape routes are clear of obstacles, fire doors are closed and keys are where they are meant to be; and only leave electric blankets on if safe to do so.

www.london-fire.gov.uk

If you discover a fire in its very early stages you may be able to prevent it spreading. However, fire spreads very quickly and even a small, contained fire can produce smoke and fumes that can kill in seconds. If you are in any doubt, do not tackle a fire, no matter how small.

Provided that the fire is in its very early stages, the room is not filling with smoke, you are confident about your safety and have been appropriately trained, use the appropriate fire extinguisher. There are four main types of fire extinguisher, each having a different coloured label.

1. Water extinguishers (red) are used on combustible material such as wood, paper and textiles. Don't use them when electricity is present or on burning fat, oil or liquids.

2. Carbon dioxide (CO_2) extinguishers (red with a black panel) are used on fires involving electrical equipment and flammable liquids. Don't use them in confined spaces, such as walk-in cupboards, as the CO_2 will replace all the oxygen available, making it impossible to breathe.

3. Spray foam extinguishers (red with a cream panel) are used on fires involving fat, oil, flammable liquids and wood, paper and textile. Don't use spray foam extinguishers when electricity is present.

4. Dry powder extinguishers (red with a blue panel) are used on fires involving electricity, flammable liquids and gases.

www.firesafe.org.uk

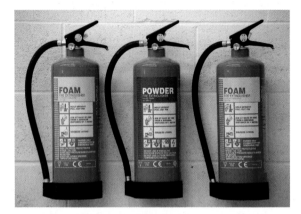

Figure 8.11 Fire extinguishers

Note: older extinguishers were painted red, black, cream or blue. They are still legal and do not need changing unless defective.

Always follow the manufacturer's instructions when using a fire extinguisher, but as a rule of thumb:

P – pull the safety pin from the handle.
A – aim the fire extinguisher nozzle at the base of the fire.
S – squeeze the trigger handle.
S – sweep the spray from side to side.

If the fire is small, such as in a frying pan or waste bin, or if clothing is on fire, you can prevent it spreading by using a fire blanket. Pull the blanket from its case and, provided it is larger that the fire, hold it up in front of you by the top corners, with your hands tucked behind. Place it over the fire and leave it in place for half an hour, to allow the material to cool down.

Case Study

 Fire

In June 2010 the *Isle of Wight County Press* reported that a small fire in the laundry room of a care home was out when firefighters arrived there, according to Isle of Wight Fire and Rescue.

1. How might such a fire have started?

2. What were the risks of it spreading and how might it have spread?

3. How would it have been extinguished?

A smoke alarm alerts people to the danger of fire, giving them time to escape. Ideally there should be one in every room. There are two types of smoke alarm:

1. Ionisation alarms, which detect fires that burn fiercely, such as deep fat fryers, before smoke gets too thick.

2. Optical alarms, which are more effective at detecting slow-burning fires, such as smouldering foam-filled furniture or overheated wiring.

Smoke alarms should be tested once a week, by pressing the test button until the alarm sounds; and the battery should be changed once a year (unless it is a ten-year alarm). Smoke alarms should be replaced every ten years.

Evidence activity

 Preventing fires from starting and spreading

Carry out a survey of your workplace to identify:

■ potential fire risks – make a note of how you would minimise or get rid of these risks to prevent fires from starting

■ measures for preventing the spread of fire – make a note of how each is used.

7.2 **Demonstrate measures that prevent fires from starting**

Practice activity

7.2 **Measures that prevent fires from starting**

This activity gives you an opportunity to show that you know how to prevent fires from starting.

Talk to your manager or employer about the potential fire risks you identified for Evidence activity 7.1, and if you are given permission, either minimise or get rid of them.

7.3 Emergency procedures to be followed in the event of a fire in your work setting

1. DO NOT PANIC! Stay calm.

2. Immediately sound the fire alarm. If there is no alarm in the vicinity, shout 'FIRE!' as loudly as you can.

3. Only attempt to control a fire if it is small and contained, you can do so safely and you have been trained.

4. Dial 999 for the fire brigade. Be prepared to give your name, address, the nature and exact location of the fire, how fast it seems to be spreading, the needs of people in the building and whether any are trapped or unable to escape.

5. Take able-bodied people out of the building or to the fire-safe stairwell via the fire exit doors. Patients in bed should stay in their rooms with the door shut and await rescue by the fire brigade.

6. Close all doors behind you and proceed in a quiet and orderly manner. Walk, don't run. Don't stop to take any personal belongings with you.

7. Do not use the lifts.

8. If you encounter smoke or any blockage along an exit route, choose an alternative path.

9. When you leave the building, move well away from the doors to allow others behind you to emerge from the exits. Do not obstruct entrances or traffic routes.

10. Do not re-enter the building for any reason until the fire brigade gives the OK.

Evidence activity

7.3 Emergency procedures in the event of a fire

Check out the fire procedure at work and, using your own words, rewrite it giving reasons why it needs to be followed.

7.4 Ensure that clear evacuation routes are maintained at all times

Health and social care settings should have clearly designated fire escape routes, with signed fire exits and fireproof doors that shut automatically in the event of a fire. Fire escape routes should be well lit, fitted with fire alarms, smoke detectors and fire fighting equipment, as well as adaptations such as handrails, and be wide enough to accommodate large groups of people and mobility aids, such as wheelchairs and walking fames. They also need to be free of obstructions at all times.

Practice activity

7.4 Ensure that clear evacuation routes are maintained at all times.

This activity gives you an opportunity to show that you know how to keep evacuation routes clear.

Keep a running log of the changes you make to maintain clear evacuation routes. Regularly update your manager or employer about the changes, to reassure them that you understand the need for clear routes and are fulfilling your responsibility to co-operate with them in relation to health and safety issues.

LO8 Be able to implement security measures in the work setting

8.1 Demonstrate the use of agreed procedures for checking the identity of anyone requesting access to premises and information

Not all callers to work settings are genuine. You need to be on your guard for bogus callers claiming, for example, to be council employees, health workers, meter readers, repairmen, salesmen, even friends and relatives of the people you work with. Bogus callers have ill-intent – the press is awash with examples of tragedies associated with intruders – and the people you work with have a right to feel safe and secure. So it is very important to check the ID of visitors and their right to enter before allowing them access to your workplace.

Different organisations have different procedures for checking a caller's ID and their right to enter. However, as a general rule:

■ Think before you open the door. Do you recognise the caller? Are they expected?

■ If there is a chain lock on the door, make sure it is on at all times. If there isn't a chain lock, or there isn't a facility to see who is there or to speak with them, ask your manager for security measures to be fitted, such as a peephole and an intercom.

■ Politely ask for proof of identity, such as an ID card. Check for a photograph, their name and their organisation's telephone number before you unlock and open the door. And check their clothing – some official callers wear a uniform with their organisation's name or logo on.

■ If they don't have an appointment, ask them to wait outside while you ring their organisation to confirm their identity. Be polite.

■ If you have any suspicions at all, do not let them in. Talk to your employer or manager, who may feel it necessary to call the police.

If, after checking their ID, you feel that their visit is legitimate, ask them to complete the visitor's book on arrival (name, who they are visiting, reason for visit, time of arrival, car number plate) and exit (time of leaving) and ensure that they wear a visitor's badge. This will indicate to others that they have a right to be in the building. Anyone who is not known and who is not wearing a visitor's badge should arouse suspicion.

Personal information may only be disclosed to someone else if the individual concerned gives consent, if there is a life and death situation, or if people need it in order to work with the individual. Therefore, if you are asked to disclose information about someone you work with, you must be satisfied that the person asking for the information has a right to know.

Different organisations have different procedures for checking a person's right to know. However, as a general rule, ask for proof of ID and documentation that demonstrates their right to know. If they have no such proof or the enquiry is over the telephone, ask questions which you believe only they could answer, for example the date of birth and family names of the person concerned. If you remain unconvinced, explain politely that you cannot disclose any information because, under the terms of the 1998 Data Protection Act, you are unsure of their identity. Suggest that they write or return with suitable ID. If you are satisfied with their ID but unsure about making a disclosure, take their telephone number and speak with your manager.

A great deal of personal information is recorded electronically on computers and on paper, for example health records and care plans. Except in the situations above, no one has the right to know what is recorded about someone else; even family members are not entitled to see information about someone you work with without their consent. Information on computers should be protected by means of a secure password, and information on paper should be protected under lock and key with a designated key holder.

 Time to reflect

8.1 Bogus callers

Think about the occasions when you have admitted someone into your home or workplace without knowing for sure who they are or that they have a right of entry. What might have been the outcome? What do you think you should have done to check their ID?

The Data Protection Act 1998 is in place to protect our right to privacy, particularly of personal information such as our ethnicity, political and religious beliefs, health, sexuality and criminal record. Your responsibility is to ensure that information about the people you work with remains confidential and secure.

 Practice activity

8.1 Demonstrate use of agreed procedures for checking the ID of anyone requesting access to premises and information.

This activity gives you an opportunity to show that you know how to use procedures for checking the ID of anyone requesting access to your workplace and information about the people you work with.

Give a short talk to your team about the procedures that your organization has in place for checking visitors' and callers' ID. Illustrate your talk with examples of occasions when you have used the procedures and why it was necessary to do so.

8.2 Demonstrate use of measures to protect your own security and the security of others in your work setting

Health and social care work settings and people's own homes are accessed by the public and are therefore potentially insecure, both for workers and for the people using the services. Your workplace will have measures in place for ensuring that nobody's security is compromised, and it is your responsibility to use these measures effectively.

You have already looked at ways of checking the ID of people requesting access to premises and information. Other measures intended to protect security include CRB checks, which identify people who may be unsuitable to work with children or vulnerable adults; and **CCTV** images, which help identify intruders, thieves, aggressive and dangerous encounters, abandoned packages that might contain explosives, and so on.

Key term

CCTV stands for closed ciruit television.

Your workplace will have procedures in place telling you how to:

■ deal with potential breaches in security, report and record breaches and support others in the aftermath of a breach

■ deal with theft, bomb scares and missing persons

■ use panic buttons, personal alarms, pagers and mobile phones in the event that you are alone, for example working in the community or in someone's home

■ manage challenging behaviour – if there is a risk of challenging behaviour in your workplace, ask for training in how to handle it.

8.3 The importance of ensuring that others know your whereabouts

Many health and social care workers work by themselves, for example outside of normal working hours. Some visit people in their own homes, collect and deliver prescriptions, and some use their car as a base.

Lone working is fraught with risks, including the worker suddenly becoming ill; the office not being available to answer queries; violent people in quiet areas and during darkness; violence from people using the service, their friends, relatives or pets; having to park in unlit, isolated areas; car accidents, break-ins and breakdowns; and accidents due to moving and handling and using equipment belonging to the people who use the service.

Case Study

8.3 Suzy Lamplugh

In 1986, British estate agent Suzy Lamplugh vanished without trace. A major problem with the investigation of her disappearance was that no one realised she was missing until hours after the incident happened. All her diary said was that she had an appointment to show a man around a house.

1. What do you think Suzy should have done before she went to her appointment?

2. How might Suzy have protected her security while she was out of the office?

Health and safety legislation requires employers and managers to be able to trace lone workers and to have policies and procedures in place to ensure they are safe:

Practice activity

8.2 Using measures to protect yourself and others

Make a list of all the measures that your workplace has in place to protect everyone's security. Annotate each with the occasions when you use them. If there are some that you never use, ask yourself why. Is it because of carelessness? Be aware that carelessness can lead to accusations of negligence and abuse.

■ Lone worker policy and procedures outline how your safety will be managed.

■ Mobile phone policy and procedures tell you how and when to use your mobile phone.

■ Communication policy and procedures tell you about checking in and out of each visit and letting the office know when you have reached home safely.

■ Staff welfare policy and procedures make sure that you are equipped with a personal safety alarm.

■ Staff learning and development policy and procedures require you to attend personal safety and awareness training.

Your main responsibility when working alone is to be aware of your surroundings and the possible threats to your personal safety. A disciplinary policy will set out procedures for disciplining you if you fail to follow measures set up to protect you.

We care because you care, Lone Worker Safety Guide, Skills for Care 2010.

 Evidence activity

8.3 The importance of others knowing your whereabouts

Make a list of all the procedures you have to follow at work and the systems you use in your private life to let people know where you are. Why is it necessary to follow these procedures and systems? What might happen if you didn't follow them?

LO9 Know how to manage stress

 Describe common signs and indicators of stress

We all experience pressure from time to time, and some of us work best under pressure – it motivates us to get on with the job! However, if the pressure builds up to the point that we can no longer cope, we become stressed. Some people thrive on stress – for them it is a positive, energising emotion. But for most, it has negative consequences. According to the HSE, around 14 million working days and £4 billion are lost to work-related stress each year.

The common signs and symptoms of stress include:

■ emotional ill health, such as feeling unable to cope, tearfulness, anxiety and depression, negativity, irritability, anger, poor concentration, difficulty in making decisions, and thoughts of suicide

■ physical ill health, such as not being able to relax, headache, insomnia, high blood pressure, palpitations, heart attack, indigestion, asthma, skin disorders, loss of libido and weight gain or loss

■ social problems, such as social conflict, unacceptable behaviour and social isolation.

 Describe signs that indicate your own stress

 Evidence activity

9.1 & 9.2 Common signs of stress

You read above that the signs of stress fall into three main categories – emotional, physical and social. Think about two or three people you know who you think become stressed from time to time. What makes you think they are stressed? Answer in terms of their emotional and physical status and their interactions with others.

Now do the same for yourself. What sort of things indicate that you are stressed?

 Analyse factors that tend to trigger own stress

To be able to manage our stress, we need to identify the factors or stressors that trigger it.

■ Emotional stressors include fear and anxiety; having to meet deadlines and make decisions; job roles and responsibilities; personality traits such as wanting to create a good impression; and feeling a sense of helplessness or lack of control.

■ Physical stressors are things that put pressure on your body, such as pain, ill-health, disability; insufficient sleep and rest; a poor diet; too much or too little exercise; and being on your feet all day. They can be chemical, such as alcohol, caffeine and nicotine; and environmental, such as noise, pollution, a lack of space and an uncomfortable temperature.

■ Social stressors include mixing with others; relationships; financial problems; coping with children and caring for elderly or infirm relatives; the **empty-nest syndrome**; and important life events such as leaving home, moving house, a new job, getting married, having a baby and bereavement.

Key term

Empty-nest syndrome is the array of feelings experienced by some parents after their children have grown and left home.

Evidence activity

 Analyse factors that trigger stress in you

Think about the things that stress you, for example certain work activities, being in a cramped space or having to make small talk with someone you don't know at a party. Now think about why they stress you. For example, why does one work activity stress you more than another? Is it because you don't like the people you are working with, because the activity is boring or you feel it could be done in a better way?

9.4 Compare strategies for managing stress

Having identified what in particular stresses you, you can start to manage your stress. According to Professor Cary Cooper, an occupational health expert at the University of Lancaster, the keys to good stress management are building emotional strength, taking control of your situation, having a good social network and adopting a positive outlook.

Professor Cooper's top ten stress-busting techniques

1. Be active. Exercise will help you get rid of pent-up energy, calm your emotions and help you think more clearly.

2. Take control. Taking control is empowering and will help you find a solution that satisfies you, not someone else.

3. Connect with people. Talking things through with a friend will help you solve your problems. In addition, a good social support network will help you see things in a different way.

4. Have some 'me time'. Earmarking a couple of days a week for some quality 'me time' will help you achieve a healthy, stress-free work–life balance.

5. Challenge yourself. Setting yourself goals, such as learning something new, builds confidence and helps you take charge of your life.

6. Don't rely on alcohol, smoking and caffeine as your ways of coping. They might provide temporary relief but in the long term they don't solve problems, they just create new ones.

7. Do some voluntary work. Helping people in situations worse than yours will help you put your problems into perspective. And do someone a favour every day. Favours cost nothing and you'll feel better.

8. Work smarter, not harder. Good time management and concentrating on tasks that will make a real difference will help you feel more fulfilled.

9. Be positive. Try to be 'glass half full' instead of 'glass half empty'.

10. Accept the things you cannot change. Changing a difficult situation is not always possible. If you can't make any changes, accept things as they are and concentrate on everything that you do have control over.

www.nhs.uk; www.stress.org.uk

Evidence activity

 Compare strategies for managing stress

Look at Professor Cooper's top ten stress-busting techniques. Are there any techniques there that you think might work for you? For example, if having to hold meetings in a small, stuffy room stresses you, can you find another room, one that is more comfortable? In other words, can you take control of the situation and remove the stress?

Assessment summary

Your reading of this chapter and completion of the activities will have prepared you to be able to engage in personal development in health, social care or children's and young people's settings.

To achieve the unit, your assessor will require you to:

Learning outcomes	Assessment Criteria
Learning outcome **1**: Show you understand your responsibilities, and the responsibilities of others, relating to health and safety by:	**1.1** identifying legislation relating to health and safety in a health or social care work setting See Evidence activity 1.1, p. 135
	1.2 explaining the main points of health and safety policies and procedures See Evidence activity 1.2, p. 135
	1.3 analysing the main health and safety responsibilities of yourself, your employer or manager and others in the work setting See Evidence activity 1.3 p. 137
	1.4 identifying specific tasks in the work setting that should not be carried out without special training See Evidence activity 1.4 p. 139
Learning outcome **2**: Be able to carry out your own responsibilities for health and safety by:	**2.1** using policies and procedures or other agreed ways of working that relate to health and safety. See Practice activity 2.1, p. 140
	2.2 supporting others to understand and follow safe practices See Practice activity 2.2, p. 140
	2.3 monitoring and reporting potential health and safety risks See Practice activity 2.3, p. 141

Learning outcomes	Assessment Criteria
Learning outcome **2**: Be able to carry out your own responsibilities for health and safety by:	(2.4) using risk assessment in relation to health and safety See Practice activity 2.4, p. 141
	(2.5) demonstrating ways to minimise potential risks and hazards See Practice activity 2.5, p. 144
	(2.6) accessing additional support or information relating to health and safety See Practice activity 2.6, p. 145
Learning outcome **3**: Understand procedures for responding to accidents and sudden illness by:	(3.1) describing different types of accidents and sudden illness that may occur in your work setting See Evidence activity 3.1, p. 146
	(3.2) explaining procedures to be followed if an accident or sudden illness should occur See Evidence activity 3.2, p. 148
Learning outcome **4**: Be able to reduce the spread of infection by:	(4.1) explaining your role in supporting others to follow practices that reduce the spread of infection See Evidence activity 4.1, p. 149
	(4.2) demonstrating the recommended method for hand washing See Practice activity 4.2, p. 149
	(4.3) demonstrating ways to ensure that your own health and hygiene do not pose a risk to an individual or to others at work See Practice activity 4.3, p. 150

Learning outcomes	Assessment Criteria
Learning outcome 5: Be able to move and handle equipment and other objects safely by:	5.1 explaining the main points of legislation that relate to moving and handling See Evidence activity 5.1, p. 151
	5.2 explaining the principles for safe moving and handling See Evidence activity 5.2, p. 152
	5.3 moving and handling equipment and other objects safely See Case study 5.3, p. 153
Learning outcome 6: Be able to handle hazardous substances and materials by:	6.1 describing types of hazardous substances that may be found in the work setting See Evidence activity 6.1, p. 154
	6.2 demonstrating safe practices for storing, using and disposing of hazardous substances and materials See Practice activity 6.2, p. 155
Learning outcome 7: Be able to promote fire safety in the work setting by:	7.1 describing practices that prevent fires from starting and spreading See Evidence activity 7.1, p. 156
	7.2 demonstrating measures that prevent fires from starting See Practice activity 7.2, p. 156
	7.3 explaining emergency procedures to be followed in the event of a fire in your work setting See Evidence activity 7.3 p. 157
	7.4 ensuring that clear evacuation routes are maintained at all times See Practice activity 7.4 p. 157.

Learning outcomes	Assessment Criteria
Learning outcome **8**: Be able to implement security measures in the work setting by:	**8.1** demonstrating the use of agreed procedures for checking the identity of anyone requesting access to premises and information See Practice activity 8.1, p. 158
	8.2 demonstrating the use of measures to protect your own security and the security of others in your work setting See Practice activity 8.2, p. 159
	8.3 explaining the importance of ensuring that others know your whereabouts See Evidence activity 8.3, p. 160
Learning outcome **9**: Know how to manage stress by:	**9.1** describing common signs and indicators of stress See Evidence activity 9.1 & 9.2, p. 160
	9.2 describing signs that indicate your own stress See Evidence activity 9.1 & 9.2, p. 160
	9.3 analysing factors that tend to trigger your own stress See Evidence activity 9.3 p. 161
	9.4 comparing strategies for managing stress See Evidence activity 9.4 p. 161

Good luck!

Web links

Health and Safety Executive	www.hse.gov.uk
BBC	www.bbc.co.uk
NHS	www.nhs.uk
Health Protection Agency	www.hpa.org.uk
Infection Control services	www.infectioncontrolservices.co.uk
London Fire Brigade	www.london-fire.gov.uk
Fire Safety Advice Centre	www.firesafe.org.uk
Stress Management Society	www.stress.org.uk

Promote good practice in handling information in health and social care settings

For Unit HSC 038

What are you finding out?

It seems impossible to open a newspaper or turn on the television without reading about some incident involving bad practice in handling information. For example, since 2007:

■ HM Revenue & Customs has lost two CDs containing the personal records and bank details of 25 million people.

■ The MoD has lost a laptop containing the passport details, National Insurance numbers, drivers' licence details, family details, doctors' addresses and National Health Service numbers of 600,000 people.

■ Hundreds of documents containing sensitive personal data such as details of benefit claims, passport photocopies and mortgage payments were found dumped on a roundabout in Devon.

■ Zurich Insurance has lost the personal details of 46,000 of its customers.

■ The health and social care sector is far from immune to bad practice. For example:

■ A USB memory stick containing information on hundreds of NHS mental health patients was found by a member of the public in Teesdale.

■ A 12-year-old boy found a USB memory stick containing sensitive information about staff and patients at a hospital in Scotland in a supermarket.

■ The personal details of 9,000 school pupils, including their names, date of birth, addresses, phone numbers and school attainment, were stolen from the home of a Barnet Council worker.

Breaches of security and confidentiality are extremely serious. Not only do they destroy confidence in organisations in which the public has entrusted its personal details, they also cause anxiety for the individuals concerned.

The reading and activities in this chapter will help you to:

Understand requirements for handling information in health and social care settings

Be able to implement good practice in handling information

Be able to support others to handle information.

LO1 Understand requirements for handling information in health and social care settings

1.1 Identify legislation and codes of practice that relate to handling information in health and social care

This UK government is committed to protecting civil liberties and personal privacy.

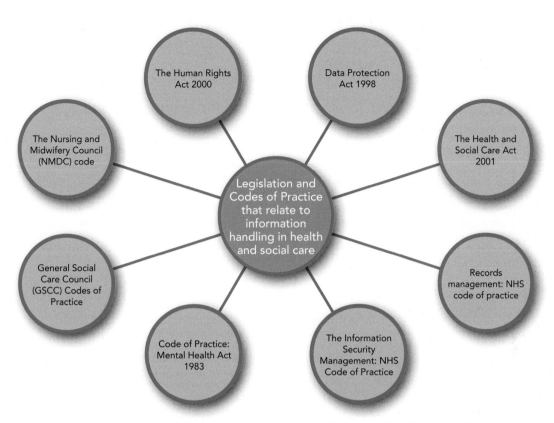

Figure 9.1 Legislation and Codes of Practice that relate to information handling in health and social care

Evidence activity

1.1 Legislation and codes of practice related to information handling

This activity gives you an opportunity to demonstrate your knowledge of legislation and codes of practice that relate to information handling in health and social care.

Choose three different care settings, for example an early years setting, a GP practice and a day care centre for people with learning difficulties. Make a list of the laws and codes of practice that govern how information must be handled within each area.

1.2 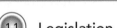 Summarise the main points of legal requirements and codes of practice for handling information in health and social care

The Human Rights Act 2000 Article 8: the right to respect for private and family life

Everyone has the right to respect from others for their private and family life, home and correspondence. The right to a private life includes the right to have information about us, such as official records, photographs, letters, diaries and medical information kept private and confidential. Unless there is a very good reason, public authorities should not collect or use information like this; if they do, they need to make sure the information is accurate.

The Information Security Management:

Article 8 of the Human Rights Act is a qualified right. This means that in certain situations, for example where public safety, security or health is at risk, or the protection of other people's rights and freedoms is at risk, personal information can be disclosed to a relevant authority.

A Guide to the Human Rights Act 1998, Third Edition, DCA 2006; www.justice.org.uk

Data Protection Act 1998

The Data Protection Act 1998 became effective in 2000 and superseded the Data Protection Act 1984 and the Access to Health Records Act 1990. The purpose of the Act is to protect the rights of individuals about whom **personal or sensitive data** is processed (collected, used and stored), disclosed and destroyed. It applies to information that is held in paper and computerised records, imaging records such as X-rays and photographs, and recordings such as video and CCTV images, telephone calls and tape recordings.

> ### Key term
>
> Personal or sensitive data is information about ethnic origin, religious and political beliefs, health, disability, criminal offences or alleged offences, sexual life and trade union membership.
> Integrity of data is to do with its accuracy and completeness.
> Access means to see, obtain or retrieve.
> Jargon is the technical language particular to a trade or profession.
> An individual is deemed competent when they have a clear appreciation and understanding of the facts, and the implications and consequences of an action.

The Act requires that security measures are put in place to retain the confidentiality and **integrity** of personal or sensitive data, and to ensure that it remains intact for as long as it is needed. In other words, people and organisations that handle personal or sensitive information must prevent:

■ unauthorised **access**, disclosure, alteration and destruction

■ accidental loss or destruction.

The Data Protection Act gives individuals the right to access information held about them except in certain situations. For this reason, any information that might be unintelligible, for example, abbreviations and **jargon**, must be explained. Representatives acting on behalf of individuals deemed **competent** to manage their affairs can see and discuss information held about the individual, provided that the individual has given consent. If an individual is deemed not

competent, the person appointed by a court to manage their affairs has the authority to give or withhold consent.

www.patient.co.uk

> ### When might a request to see information be refused?
>
> Types of information held about an individual that might not be given to them include:
>
> - records that contain information about other people, unless they have given their permission
>
> - information that has been received from third parties, unless they have given their permission
>
> - information that could affect their or somebody else's emotional or mental stability
>
> - records relating to work where legal proceedings have taken place
>
> - records where disclosure could affect crime prevention, detection, apprehension or prosecution of offenders.

www.dwp.gov.uk

Anyone who handles personal or sensitive data must comply with the Data Protection Act 1998 and the eight Data Protection Principles.

> ### Data Protection Principles
>
> The 8 Data Protection Principles require that personal or sensitive information is:
>
> 1. processed fairly and lawfully – for example, don't collect and use someone's personal information unless they have given you permission or you are confident that you are entitled to handle it
>
> 2. only used for the purpose for which it was obtained
>
> 3. adequate, relevant and not excessive – only collect and use as much information as you need
>
> 4. accurate, up to date and necessary – correct errors promptly and never handle personal or sensitive information that you do not need for your work
>
> *contd*

5. only kept for as long as needed – delete or destroy information when it is no longer needed.

6. processed in accordance with the individual's rights – for example, we have a right to know how our information is being used, to have any errors corrected, and to prevent information about us being used for advertising or marketing

7. kept secure at all times and protected from unauthorised access, disclosure, alteration and destruction

8. not transferred outside of the European Economic Area (EEA) unless the individual concerned has given consent and you are confident that you are entitled to transfer it.

Key term

The European Economic Area (EEA) is an economic association of European countries.

Research & investigate

1.2 Collecting information

1. Who do you collect information about at work?

2. What information do you collect?

3. How do you know that you can collect it?

4. Why do you need the information?

Time to reflect

1.2 How would you feel if …

• your personal correspondence, for example letters, emails, texts, were opened and read by other people?

• someone put photographs of you on a website without asking your permission?

• your GP told your employer about your medical history?

In 1997, Dame Fiona Caldicott carried out an investigation into the handling of patient information by health and social care service providers. As a result, six Caldicott Principles were identified to help them comply with the Data Protection Act. In summary, the Caldicott Principles require that anyone who handles personal or sensitive data that can be identifiable with a particular person must:

1. be able to justify its use – for example, it would be unjustifiable to let someone's ethnic background dictate whether to prescribe them medication for a failing memory, but it would be important to ensure that a female care worker is available to help female patients with intimate care if their religion and cultural traditions require same-sex care

2. not use it unless it is absolutely necessary – for example, it is absolutely unnecessary to know about someone's criminal record when helping them use the toilet, unless their record includes a history of sexual offence

3. use the minimum amount of information necessary – you don't need to know lots of information about someone's personal life when helping them choose from a menu, but it would be an advantage to know about their health and religious beliefs as these may dictate their dietary needs

4. ensure that access to it is on a strict 'need-to-know' basis – on no account should you disclose information about people without their consent or proper authorisation, nor should you disclose information to anyone who does not need that information to carry out their job

5. ensure that everyone with access to it is aware of their responsibilities, including ensuring that any personal data they see or hear goes no further, either by word of mouth or by unauthorised viewing of information, for example on a computer printout or computer screen

6. understand and comply with the law – you can be prosecuted for unlawful action under the Act and be fined if you use or disclose information improperly.

Case Study

1.2 Applying the Caldicott Principles

An early years setting holds information on children in order to support their development, monitor their progress, provide appropriate pastoral care and assess how well the setting as a whole is doing. This information includes contact details, attendance information, characteristics such as ethnic group, special educational needs and any relevant medical information. From time to time it is necessary to pass on some of this data to local authorities and official agencies, such as QCA and Ofsted. In particular, at age five an assessment is made of all children (the Foundation Stage Profile), and this information is passed to the local authority and receiving maintained school.

How is this setting complying with the Caldicott Principles as regards:

1. justifying its use of data?

2. not using data unless it is absolutely necessary?

3. using the minimum amount of information necessary?

4. ensuring that access to data is on a strict 'need-to-know' basis?

5. ensuring that everyone with access to the data is aware of their responsibilities?

6. understanding and complying with the law?

The Children Act 2004

The Children Act states that organisations have a duty to safeguard and promote the welfare of children and young people. Information sharing among care agencies enables them to work efficiently and effectively, but it must also comply with laws relating to confidentiality, data protection and human rights. Safeguarding Children Boards use The Children Act to develop policies and procedures related to information sharing, thereby complying with legislation and ensuring the safety and well-being of the child or young person.

The Health and Social Care Act 2008

The Health and Social Care Act gives the Secretary of State for Health the power to authorise health and social care service providers to disclose information about people in the interests of improving patient care or in the wider public interest, to monitor communicable diseases and for medical research.

Codes of Practice relating to handling information in health and social care are based on legislation, professional body standards and professional best practice.

Records Management: NHS Code of Practice

Records are valuable because of the information they contain. However, information is only useful if it is correctly recorded in the first place, regularly updated and easily accessible when needed. The *Records Management: NHS Code of Practice* describes different actions and responsibilities for effective collection, use and storage of all types of NHS records, and for their maintenance and disposal.

The Information Security Management: NHS Code of Practice

This applies to all organisations, including local authorities, that handle NHS information. Its purpose is to guide them in maintaining the security of information that they handle.

Code of Practice: Mental Health Act 1983

This requires that information to help them understand why they are in hospital or subject to guardianship is given to patients detained under the Mental Health Act and, unless they object, to their nearest relatives. It also states that, 'ordinarily, information about a patient should not be disclosed without their consent. Occasionally it may be necessary to pass on particular information to professionals or others in the public interest, for instance where personal health or safety is at risk.'

Research & investigate

 Disclosing information

- Who do you disclose information to?

- What information do you disclose?

- How do you know that you can disclose it?

- Why do other people and organisations need the information you give them?

General Social Care Council (GSCC) Codes of Practice

These set out the standards of practice that everyone who works in social care should meet. With regard to handling information, the Codes state that:

■ Social care employers must have written policies in place to help social care workers meet the GSCC's Code of Practice for Social Care Workers, including policies on confidentiality.

■ Social care workers must:

■ protect the rights of the people they support, including their right to privacy

■ respect confidential information and be able to explain their workplace's policies about confidentiality to the people they support, their family and friends

■ not abuse the trust of the people they support or the access they have to any personal information about them

■ maintain clear and accurate records as required by procedures established for their work.

General Social Care Council, 2002

The Nursing and Midwifery Council (NMC) code

This sets out the standards of conduct, performance and ethics that nurses and midwives must apply in their work. With regard to handling information, the code requires them to:

■ respect people's right to confidentiality

■ ensure that people are informed about why and how information is shared by people providing their care

■ disclose information if they believe someone may be at risk of harm

■ keep clear and accurate records and not tamper with original records in any way

■ ensure entries in records are clearly and legibly signed, dated and timed

■ ensure all records are kept securely.

Nursing & Midwifery Council, 2008

Evidence activity

 Legal requirements and codes of practice for handling information

Identify two pieces of legislation and two codes of practice that regulate the way personal and sensitive information is handled where you work. For each, sum up how they affect your work.

LO2 Be able to implement good practice in handling information

2.1 Describe features of manual and electronic information storage systems that help ensure security

Manual information storage systems

Manual information storage includes:

■ paper or card health records, case notes, care plans, pupils' files, assessment records, special educational needs data, staff records, registers, reports, computer printouts and administrative records such as letters, invoices and minutes from meetings

■ imaging records such as X-rays, CCTV film, photographs and slides

■ audio recordings such as telephone calls and tape recordings.

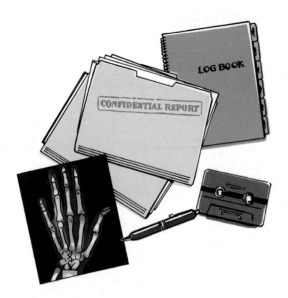

Figure 9.2 Manual information storage systems

Manual information should be held in named folders to make filing and access easy. The information within a folder should, if possible, be copied, and copies stored in a separate, secure location, for example on a USB flash drive (memory stick), as a precaution against loss.

An authorised person or the designated 'data owner' should take responsibility for ensuring that manual information is secure. All information should be annotated with its level of security, and confidential information must identify who is authorised to have access. There are three levels of security:

1. Low security means that the information can be accessed by the public, for example policies and procedures and an organisation's website.

2. Medium security means that the information is not readily accessible but may be disclosed in certain circumstances, for example basic personal information such as class lists.

3. High security means that the information contains personal and sensitive identifiable information and access is on a 'need-to-know' basis only.

Secure storage requires arrangements to be in place to make sure that:

■ information remains confidential

■ there is no risk of physical deterioration due, for example, to fire from electronic, electric and kitchen equipment, or water from sinks, toilets, pipes, radiators.

Research & investigate

(2.1) Manual storage of information

- Where is manual information stored at your workplace?

- Who can have access to this information and why?

Storage facilities for medium- and high-risk information, such as filing cabinets, cupboards and stores should be kept under lock and key, and keys and keypad number sequences held by the designated data owner or a named key holder. Access to information should be given on a need-to-know basis and a tracking record maintained of who has had access, when and why. If information is removed from storage a record should be made of when it was returned. Tracking systems can be either paper-based or electronic, such as when records are scanned in and out of storage.

When information stored manually is no longer needed, it should be dealt with as appropriate. Closed or inactive files may have to be retained for some time, in which case appropriate storage facilities will be required. Some information will need to be permanently preserved by **archiving**, some retained for review and some destroyed. Low-security information should be recycled; medium- and high-risk information should be shredded, pulped or incinerated.

Key term

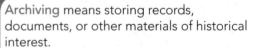

Archiving means storing records, documents, or other materials of historical interest.

Electronic information storage systems

Information can also be stored (saved) electronically on a computer's hard disk drive, an external hard drive, USB memory stick, CD or DVD, using programmes such as Word, Excel, PowerPoint and Outlook. Programmes provide the template for creating documents such as:

■ word documents, for example letters and reports

- spreadsheets, for example to record and monitor physiological measurements
- presentations, for example for training
- email, for sharing information.

Research & investigate

2.1a Storage of electronic information

- Where is electronic information stored at your workplace?
- Who can have access to this information and why?

The documents produced using these programmes are put into folders, which are the equivalent of the manual folders stored in filing cabinets and cupboards. Folders containing documents that are personal and sensitive need to be stored securely.

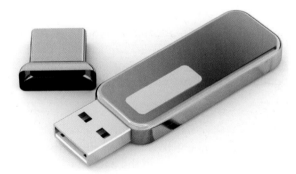

Figure 9.3 Electronic information storage systems

Encryption is the scrambling and transforming of information from an easily readable and understandable format (plaintext) into an unintelligible format that seems to be useless (ciphertext). The Data Protection Act requires organisations that use portable electronic information storage systems, such as laptops, handheld computers and USB memory sticks, to encrypt personal and sensitive information and regularly review and update the encryption to make sure it remains effective. The Act also requires that organisations have policies regarding the use and security of portable systems and that they ensure that their staff are properly trained in these.

Taking portable electronic information storage systems off site carries a risk of theft and unauthorised access to and modification of information.

Ten top tips for ensuring the security of information stored in equipment you take off site

1. Follow your organisation's home working and portable computing policies.
2. Know and understand how to use the equipment.
3. Keep it with you at all times.
4. If you have to leave it unattended, lock it up and store it in a secure place.
5. Take great care when using it in a public place to ensure that information is not overseen.
6. When travelling on public transport, carry laptops as hand luggage.
7. If you use a car, ensure that the equipment is not left on display. Lock it in the boot but do not leave it in the boot overnight.
8. Do not modify any stored information without authorisation.
9. Sending information over the internet could be classified as a breach of security, so never send identifiable information via email or devices such as Blackberries. In fact, never send information electronically that you would not put on the back of a postcard.
10. Do not use the equipment for your personal use, especially for internet access and emailing.

Research & investigate

2.1b Portable electronic information storage systems

- What portable electronic information storage systems are used at your workplace?
- Describe the policies and procedures that govern the way they are used off site.

If computer equipment has to go off site for service, repair or recycling, all information should be backed up, for example on a USB memory stick, and then removed. Normal deletion doesn't actually delete information, it simply removes the 'address' indicating where the files are stored. This means that data recovery software can be used to 'undelete' deleted files. It is better to use data destruction software or software that overwrites everything. The same applies to when computer equipment has to be discarded – remove all sensitive data first; alternatively, physically destroy the hard drive.

Computer viruses cause severe loss and destruction of information; antiviral software is highly recommended. Firewalls help prevent attacks against computers while connected to the internet, but viruses can arrive within files attached to emails. Some of these viruses (Trojans) contain programmes that allow an outsider to access and take control of computers over the internet. For this reason, never open files attached to emails from people you don't know. If you do know the sender but have even the slightest doubt, check to confirm that they have sent it.

Research & investigate

2.1c Secure storage and deletion of electronic information

How does your workplace ensure that electronically stored information is:

- not accidentally lost or destroyed?

- securely dealt with when no longer needed?

Anyone given authority to access electronic information should have a secure **username and password**. Used correctly, usernames and passwords ensure the security of personal and sensitive information. If you have authority to access information on a computer:

■ Keep your username secret. *Never* allow anyone else to use it, and don't allow the computer to save it, particularly if you share the computer with other people.

■ Keep your password secret. If you think someone might have watched you keying it in, change it immediately. Don't be obvious in your choice of password, for example don't use your name, birthday or anything else that someone might guess. Change it frequently and if you have to write it down, disguise it. Use a different password for every computer username allocated to you.

Key term

A username and password are the names that someone uses for identification purposes when logging on to a computer.

Time to reflect

2.1 Have you ever ...

Have you ever shared any of your personal ID, for example your PINs or computer usernames and passwords, with anyone else? What might be the outcome of sharing such information?

Dos and Don'ts of using electronic information storage systems to access, store and share sensitive and personal information

Do:

■ log in with your username and password.

■ position your monitor so that it cannot be overseen.

■ log out if you have to leave your computer unattended and when you have finished using it.

■ **back up** all the information you save, and store backup devices securely.

■ encrypt all the information you save on portable storage systems.

Key term

To back up means to copy saved information so that it is preserved in the event of equipment failure.

Don't:

■ Take computer equipment off site unless you have permission. If you do, make sure you know how to use the equipment and that you follow your organisation's homeworking and portable computing policies.

■ Store information in programmes that are connected to the internet, for example social networking websites and organisational intra- and internet web pages.

■ Send information via email unless it is encrypted.

■ Send sensitive information contained in portable storage systems, even if it is encrypted.

■ Rely on the delete button to erase information no longer needed. Use appropriate data destruction software.

Evidence activity

2.1 Features of storage systems that help ensure security

Think about the manual and electronic storage systems that you use at work. Describe how each ensures security of the information it stores.

2.2 Demonstrate practices that ensure security when storing and accessing information

2.3 Maintain records that are up-to-date, complete, accurate and legible

Good practice in health and social care relies on **multidisciplinary teamwork**. To ensure that the team is able to support people efficiently and effectively, it needs up-to-date, complete, accurate and legible records. Records that health and social care workers contribute to include health records, case notes, care plans; pupils' files, assessment records and special educational needs data; staff records; registers; and correspondence with the people they support, their relatives and representatives, and other members of their team.

 Practice activity

2.2 Ensuring security when storing and accessing information

Complete the following tables to show how you ensure security when storing and accessing information.

Manual information storage systems

Precautions I take to prevent unauthorised: • access to information • disclosure of information • alteration of information • destruction of information.	
Precautions I take to prevent accidental loss or destruction of information.	

Electronic information storage systems

Precautions I take to prevent unauthorised: • access to information • disclosure of information • alteration of information • destruction of information	
Precautions I take to prevent accidental loss or destruction of information.	

Key term

Multidisciplinary teamwork is when members of different professions work together.

A good record contains enough information to allow another professional to maintain continuity of care and help the individual develop and progress. It should be professionally written but, because The Data Protection Act gives individuals the right to access information held about them, it should contain explanations of information that they, their relatives or representatives might find difficult to understand.

The content of a report should therefore be complete. It should include, so far as is relevant to the situation, up-to-date details about the individual's:

■ age, sex, address, physical and intellectual ability; social, cultural and religious beliefs, values and preferences, life experiences and achievements.

■ health and social care needs, planned investigations or interventions, and information that they and their relatives and representatives have been given, for example details of the risks and benefits of different treatments and activities

■ treatment, for example the type and dosage of prescribed and **complementary and alternative medicine (CAM)** that they are taking, support groups they attend

■ response to different treatments and interventions

■ consent, for example, to medication or disclosure of their personal information

■ wish to refuse all or some forms of medical treatment in advance of loss of mental capacity, also known as their Living Will or Advance Directive.

www.medicalprotection.org; www.direct. gov.uk

It should also contain up-to-date contact details for relatives, friends and representatives, their **Lasting Power of Attorney** and contacts in the event of an emergency.

■ Time to reflect

2.3 What if …

What might be the outcomes for an individual if, for example, their and their relative's contact details, medication, consent to disclosure of personal information, and so on, were not kept up to date?

The completeness of a report can be diminished if it is tampered with or if alterations are not made properly. Mistakes or inaccuracies on electronic records should be remedied using a **tracking** device, and should be annotated with the date and author of the alteration.

Mistakes or inaccuracies on manual records should be remedied by adding a signed and dated note in ink. If an individual asks you to alter information about them because it is incorrect, include a note to say that you have altered it at their request. If the incorrect information would be harmful to them, delete it but insert a signed and dated note to explain what has happened and why.

In addition to ensuring that content is complete, you must ensure that records are accurate.

■ Write up notes as soon after an event as possible, before you forget exactly what was said or what happened.

■ Bear in mind that in some situations, information about an individual given by a third party, for example a relative, police officer or translator, may not be the same as that given to you by the individual themselves. We all see things differently and have different stories to tell as a result. Make a note of the person's name and position in the event that information needs clarifying.

■ Subjectivity takes away from accuracy. Records must be objective, that is, based on fact, so don't include your opinions, especially if they are likely to insult or cause distress.

Key term

Complementary and alternative medicine (CAM) is the term for health care products and practices that are not part of standard, scientific care.
Lasting Power of Attorney is the responsibility an individual gives to someone they trust to make financial and health decisions on their behalf at a time in the future when they lack the mental capacity to make decisions or no longer wish to make those decisions themselves.
Tracking is a process that highlights any alterations made to a document.

Case Study

(2.3) The truth, the whole truth and nothing but the truth

Mary lives in a sheltered housing complex. She has progressive Alzheimer's disease but the authorities are confident that she is able to live in her own flat at the present time. A neighbour frequently sees her wandering in her nightie around the gardens late at night and others, including the warden, are growing increasingly frustrated with Mary's fast declining memory, the health and safety risks she poses to them and herself as a result, and her growing dependence on everyone for everyday support.

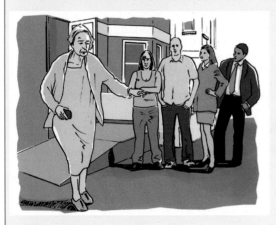

Figure 9.4 Mary

Mary's neighbours and the warden have organised a meeting with social services, in order to spell out their concerns. The warden's written report is as follows:

'Mary X is a nuisance. She is quite doolally and it won't be long before she blows the place up. The other residents are sick to death of having to look out for her when she does nothing for them in return. She can't look after herself any more and should be put in an old folk's home.'

Should the content of this report be relied on for accuracy? If not, why not?

Records must also be **legible**.

Key term

Legible means clear, readable, understandable.

- If you can't write legibly, use a computer or have someone write on your behalf. In this situation, dictate what you want to say and sign to show that the record accurately reflects what you have said.

- Be careful with abbreviations and jargon. Only use them if you can explain, in words of one syllable, what they mean.

- Sign each entry with the date, time and your status.

Practice activity

(2.3) Maintain records that are up-to-date, complete, accurate and legible

This activity gives you an opportunity to demonstrate that you can maintain good and appropriate records.

Photocopy half a dozen records, making sure to anonymise them, to which you have contributed and which demonstrate your ability to ensure records are up-to-date, complete, accurate and legible.

LO3 Be able to support others to handle information

(3.1) Support others to understand the need for secure handling of information

Maintaining security of information at work is everyone's responsibility.

How can you help others to understand the need to handle information securely? First and foremost, set an example. By following procedures based on relevant legislation and by being seen to handle information in accordance with professional codes of ethics and good practice, you will encourage colleagues to carry out their responsibilities to consistently high standards. Secondly, monitor their handling of information, offering advice and guidance where necessary.

Make everyone aware that they have a duty under the Data Protection Act to keep personal and sensitive information confidential. Posters on notice boards and easy access to policies and guidance documents should prompt colleagues about their responsibilities. And show respect for the right to privacy of the people you support. The experience of having our rights protected helps ensure that we fulfil our duty to respect other people's rights.

Time to reflect

3.1 Respecting people's rights

Has your private information ever been shared by someone without first seeking your permission? How did or would you feel? Would you or have you ever done the same to anyone else? How do you think they would feel? Do you think it is right to share information without first getting permission?

Encourage colleagues to become more security aware and to understand the possible consequences of failing to follow best practice. There are many ways in which workers can update their knowledge and skills in relation to secure information handling, for example through meetings and discussions, in-service training activities and attendance at professional events, and experiential, on-the-job learning. In addition, specialist journals, online information sources, e-learning and open learning programmes can provide opportunities for improving best practice.

Be aware of sources of information, referral, advice and guidance that can help you handle information securely, and share these resources with your colleagues.

Ensure that personal and sensitive information is labelled. This helps people handling it to understand the need to keep it secure and deal with it appropriately when it is no longer needed.

Encourage colleagues and the people you support to be on the alert for risks to security of information. Hazards include fire and water, impostors and thieves, computer hackers and lack of training. Ensure that colleagues can recognise hazards and are able to deal with associated risks, such as:

■ fire and water damage

■ requests for information from people who do not have a need to know

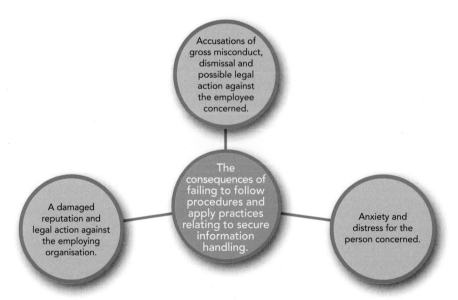

Figure 9.5 The consequences of failing to follow procedures and apply practices relating to secure handling

■ accidental or unauthorised loss of information due to, for example, not backing up, not encrypting information that is to leave the premises, and insecure transport and storage of equipment when off the premises

■ failure to deal with information appropriately when it is no longer needed

■ failure to report security concerns and breaches to the appropriate person without delay.

Practice activity

 Support others to understand the need for secure handling of information

This activity gives you an opportunity to demonstrate that you are able to support others to understand the need for secure handling of information.

■ Why is it important to handle information securely?

■ Make a list of the ways that you currently help colleagues and those you support to understand the need to handle information securely.

■ How can you develop their understanding?

Support others to understand and contribute to records

You read earlier that health and social care records need to be up to date, complete, accurate and legible. Anything else would make it difficult for professionals to work together to ensure continuity of care and appropriate support.

How can you support others to understand and contribute to records? Most importantly, by ensuring that you set a good example in the production and maintenance of records. Secondly, by raising their awareness of the consequences of records that are out of date, incomplete, inaccurate or illegible. Deficient, badly written records can result in an individual being given the wrong treatment or the wrong advice and information, with disastrous, possibly fatal, results for them and a formal complaint or even court proceedings against the worker and their employer.

Support your colleagues in their understanding of how the 8 Data Protection Principles underpin the production of good records. When collecting information, make sure they can explain to the individual concerned:

■ why they need the information

■ that they will only collect information if given permission and only use it for the purpose for which it is collected

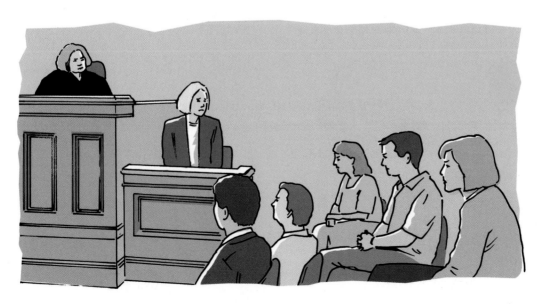

Figure 9.6 The consequences of failing to maintain up-to-date, complete, accurate and legible records

- that the information will remain secure and not be shared with anyone except people with a need to know, for example, other professionals involved in their care and support

- that the information will only be kept for as long as is necessary

- that the individual has a right to see any information collected about them, to make sure it is correct.

Support your colleagues in their knowledge of how to contribute to records. Make sure that they know to:

- only collect as much information as is needed and is relevant

- obtain the individual's agreement for their information to be shared with people with a need to know

- follow security procedures when accessing and storing/saving information

- write their contributions up promptly, before any detail is forgotten

- write professionally but with regard for people for whom jargon and abbreviations would be difficult to understand

- ensure that verbal contributions are in line with security procedures, for example made in privacy and to the appropriate person.

- contribute information that is accurate, objective and factual – prejudices, personal values and opinions have no place in record keeping

- consult with the appropriate people to make sure records stay up to date and free from error

- record and report any difficulties they have in accessing and updating records and reports.

Ten top tips to support individuals you work with to understand and contribute to their records

1. Use **interpersonal skills** to put them at ease while you explain your need for information and while you collect it.

Key term

Interpersonal skills are the positive people skills that nurture effective communication and relationships.

2. Have regard to their age, sex, cultural and religious background as this can affect who they will speak with, especially when the subject is of a personal, intimate nature.

3. Use the method of communication with which they are most comfortable.

4. Explain that the information you collect will be stored securely.

5. Explain that others in the care team may need to see the information you collect but that you will seek their permission before you share it.

6. Explain that they have a right to see any information held about them.

7. Be patient, give them time to think about their answers and use active listening skills to show you are interested and want to understand everything they tell you.

8. Don't interrupt and don't put answers into their heads. Let them tell you what they want to say, not what they think you want them to say.

9. Check your understanding by asking questions, summarising what they tell you, restating it in your own words.

10. Check that they agree to you sharing the information they have given you with relevant people.

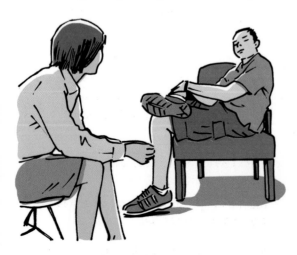

Figure 9.7 Who's asking?

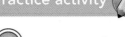

Practice activity

(3.2) Support others to understand and contribute to records

- Why is it important to contribute to records?
- Make a list of the ways that you currently help colleagues and those you support to understand and contribute to records.
- How can you develop their skills and understanding?

Assessment summary

Your reading of this chapter and completion of the activities will have prepared you to be able to engage in promoting good practice in handling information.

To achieve the unit, your assessor will require you to:

Learning outcomes	Assessment Criteria
Learning outcome **1**: Understand requirements for handling information in health and social care settings by:	**1.1** identifying legislation and codes of practice that relate to handling information in health and social care See Evidence activity 1.1, p. 167
	1.2 summarising the main points of legal requirements and codes of practice for handling information in health and social care See Evidence activity 1.2, p. 171
Learning outcome **2**: Be able to implement good practice in handling information by:	**2.1** describing features of manual and electronic information storage systems that help ensure security See Evidence activity 2.1, p. 175
	2.2 demonstrating practices that ensure security when storing and accessing information See Practice activity 2.2, p. 175
	2.3 maintaining records that are up-to-date, complete, accurate and legible See Practice activity 2.3, p. 177

Learning outcomes	Assessment Criteria
Learning outcome **3**: Be able to support others to handle information by:	**3.1** supporting others to understand the need for secure handling of information See Practice activity 3.1, p. 179
	3.2 supporting others to understand and contribute to records See Practice activity 3.2, p. 181

Good luck!

Web links

Justice – legal and human rights organisation   www.justice.org.uk
Health information for patients   www.patient.co.uk
Department for Work and Pensions   www.dwp.gov.uk
Medical Protection Society   www.medicalprotection.org
Public Services website   www.direct.gov.uk

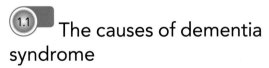

10 Understand the process and experience of dementia

For Unit DEM 301

What are you finding out?

Dementia is a **syndrome** that is associated with an ongoing decline of the brain and its abilities. These include thinking, language, memory, understanding and judgement. The consequences are that people become progressively less able to care for themselves.

Dementia is a common condition that currently affects over 800,000 people in the UK, and this number is set to rise considerably as more people live longer. Its **incidence** increases with age. About 1.5% of men and women aged 60–65 years are affected, while at age 85 and over, the figure is 20% and 28% for men and women respectively. Sixty thousand deaths a year are directly attributable to dementia, which costs the UK economy £23 billion per year, more than cancer and heart disease combined.

www.dementia2010.org

It is very important that individuals who are diagnosed as having dementia have their particular needs recognised and understood. Person-centred care, which values people regardless of their needs, treats them as individuals, understands the world from their perspective and provides a positive social environment, aims to improve quality of care and quality of life for them and their carers.

www.personcenteredcareadvocate.org

The reading and activities in this chapter will help you to:

- Understand the neurology of dementia

- Understand the impact of recognition and diagnosis of dementia

- Understand how dementia care must be underpinned by a person-centred approach.

Key terms

Incidence means occurrence.
A syndrome is a group of related symptoms.

LO1 Understand the neurology of dementia

1.1 The causes of dementia syndrome

Dementia syndrome is a group of related symptoms that are associated with a progressive decline of the brain, due to disease, and of intellectual functions that are needed for everyday living, such as memory. There are over 100 different types of dementia, some of which are described next.

Alzheimer's disease

This is a condition of the brain in which **plaques** and **tangles** develop in the brain, leading to the death of brain cells. There is also a shortage of **neurotransmitters**. It is a progressive disease, which means that over time, more and more parts of the brain become damaged, resulting in increased severity of symptoms. It is thought to be caused by a combination of factors, including age, genetic inheritance (people with Down's syndrome are at an increased risk of developing Alzheimer's disease), environmental factors, diet and overall general health. In some people, the disease may develop silently for many years before symptoms appear.

Key terms

Neurotransmitters are chemicals that are involved with the transmission of messages between nerve cells.
Plaques are insoluble protein deposits that build up around nerve cells.
Tangles are insoluble twisted protein fibres that build up inside nerve cells.
A neurological disease is a disease of the nervous system.

Vascular dementia

This is the second most common form of dementia after Alzheimer's disease. It is caused by problems in the supply of blood to the brain. Blood is delivered through a network of blood vessels called the vascular system. If the vascular system in the brain becomes damaged, for example because of high blood pressure, heart problems, high cholesterol and diabetes, and blood cannot reach the brain cells, the cells will eventually die, leading to the onset of vascular dementia.

Dementia with Lewy bodies (DLB)

This is a form of dementia that is similar to both Alzheimer's and Parkinson's diseases. Lewy bodies are tiny, spherical protein deposits found in nerve cells. Their presence in the brain disrupts the brain's normal functioning, including that of important neurotransmitters. Lewy bodies are also found in the brains of people with Parkinson's disease, a progressive **neurological disease** that affects movement. Some people who are initially diagnosed with Parkinson's disease later go on to develop a dementia that closely resembles DLB.

Fronto-temporal dementia

This covers a range of conditions, including Pick's disease, frontal lobe degeneration and dementia associated with motor neurone disease. All are caused by damage to the frontal lobe and/or the temporal parts of the brain, which are responsible for our behaviour, emotional responses and language skills.

Korsakoff's syndrome

This is caused by lack of vitamin B1 (thiamine), which affects the brain and nervous system. Thiamine deficiency is often seen in heavy drinkers because:

■ they have poor eating habits, so their nutrition is inadequate and does not contain essential vitamins

■ alcohol can damage the stomach lining, inhibiting the body's ability to absorb vitamins from food.

Creutzfeldt-Jakob disease (CJD)

This is the best known of a group of diseases called prion disease. Prions are proteins found in the central nervous system, and in prion disease they form clusters in the brain. When brain cells die, they cause spongiosis or holes in the brain, which makes the brain look like sponge when viewed under the microscope. This results in dementia.

Mild cognitive impairment (MCI)

Mild **cognitive impairment** (MCI) is the term used to describe the condition of people who have some problems with intellectual functioning but do not actually have dementia.

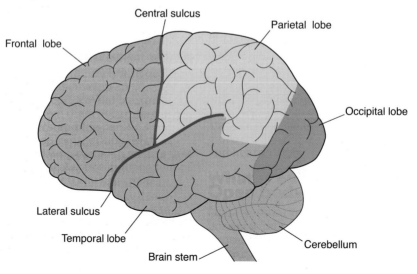

Figure 10.1 The brain

People are usually not diagnosed with dementia until their symptoms begin to affect their life. Identifying people with MCI is important because they can be prescribed medication to improve their symptoms and slow down the progression of dementia. Delaying the onset of dementia by five years would reduce deaths directly attributable to dementia by 30,000 a year.

> ## Key term
>
> Cognitive impairment means difficulty in carrying out intellectual functions, such as learning, thinking and remembering.

People with AIDS (Acquired Immune Deficiency Syndrome) sometimes develop cognitive impairment, particularly in the later stages of their illness. AIDS is caused by the presence of HIV (Human Immunodeficiency Virus) in the body. HIV attacks the body's immune system, making the person more susceptible to infection. HIV-related cognitive impairment can be caused by:

- the direct impact of HIV on the brain

- infections that exploit the weakened immune system.

Time to reflect

1.1 Dementia statistics

According to The Alzheimer's Society:

- Two-thirds of people with dementia live in the community while one-third live in a care home.

- Sixty-four per cent of people living in care homes have a form of dementia.

- Two-thirds of people with dementia are women.

- One third of people over 95 have dementia.

- There are over 16,000 younger people with dementia in the UK. A younger person is an adult of 65 and under who, for example, has dependent children or is in work at the time of diagnosis.

contd.

Time to reflect

How do these figures compare with the people you know and work with who have dementia? For example, if you work in a care home, do two-thirds of the individuals have some form of dementia? And are two-thirds of the people you know with dementia women?

Evidence activity

1.1 Describe a range of causes of dementia syndrome

This activity enables you to demonstrate your knowledge of the causes of dementia syndrome.

- Write a series of case studies about people with dementia, in which you describe the cause of their condition. Describe at least three different types of dementia and, if you use people you know or support at work, make sure you maintain their confidentiality.

- Present your case studies to colleagues in order to improve their knowledge and understanding of dementia syndrome.

1.2 Types of memory impairment commonly experienced by individuals with dementia

Memory is the ability to store, retain and recall information. The two main types of memory are short-term memory (STM), which has a fairly limited capacity, about 30 seconds; and long-term memory (LTM), into which important information is gradually transferred from the short-term memory. For long-term memories to survive, we have to recall or practise them from time to time.

We all forget things occasionally, such as someone's name, where we left the keys, where we parked the car; and we can usually attribute such lapses to tiredness, stress, overwork, ill health, the side effects of certain medications, even to the 'senior moments' of advancing years! However, memory problems that get progressively worse and that impact on everyday life can be an early sign of dementia.

There are four areas in which people with memory loss may have difficulty:

1. Remembering new information – people with damage to the part of the brain that allows new information to be absorbed often find it hard to take in and remember new things. This means that if they deny having heard some information before, for example the date of an appointment, when to expect a visitor, or to eat, drink and take their medication, they may well be telling the truth.

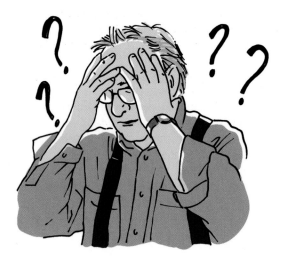

Figure 10.2 Where did I put my keys?

2. Remembering or recalling recent events – the inability of the brain to recall recent events is known as short-term memory loss. Long-term memory, of things that happened in the past, is far more clear and detailed, so much so that people with dementia often spend their time 'living in the past'. This accounts for their inappropriate behaviour, such as child-like or sexual behaviour. However, even long-term memories eventually decline.

3. Remembering places and people, even their own reflection; things they have heard, seen or read; and the names of friends and everyday objects. When people cannot remember who they are, they lose their sense of self and self-awareness, becoming seemingly selfish, with a lack of feeling for others.

4. Separating fact from fiction – people with dementia can lose sight of the difference between fact and what they imagine to be the truth, leading to, for example, assertions that a visitor has called, or accusations of theft when something has simply been misplaced.

Evidence activity

1.2 Types of memory impairment common with dementia

This activity enables you to demonstrate your knowledge of the types of memory impairment commonly experienced by individuals with dementia.

Talk to people who have been diagnosed with dementia and also to their carers, family and friends, to find out what the people with dementia tend to forget, how their failing memory impacts on their everyday life and how they feel as a consequence. How does this compare with what you forget and the memory lapses of others who have not been diagnosed with dementia?

1.3 How individuals process information with reference to their abilities and limitations

Dementia is associated with the decline of the brain's capacity to process information. This decline can have far-reaching affects on an individual's ability to carry out day-to-day activities, communicate, make sense of the world and make judgements.

Decline of information processing affects day-to-day activities such as:

■ putting letters and words together in order to read and write

■ combining numbers to make calculations

■ coordinating movements, for example to dress, use a knife and fork, walk

■ locating objects within a space, for example to pick something up. And the inability to locate oneself within a space causes confusion and disorientation

■ thinking, planning and learning new tasks – if the areas of the brain that are critical for these skills become damaged, plans of action and ways of doing things get 'lost' or 'unlearnt', and tasks such as shopping and cooking become almost impossible; in addition, damage can cause people to get 'stuck' on what they are doing – this is known as **perseveration**

■ performing particular activities, for example to get out of bed and maintain social contacts, because of **apathy**.

Key terms

Apathy is lack of motivation or 'get up and go'.
Perseveration means to use the same words and behaviours over and over again, without any specific purpose.
The communication cycle involves having an idea, expressing it such that others can understand, and receiving and understanding others' responses.
Non-verbal communication (NVC) is body language.

The **communication cycle** requires the brain to process a great deal of information. Initially dementia limits a person's ability to find the right words for what they want to say. They may use an incorrect word or not find any word at all and, as time passes, become unable to understand or respond to what others are saying. There may come a time when they can hardly communicate through language at all. On the other hand, **non-verbal communication (NVC)** remains important. People with dementia remain able to express themselves using, for example, facial expressions, movement and body posture, and they also retain the ability to read body language.

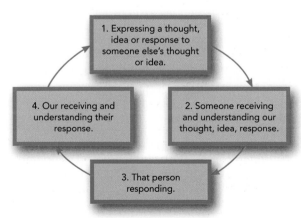

Figure 10.3 The communication cycle

In order that we can make sense of the world around us, the brain has to process information from the **visual system**. This is known as visuoperception, and visuoperceptual mistakes can cause someone with dementia to misinterpret their environment and what is in it. 'Visual mistakes' include:

■ misperceptions, for example mistaking a dark stain on the carpet for a cat

■ misidentifications, for example the inability to distinguish between a wife and daughter

■ misnaming what is seen, for example referring to a collection of supermarket trolleys as robots

■ illusions and visual and auditory hallucinations.

Other visual difficulties include **perceiving** colour, depth and movement; detecting a contrast between colours (contrast sensitivity); and recognising faces and objects.

Key terms

Perceiving means understanding.
The visual system is the eyes, optic muscles, retinas and optic nerve.

Time to reflect

1.3 How would you feel if …

Imagine that you couldn't remember how to get dressed, find the right words to describe how you feel or answer a question, or that you started seeing things that didn't exist. How would you feel, especially if you lived alone, were the breadwinner supporting a family or were elderly and caring for an elderly relative?

Dementia affects the ability of the brain to process information so that we have insight and can make choices and judgements. For example:

■ A failure of insight, for example into danger, means that people with dementia are easily exploited, doors are left unlocked, the gas is not lit and the tap not turned off.

■ If a person chooses not to maintain their personal hygiene, they put their dignity and health at risk.

■ If a person loses their sense of time, they find it hard to judge how much time has passed, missing appointments and visits; and if they cannot remember what they have done, they find it hard to anticipate what will happen next.

In addition, an inability to judge the appropriateness of their behaviour means that people with dementia may be rude or lose their inhibitions, such as removing their clothes or exposing their genitals in public.

www.alzheimers.org.uk

'Living well with dementia: A National Dementia Strategy', DH 2009

Evidence activity

1.3 The way individuals process information

This activity enables you to demonstrate your understanding of the way individuals process information with reference to their abilities and limitations.

Mary is 92, was diagnosed with Alzheimer's disease 10 years ago and lives in a residential care home. She is incapable of making any decisions; she can feed herself and use the toilet on her own, but she cannot dress or bathe herself and is increasingly unable to walk unaided; she has no conversation and no comprehension of time; she misinterprets what she sees, for example she mistakes her sons for her father, and she is increasingly unable to recognise the faces of people she sees on a regular basis.

What reasons can you give for Mary's limitations and decline in abilities?

1.4 Factors that can cause changes in an individual's condition that may not be attributable to dementia

Many of the problems you have read about so far do not inevitably foretell a diagnosis of dementia. Communication problems are not necessarily attributable to dementia. They may be caused by pain, illness, such as stroke, or the side effects of medication; poor sight, when a lens prescription is no longer correct; poor hearing, when hearing aids are not working properly; or ill-fitting dentures, which make speaking difficult.

Visual problems are not necessarily attributable to dementia either. The normal ageing process affects sight and visuoperception but, while most people as they get older are able to adjust to their changing vision, solve visual problems and learn to compensate for visual changes, people with dementia are unable to do this.

You read above that dementia can cause visuoperceptual mistakes, including hallucinations. The normal ageing process, as well as alcohol and recreational drugs, can also cause hallucinations, and alcohol and drugs, including medication, can have visual side effects.

Many people with dementia develop a compulsion to walk about or leave home, seemingly aimlessly or for a variety of reasons, for example, because they:

■ are confused about the time and think that when they wake in the night it is time to get up and get on with the day

■ feel a need to search for someone or something related to their past

■ feel lost and disorientated and need to find somewhere they know

■ have forgotten that they should not go out or to wait for someone to take them out.

However, many people who don't have dementia also develop a need to walk about, to relieve pain, boredom or stress, to use up energy, or to stay independent.

People with dementia can experience mood swings and behave aggressively, because, for example, they are frightened or frustrated, find it difficult to make decisions, or have lost their inhibitions and understanding of appropriate social behaviour. But mood swings and challenging behaviour are not peculiar to dementia. Drugs, medication and alcohol, the frustrations associated with increasing age, disability and poor health, having to share accommodation with people we don't like, having to comply with authority, and so on and so forth, can all trigger hostility and aggression.

Time to reflect

1.4 A false diagnosis

Think about an occasion when you have had problems:

- communicating, for example because you were on your mobile phone and unable to 'read' the other person's body language or there was too much noise for you to hear them properly

- seeing things as they really are, for example because you'd had too much to drink and your hand missed your glass as you reached for it

- containing your angst, for example because you had to work with a difficult individual or you couldn't remember where you'd left your car keys.

How would you feel if your GP told you that he thought you might have dementia?

People with dementia can have eating problems, for example they may forget or, if being fed, refuse to open their mouth, or they may spit or throw their food about. But eating problems also occur when chewing and swallowing are painful, if people are depressed or have an eating disorder, or when they are faced with food and drink that they don't enjoy.

Other conditions that have similar symptoms to dementia include:

- infections

- severe constipation

- depression

- taking medication incorrectly or that has not been prescribed

- vitamin and thyroid deficiencies

- brain tumours.

www.alzheimers.org.uk; www.dementiauk.org

Evidence activity

1.4 Other factors not attributable to dementia

This activity enables you to demonstrate your understanding of how other factors, that may not be attributable to dementia, can cause changes in a person's condition. *contd.*

Evidence activity

Look back at Evidence activity 1.3, in which Mary was described as unable to make decisions, dress or bathe herself, make conversation, understand time, interpret what and who she sees, and recognise faces. In addition, she is increasingly unable to walk unaided.

Had you not known that Mary has Alzheimer's disease, and given the fact that she is 92 and institutionalised in her way of living, would you necessarily attribute her limitations and abilities to dementia? If not, why not? What alternative factors could be the cause of her condition?

1.5 Why the abilities and needs of an individual with dementia may fluctuate

As you know, dementia is a progressive decline in the ability to remember and process information. However, everyone is different and people with dementia experience it differently, in their own way, depending on, for example, their physical make-up, emotional resilience and the support they receive.

www.lbda.org; www.pdsg.org.uk; www.nursingtimes.net; www.alzheimers-research.org.uk

Evidence activity

1.5 Fluctuations in abilities and needs

This activity enables you to demonstrate your understanding of why the abilities and needs of an individual with dementia may fluctuate.

Write a case study of someone you know who has dementia, in which you describe and give the reasons for their fluctuating abilities and needs. If the individual you write about is someone you work with, be sure to maintain confidentiality.

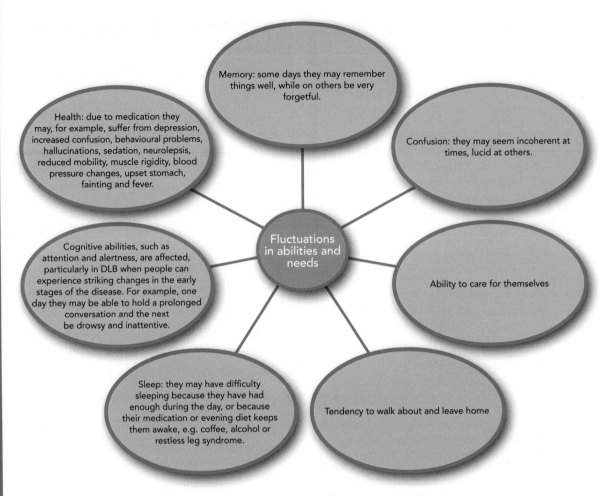

Figure 10.4 Fluctuations in abilities and needs experienced by people with dementia

LO2 Understand the impact of recognition and diagnosis of dementia

2.1 The impact of early diagnosis and follow-up to diagnosis

Dementia is diagnosed by specialist professionals through: an assessment, usually a conversation, with the person being diagnosed and the people they are close to; a physical examination; memory tests, such as the Mini Mental State Examination (MMSE), a commonly used test for concerns about memory problems; and/or brain scans.

The value of early diagnosis of dementia is that it:

■ enables other, treatable, conditions to be ruled out

■ enables **interventions** to be put in place, to improve quality of life and delay or prevent the person having to go into a residential care home

■ allows the person with dementia and their carer to plan and make arrangements for the future.

At the time of writing (July 2010), only about one-third of people with dementia ever receive a formal diagnosis; people aren't diagnosed accurately; or the diagnosis is too late for effective intervention and for people to make choices. There are many reasons for this, including low public awareness of the condition, the **stigma** of having the condition, and GP knowledge and attitudes.

Key terms

Interventions are measures whose purpose is to improve health or alter the course of disease.
Stigma means shame, disgrace.

Case Study

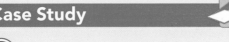

2.1 Attitudes to dementia'

'The consultant said it's dementia and I just burst into tears because I was so … I half expected it, but it's still a terrible shock.' (Carer)

'We had gone to him [the GP] for a lot of things and he was telling [the person with dementia] that it was in his mind, he hadn't got these problems, he needed to pull himself together.' (Carer)

[source] 'Living well with dementia: A National Dementia Strategy', DH, 2009

1. What sort of attitudes are being shown here by the carers and the GP?

2. Why do you think these attitudes to dementia prevail?

3. What is your response to attitudes like these?

For some people, being diagnosed with dementia when it is in its early stages can be distressing, particularly if they are still in work or have dependent children. For others, it can be a relief to know what is causing their symptoms.

Terry Pratchett, a well-known author, was only 59 when he was diagnosed with Alzheimer's disease. An article written by him for the *Daily Mail* in October 2008 (www.dailymail.co.uk) headlined, 'I'm slipping away a bit at a time... and all I can do is watch it happen'. Below is a selection of his reactions to his early diagnosis as printed in the article.

'I regarded finding I had a form of Alzheimer's as an insult.

'When, in *Paradise Lost*, Milton's Satan stood in the pit of hell and raged at heaven, he was merely a trifle miffed compared to how I felt that day. I felt totally alone, with the world receding from me in every direction, and you could have used my anger to weld steel.

'I remember on that day of rage thinking that if I'd been diagnosed with cancer of any kind, at least there would have opened in front of me a trodden path. There would have been specialists, examinations, there would be in short, some machinery in place.

'I was not in the mood for a response that said, more or less, "go away and come back in six years".' (He had been told by one specialist that he was too young, at 59, to have Alzheimer's.)

'My wife said: "Thank goodness it isn't a brain tumour," but all I could think then was: "I know three people who have got better after a brain tumour. I haven't heard of anyone who's got better from Alzheimer's." '

Other, more positive responses to early diagnosis include:

'It was as if the thunder clouds had been taken away because they had given an answer to me, why I was treating my family so like a louse that I was.' (Person with dementia)

'I was really relieved that what I was trying to convince people of had been verified.' (Person with dementia)

'I need to make those decisions while I have the mental capacity to be able to do that and to understand the implications of it before I get too far down the line. So it has given me the time to think about that.' (Person with dementia)

Living well with dementia: A National Dementia Strategy', DH, 2009

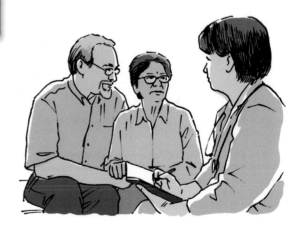

Figure 10.5 Early diagnosis

Follow-up to diagnosis involves treatment, care and support. By far the best treatment is to ensure that people with dementia are physically healthy, comfortable, well cared for and have an opportunity to participate in interesting and stimulating daily activities. Antipsychotic drugs are often prescribed for the treatment of memory loss, mood disorders, behavioural problems, psychiatric problems and sleep disturbance, but ought to be avoided unless really necessary.

Unless they are well supported, many people and their carers flounder socially and emotionally after a diagnosis. You have read that there is a stigma attached to having dementia. As Terry Pratchett said, 'It is a strange life when you "come out". People get embarrassed, lower their voices, get lost for words.' And, 'It seems that when you have cancer you are a brave battler against the disease, but when you have Alzheimer's you are an old fart. That's how people see you. It makes you feel quite alone.'

Time to reflect

2.1 What do you think?

What do you think about dementia? How do you treat people who have the condition? Has reading this chapter altered your view point at all? Has it made you think twice about your treatment of people with dementia?

It is critically important that people with dementia and their carers are supported by:

■ peer and support groups that offer social and emotional support and reduce social isolation

■ specialist advisors, who can offer good-quality, accessible and appropriate information about dementia and the support services available as the condition develops.

Support services for people with dementia should help them to:

■ have as good a quality of life as their limitations allow

■ live as normal a life as possible, whether in their own home or in a residential care home

■ readjust to living at home after a period away, for example in hospital or **respite care**.

Key term

Respite care is care that gives families a short break from the duties of constant care.

Support services for carers should help them to:

■ continue caring for the person with dementia in their own home for as long as they can

■ maintain their relationship with the person they care for – caring for someone with dementia can be very stressful and take an emotional and physical toll

■ feel fulfilled and satisfied in their caring role.

Case Study

2.1 Getting support

'Most important of all to be given all the information they need: not about what's just happened but about what is likely to happen and where you can go for assistance.' (Carer)

[source] 'Living well with dementia: A National Dementia Strategy', DH, 2009

Why do you think information about what is likely to happen and where to go for assistance is so important?

Evidence activity

2.1 The impact of early diagnosis and follow-up to diagnosis

This activity enables you to demonstrate your knowledge of the impact of early diagnosis and follow-up to diagnosis.

Prepare a presentation to give to your colleagues about:

■ the way people feel when they or their loved ones have been diagnosed with dementia

■ post-diagnosis support and its importance.

2.2 The importance of recording possible signs or symptoms of dementia in an individual in line with agreed ways of working

You are now familiar with a range of signs and symptoms that either describe dementia or point to the possibility that an individual is in its early stages. It is extremely important that you record any signs or symptoms you observe in the people you support, in order that:

■ Assessments can be made to establish what might be causing or influencing your observations, such as changes in health, side effects of medication and the effects of their environment

■ Changes in needs can be identified, both of the people concerned and, if they live in their own home, their carers. According to the Carers (Equal Opportunities) Act 2004, carers have a right to be offered an assessment of their needs, and any changes in the needs of the people they support will impact on theirs.

www.direct.gov.uk; www.carers.org

■ Care plans can be written or reviewed to ensure that changing needs are met, including how to manage increased safety needs and challenging behaviour.

■ The need for dementia care training can be identified and training offered to everyone concerned.

■ Appropriate support services provided by **inter-agency working** can be put in place.

Key term

Inter-agency working is the coming together of agencies or organisations that have a shared interest in supporting people who have care needs.

It is equally important that you follow your organisation's procedures and agreed ways of working with regard to recording possible signs or symptoms of dementia. Failure to do so could mean that your observations are not acted on, needs not met and appropriate support withheld.

Evidence activity

 The importance of recording possible signs or symptoms of dementia

This activity enables you to demonstrate your understanding of the importance of recording possible signs or symptoms of dementia in an individual in line with agreed ways of working.

Check out your workplace's procedures and agreed ways of working for recording possible signs and symptoms of dementia. Why are you required to follow these ways of working? What could happen if you failed to record your observations as required?

 ## 2.3 The process of reporting possible signs of dementia within agreed ways of working

When reporting possible signs of dementia, make sure you remain totally objective. Only report what you actually observed, not your personal, subjective thoughts or feelings about what might have been observed. And never embroider the truth for the sake of a good story. In doing so, you may incorrectly attribute other factors, such as absentmindedness or apathy, to dementia.

If you are required to make a written report of your observations, for example in care plans, reports, daily logs, handover reports, make sure your writing is legible and that you use language that can be read and understood by everyone concerned. Other professionals will need to see what you have written, so use clear, objective and appropriate language. And remember that the people you support have every right to read what you say about them, so it isn't clever to use jargon they would not understand.

Never use labels, negative statements or stereotypical language to describe people with dementia or their signs and symptoms. Traditional attitudes towards dementia have resulted in it being stigmatised. Your role is to fight negative attitudes and help people to think positively about the condition and its **prognosis**.

Key term

A prognosis is a prediction about how something will develop.

Again, make sure you understand and follow your organisation's procedures and agreed ways of working with regard to reporting possible signs of dementia.

Evidence activity

 2.3 The process of reporting possible signs of dementia

This activity enables you to demonstrate your understanding of the process of reporting possible signs or symptoms of dementia in an individual in line with agreed ways of working.

contd.

Evidence activity

contd.

Check out the process that your organisation requires you to follow in the event that you observe possible signs of dementia. What is the reason for this process? What could happen if you failed to follow this process?

2.4 The possible impact of receiving a diagnosis of dementia on the individual and their family and friends

You read earlier about the impact of early diagnosis of dementia on individuals and their family and friends. Terry Pratchett's moving experiences as a younger person with dementia, as well as those quoted in the Department of Health's National Dementia Strategy, help us to empathise with what it must be like to know that one's mental powers are going to 'slip away a bit at a time'.

The impact of diagnosing dementia can be softened by breaking the news sensitively and focusing on strengths and skills that remain and can be used, rather than on lost skills and weaknesses. Respect for an individual's strengths and skills promotes their feelings of:

■ Inclusion – as Terry Pratchett said, 'When you have Alzheimer's you are an old fart. That's how people see you. It makes you feel quite alone.' That was in 2008. Much work has been done since to raise the profile and understanding of dementia. As a result, people who have dementia and their carers are beginning to feel less **ostracised** and increasingly included.

■ Empowerment – the recognition that having dementia does not undervalue people's strengths is empowering and builds self-confidence and esteem.

■ Participation – the acknowledgment that people with dementia have useful skills to offer and have not been 'written-off' encourages their involvement in day-to-day life. This in turn helps maintain independence and everyday skills.

Key term

Ostracised means excluded or ignored.

Research & investigate

2.4 Strengths and skills

Talk to people with dementia and to their carers. Find out what strengths and skills the people with dementia have and whether or not they are acknowledged. How do they feel as a result? How would they like things to be improved?

The impact of diagnosis can also take the wind out of the sails of family and friends. It can be a shock if they attach a stigma to the diagnosis, and it can devastate their quality of life, especially if the individual concerned is still young and the main breadwinner. Caring is hard work, especially if carers are frail and getting on, or have a tendency to put the needs of the person with dementia before their own. This can impact on their physical and emotional health and the time and energy they have to give to others in the family, their friends and themselves. Stopping work, or combining work with care, has financial implications and can impact on any chance of developing a career. Claiming benefits goes against many people's principles. And they might not be equipped to care, for example, they may not have the practical skills or the appropriate personality.

Evidence activity

2.4 Possible impact of receiving a diagnosis of dementia

This activity enables you to demonstrate your knowledge of the possible impact of receiving a diagnosis of dementia on the individual and their family and friends.

Write an information sheet to be read by people who make diagnoses of dementia, which:

■ informs them of the impact a diagnosis can have on everyone concerned

■ suggests how a diagnosis might be made such that it is received more positively.

LO3 Understand how dementia care must be underpinned by a person-centred approach

3.1 Person-centred and non-person-centred approaches to dementia care

Person-centred dementia care is an **ethical** approach to caring for people living and dying with dementia.

> ### Key term
>
> Ethical means principled, moral.

Person-centred dementia care requires service providers to plan and care for an individual according to their assessed physical, intellectual, emotional, social and spiritual needs. To assess needs, they need to fully explore the individual's background, including their:

- likes, dislikes and expectations
- personal experiences and achievements
- attitudes, values and beliefs
- preferences, for example dietary, dress, personal space and method of communication.

Ten top tips for delivering person-centred dementia care

1. Know and understand the process and experience of dementia.
2. Ensure that the person with dementia is physically healthy, comfortable and safe.
3. Value their individuality.
4. Treat them with dignity and respect.
5. Accept that they have the capacity to communicate, and encourage communication.
6. Know what motivates them and try to understand the world from their perspective.
7. Empower them by supporting them to make their own choices and stay independent.
8. Provide an intellectual environment that meets their interests, and encourage participation in activities.
9. Provide a social environment that they will enjoy, and encourage social involvement.
10. Ensure they have an opportunity to worship as they choose and express themselves spiritually.

Non-person-centred dementia care, the alternative approach, focuses on ensuring that individuals get through certain tasks each day, for example, getting up, eating, going to the toilet, bathing and going to bed. This usually involves having inflexible rules and timetables, with individuals spending long hours alone so that staff can get their jobs done. It ensures that basic physical needs are met, but it doesn't consider intellectual, emotional, social and spiritual needs.

Person-centred dementia care has been written into British national policy and performance targets, such as the National Service Framework for Older People, for a number of years. More recently (2009), a study carried out by Australian researchers has confirmed its benefits. Agitation is a characteristic of dementia and involves shouting, pacing, hitting, hiding things or crying. The researchers showed that people with dementia in residential care homes become less agitated while receiving person-centred dementia care than those who receive non-person-centred dementia care.

National Service Framework for Older People, DH, 2001
www.guardian.co.uk

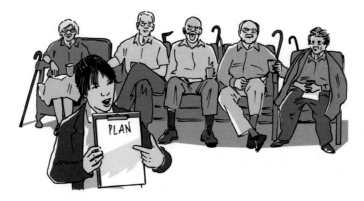

Figure 10.6 Non-person-centred dementia care

3.1 Person-centred vs non-person-centred approaches

This activity enables you to demonstrate your knowledge of the differences between a person-centred and non-person-centred approach to dementia care.

Complete the table below to show the difference between care that takes all of an individual's needs into account and care that is non-person-centred.

Characteristics of dementia	Person-centred care approach	Non-person-centred care approach
Failing memory		
Perseveration		
Communication problems		
Apathy		
Wandering		
Incontinence		

3.2 Different techniques that can be used to meet the fluctuating abilities and needs of the individual with dementia

There are numerous techniques used to support the fluctuating abilities and needs of people with dementia. However, a person-centred approach to care requires that techniques are chosen to meet the needs of the individual concerned.

Improvements and repairs, for example rewiring and improved heating systems, widened doors for wheelchairs and specially designed shower facilities, help people with dementia to stay in their own home. Aids and adaptations, such as adapted cutlery, non-spill cups, bath seats, raised toilet seats, grab rails, ramps, wheelchairs and walking frames help people to stay independent. Incontinence aids, such as waterproof bedding, absorbent undersheets and incontinence pads and pants, help retain dignity.

Memory aids include: calendar clocks; clocks with large faces; dosset boxes, which have a pill compartment for each day of the week as a reminder to take medication; labels on cupboards or rooms as a reminder of where things are; diaries, notebooks and notice boards can remind of important birthdays and phone numbers, appointments and things to do.

Assistive technology includes devices that help locate missing objects, such as keys, systems that trigger a response if the front door is opened and the person doesn't return within a given amount of time, and sensors worn on the wrist that detect if the person falls.

Boredom and frustration are common causes of challenging behaviour in people with dementia. However, behaviour can improve radically if they are occupied and stimulated with activities of their choice. Exercise, for example walking and swimming, has a calming effect, helps develop a healthy appetite and promotes sleep; and exercise classes can meet social needs. Reminiscence therapy can help trigger distant, pleasant memories, for example talking about the past, looking through old family photograph albums, listening to music, visiting old haunts and making a memory box containing objects that mean something to the person.

Time to reflect

3.2 Help yourself!

Sometimes it seems that life never stands still, we are all so busy! However, access to technology, aids and adaptations, opportunities for social interaction and intellectual stimulation make life less complicated and help us cope. What techniques do you use at work and in your personal life, to make your life more manageable?

Keeping active and staying involved help maintain existing skills, give pleasure and boost confidence and independence. For example, craft activities, such as knitting and scrapbooking, crosswords and puzzle book, card and board games; general household activities such as washing and drying up, cooking, setting the table, making the bed, getting dressed, gardening; listening to the radio and going to church, a day centre or the pub.

Techniques for coping with unusual behaviour, such as perseveration, restlessness, shouting, screaming and loss of inhibition include acknowledging that the person does not intend to be difficult but that they might be frustrated or simply trying to communicate. Distraction techniques can work; alternatively, if the behaviour becomes really difficult to manage, suitably qualified professionals can advise.

Evidence activity

3.2 Different techniques that can be used with individuals with dementia

This activity enables you to demonstrate your knowledge of different techniques that can be used to meet the fluctuating abilities and needs of the individual with dementia.

Produce an observation sheet/checklist for a Dementia Care Support Worker, which identifies a range of techniques aimed at meeting the diverse needs of people with dementia and which she or he could use when assessing and reviewing an individual's changing needs.

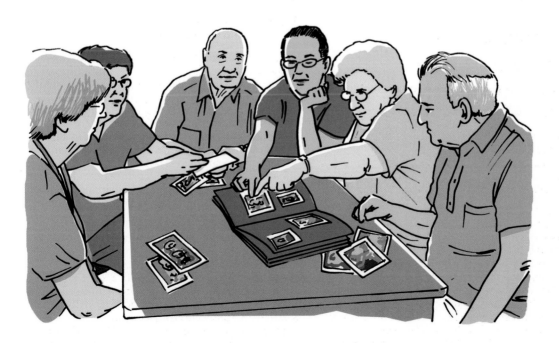

Figure 10.7 Reminiscence therapy

3.3 Myths and stereotypes related to dementia and their affect on the individual and their carers

Time to reflect

3.3 Myths and stereotypes

A myth is a legend or fable, a fairy story. What myths have you heard about dementia?

A stereotype is a way of pigeonholing people, grouping them together based on shared aspects of their appearance and behaviour. What stereotypes have you heard about people with dementia?

Do you think the myths and stereotypes you have heard are based on fact?

One of the most common myths about dementia is that it is a consequence of ageing and that nothing can be done about it. In fact, while age is an important risk factor and about 20% of people over 80 have got dementia, it is not a part of the normal ageing process. And although there is no cure, there is a great deal of support and information for people with dementia and their carers, as well as drugs for the treatment of memory loss, mood disorders, behavioural problems, psychiatric problems and sleep disturbance.

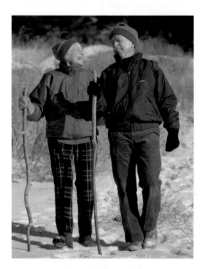

Figure 10.8 Normal ageing

Another common myth is that a poor memory is part of getting old. The truth is that mental processing does slow down as we get older, but wisdom increases, compensating for changes in speed and flexibility of thought, reasoning, making judgements and so on. Poor memory that interferes with everyday life is not normal at any age and should be investigated.

You may have heard that Alzheimer's runs in families. It does sometimes – there are some very rare cases, usually in younger people, that are known to be inherited and are passed on by a single gene. In these very rare cases, the probability that close family members will develop Alzheimer's disease is one in two. However, most cases of Alzheimer's disease are not inherited, although if you have a family history of the disease you are about three times more likely to develop it than someone where there is no family history.

Key term

A **gene** is the basic biological unit of inheritance.

Research & investigate

3.3 Running in the family

Investigate the family history of people you know who have dementia. Does there seem to be a family link? If you think there is, explain your reasoning.

There is talk that eating meat and food cooked in aluminium saucepans can increase the risk of developing Alzheimer's, but there is no convincing evidence that this is true. Similarly, there is no evidence to suggest that taking **HRT**, **Ginkgo biloba** or aspirin protects against dementia. However, research does tell us that a healthy lifestyle, especially one that protects against heart disease and stroke – a well-balanced diet, regular exercise and not smoking – reduces the chance of developing dementia.

www.alz.co.uk; www.alzheimers-research. org.uk

Key terms

HRT is an acronym for Hormone Replacement Therapy.
Ginkgo biloba is a herb used for its medicinal properties.

The stereotypes associated with dementia paint such a bleak picture that it is no surprise there is a stigma attached to the condition. 'It's as though that's it, you are dribbling and nodding, and that's Alzheimer's. That's the picture of Alzheimer's. But we are all sitting here talking perfectly normally. We have got Alzheimer's of some form, we are not nodding and dribbling.' (Person with dementia)

'Living well with dementia: A National Dementia Strategy', DH, 2009

Negative stereotypes and myths are due to a lack of public and professional awareness and understanding of dementia. Their effect is that many people with dementia and their carers are afraid to talk about what is happening, don't know that help is available, avoid getting help, don't get help quickly enough and are not diagnosed correctly. They face discrimination and become socially excluded.

 Evidence activity

(3.3) Myths and stereotypes related to dementia

This activity enables you to demonstrate your knowledge of how myths and stereotypes related to dementia may affect the individual and their carers.

Produce a poster for display in a public area that highlights various myths and stereotypes associated with dementia and describes why they are unfounded.

(3.4) Ways in which individuals and carers can be supported to overcome their fears

Myths, stereotypes, anecdotes of other people's negative experiences and a general lack of public and professional awareness and understanding of dementia can make people afraid of getting dementia, especially if they are in their later years and it seems to run in their family. In fact, people over 65 are more worried about developing dementia than cancer, heart disease or stroke. Additionally, people can be afraid that a loved one will develop the disease and worry about how they will cope with being a carer.

Dementia awareness campaigns aim to improve public and professional awareness and understanding of dementia. Some of these campaigns are targeted at specific groups of

people, such as children and young people as part of their Citizenship Education, and health and social care workers, including GPs, who lack the skills to identify and care for people with dementia. Not only do these campaigns raise awareness that dementia is a disease, is common and is not an inevitable consequence of ageing, they provide information on how to seek help and what help and treatment is available. They also tackle stigmas and misapprehensions by emphasising that:

■ someone with dementia is no less a person because they have dementia

■ dementia is not an immediate death sentence – there is life to be lived with dementia and it can be of a good quality

■ people with dementia can, and can continue to, make a positive contribution within their family and to their communities.

Dementia awareness campaigns encourage healthy lifestyles and promote health checks. They therefore focus on prevention rather than cure, which has a positive effect, helping people overcome their fears about developing the disease or caring for someone who has been diagnosed.

The media, for example film, TV and the press, have a role to play in helping people overcome their fears of dementia. They help run dementia awareness campaigns; they also give celebrities the opportunity to use their status to raise awareness and recognition of issues that are too often kept in the shadows. You have read about Terry Pratchett, who has helped enormously to raise awareness about dementia, what he called his 'embuggerance'. Monty Python star Terry Jones, Kylie Minogue and Anastacia have also used their celebrity profile to raise awareness of cancer and spur the general public into action.

Good-quality, personalised respite breaks can recharge batteries and empower people to face up to and overcome their fears. And support groups help dispel fear by giving people with dementia and their carers an opportunity to learn about the disease, swap stories and share positive experiences. Talking about the bad times can also be therapeutic – a problem shared is a problem halved.

'It was organised by various people from the Alzheimer's Society and carers, and they explained what kinds of dementia there were, and what happens, and how you can help it by healthy living and all this; it was really good.' (Carer)

'Today I have met people who are in very much the same boat as I am with things they can and can't do … so for me it's a relief, a bloody relief to find that there are other people in the same boat as me.' (Person with dementia)

'Living well with dementia: A National Dementia Strategy', DH, 2009

Evidence activity

(3.4) Supporting individuals and carers to overcome their fears

This activity enables you to demonstrate your knowledge of how individuals and carers can be supported to overcome their fears.

Research dementia awareness campaigns that are taking place locally and nationally, dementia care support groups, charitable organisations such as the Alzheimer's Society, care settings for people with dementia and so on. In what ways do campaigns and these organisations support people to overcome their fears about dementia?

Assessment summary

Your reading of this chapter and completion of the activities will have prepared you to demonstrate your learning and understanding of the process and experience of dementia. To achieve the unit, your assessor will require you to:

Learning outcomes	Assessment Criteria
Learning outcome **1**: Understand the neurology of dementia by:	**1.1** describing a range of causes of dementia syndrome. See Evidence activity 1.1, p. 185
	1.2 describing the types of memory impairment commonly experienced by individuals with dementia. See Evidence activity 1.2, p. 186
	1.3 explaining the way that individuals process information with reference to the abilities and limitations of individuals with dementia. See Evidence activity 1.3, p. 188
	1.4 explaining how other factors can cause changes in an individual's condition that may not be attributable to dementia. See Evidence activity 1.4, p. 189
	1.5 explaining why the abilities and needs of an individual with dementia may fluctuate. See Evidence activity 1.5, p. 189

Learning outcomes	Assessment Criteria
Learning outcome 2: Understand the impact of recognition and diagnosis of dementia by:	(2.1) describing the impact of early diagnosis and follow-up to diagnosis. See Evidence activity 2.1, p. 192
	(2.2) explaining the importance of recording possible signs or symptoms of dementia in an individual in line with agreed ways of working. See Evidence activity, 2.2 p. 193
	(2.3) explaining the process of reporting possible signs of dementia within agreed ways of working. See Evidence activity, 2.3 p. 193
	(2.4) describing the possible impact of receiving a diagnosis of dementia on • the individual • their family and friends. See Evidence activity 2.4, p. 194
Learning outcome 3: Understand how dementia care must be underpinned by a person-centred approach by:	(3.1) comparing a person-centred and a non-person-centred approach to dementia care. See Evidence activity 3.1, p. 196
	(3.2) describing a range of different techniques that can be used to meet the fluctuating abilities and needs of the individual with dementia. See Evidence activity 3.2, p. 197
	(3.3) describing how myths and stereotypes related to dementia may affect the individual and their carers. See Evidence activity 3.3, p. 199

Learning outcomes	Assessment Criteria
Learning outcome **3**: Understand how dementia care must be underpinned by a person-centred approach by:	(3.4) describing ways in which individuals and carers can be supported to overcome their fears. See Evidence activity 3.4, p. 200

Good luck!

Web links

BBC website – interactive brain map	www.bbc.co.uk/science/humanbody/body/
Alzheimer's Research Trust, Oxford University Report 2010	www.dementia2010.org
Educating and advocating for person-centred care	www.personcenteredcareadvocate.org
Alzheimer's Society	www.alzheimers.org.uk
Dementia UK	www.dementiauk.org
Lewy Body Dementia Association	www.lbda.org
Pick's Disease Support Group	www.pdsg.org.uk
Nursing Times	www.nursingtimes.net
Alzheimer's Research Trust	www.alzheimers-research.org.uk
Government website for public services	www.direct.gov.uk
Princess Royal Trust for Carers	www.carers.org
guardian.co.uk (newspaper)	www.guardian.co.uk
MailOnline (newspaper)	www.dailymail.co.uk
Alzheimer's Disease International	www.alz.co.uk

For Unit IC 01

What are you finding out?

Infection is caused by **pathogens**. Not all infectious diseases are transmissible but some, such as influenza, MRSA, *C. difficile* and norovirus have the potential to spread from one person to another. Understanding how pathogens behave and spread is crucial to their prevention and control.

Users of health and social care services are physically and emotionally vulnerable to infection. For example:

■   Influenza vaccination is recommended for all elderly people in the UK aged 65 and over, as well as people in at-risk groups, such as those suffering from respiratory problems like asthma and COPD (Chronic obstructive pulmonary disease)

■   During the year to March 2010, just over half of reported cases of MRSA (meticillin-resistant *Staphylococcus aureus*) and *C. difficile* (*Clostridium difficile*) in England and Wales were contracted by patients while in hospital.

■   In January 2010, norovirus, which thrives in schools, care homes and hospitals was claimed to have infected 500,000 victims per week, particularly elderly people and those with pre-existing health problems.

Infection prevention and control is therefore key to the work of health and social care employers and employees, who have a responsibility to comply with relevant legislation and regulatory and professional body standards. Health and social care employees also have a responsibility to understand the importance of infection control and risk assessment procedures, of personal protective equipment (PPE) and of maintaining good personal hygiene.

www.rcn.org.uk;
www.healthcarerepublic.com;
www.hpa.org.uk; www.dailymail.co.uk

The reading and activities in this chapter will help you to:

■   Understand roles and responsibilities in the prevention and control of infections

■   Understand legislation and policies relating to prevention and control of infections

■   Understand systems and procedures relating to the prevention and control of infections

■   Understand the importance of risk assessment in relation to the prevention and control of infections

■   Understand the importance of personal protective equipment (PPE) in the prevention and control of infections

■   Understand the importance of good personal hygiene in the prevention and control of infections.

Key term

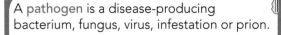

A pathogen is a disease-producing bacterium, fungus, virus, infestation or prion.

LO1 Roles and responsibilities in the prevention and control of infections

Many infectious diseases have the capacity to spread rapidly and with dire effects within health and social care settings. Infection is a major cause of illness and hospitalisation among people living in residential care homes, and healthcare-associated infections (HCAIs) may be serious, even life threatening. Many of these infections can worsen underlying medical conditions, and some HCAIs are resistant to antibiotics. For these reasons, both employers and employees have very clear roles and responsibilities in ensuring the prevention and control of infections.

Research & investigate

 Superbugs

According to www.bbc.co.uk, on 11 August 2010, a new superbug that is resistant to even the most powerful antibiotics has entered UK hospitals. Experts warn that it could produce dangerous infections that would spread rapidly from person to person and be almost impossible to treat.

Research the press and the internet for other superbugs that have threatened health around the world recently. In what ways have they affected the people you support?

Your roles and responsibilities in relation to the prevention and control of infection

As a health and social care worker you have roles and responsibilities in relation to infection prevention and control, including to:

■ cooperate with your employer in preventing and controlling infection

■ know and understand your organisation's infection prevention and control policies and procedures

■ follow infection control procedures and apply standard infection control principles to all situations all of the time

■ know how to get advice on the prevention and control of infection and to stay up to date in your knowledge and understanding of the subject

■ make your manager aware of any difficulties you have in following procedures

■ report breaches in good practice and take corrective action as appropriate.

You also have a responsibility to be on your guard for potential outbreaks of infection or resistance to antibiotics and to inform your employer if you have any concerns.

Some job roles have an overall responsibility for infection prevention and control, such as Infection Control Champion, Infection Control Lead and Infection Control Link Person. Staff in these positions have a particular interest and up-to-date knowledge and expertise in infection prevention and control. Because of their experience, they are role models and a source of information and advice for colleagues, delivering training and promoting and maintaining safe practice. They work with patients, their relatives and friends, providing information on infection prevention and control. They liaise with relevant health authorities, as appropriate, and their good communication skills enable them to influence and introduce any necessary changes in work practice.

Evidence activity

 Your roles and responsibilities regarding infection prevention and control

This activity gives you the opportunity to demonstrate your understanding of your roles and responsibilities in relation to the prevention and control of infection.

What are your roles and responsibilities in relation to infection prevention and control? Why is it important that you fulfil your roles and responsibilities in your work?

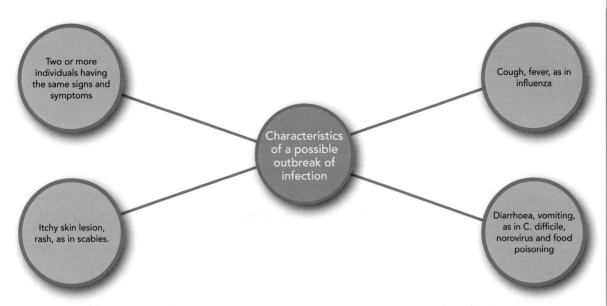

Figure 11.1 Characteristics of a possible outbreak of infection

1.2 Your employer's responsibilities in relation to the prevention and control of infection

Policies set out the arrangements that an organisation has for complying with legislation. Employers must have written policies describing the measures they take to prevent and control infection in order to uphold the law.

Procedures describe the activities that need to be carried out for policies to be implemented. Employers should have accessible (easily located, understandable, straightforward and manageable) infection prevention and control procedures that ensure a safe environment and safe working practices. They should also have a system for ensuring that you understand and follow those procedures. Failure of your employer to minimise the risk of infection and to protect you, your colleagues, the individuals you support and their family and friends against infectious disease constitutes neglect.

Employers have a responsibility to regularly produce infection prevention and control reports describing:

■ policies and procedures that are in place and how they are monitored

■ any outbreaks of infection that have taken place and the action taken to rectify problems

■ education and training that has taken place

■ planned improvements.

The purpose of infection prevention and control reports is to reduce infections and ensure improvements in infection prevention and control.

Employers have a responsibility to obtain and share with staff up-to-date advice and information about infection prevention and control from suitably qualified and competent individuals. People who can offer advice include the specialist job roles you read about earlier, general practitioners (GPs), Health Protection Nurses (HPNs), **Royal College of Nursing (RCN)** Nurse Advisers for Infection Prevention and Control, Community Infection Control Nurses (CICNs) and Environmental Health Practitioners (EHPs).

www.rcn.org.uk; www.cieh.org

Key term

The Royal College of Nursing (RCN) represents nurses and nursing, promotes excellence in practice and shapes health policies.
A Health Protection Unit (HPU) is a local centre of the Health Protection Agency (HPA).
Isolation nursing is the physical separation of an infected patient from others.

Employers have a responsibility to report suspected outbreaks of infection, changes in resistance to antibiotics and notifiable diseases to the local **Health Protection Unit (HPU)**. Typical characteristics of a notifiable disease include:

- it is potentially life threatening

- it spreads rapidly

- it cannot be easily treated or cured, for example there is no vaccine or antibiotics available.

Note: At the time of writing (July 2010), the HPA, which has responsibility for dealing with public health issues such as infectious diseases, is to transfer its workload to the Secretary of State for Health.

www.hpa.org.uk

Employers have a responsibility to ensure that people with infectious disease are nursed in **isolation**.

Notifiable diseases

Acute encephalitis, acute poliomyelitis, anthrax, cholera, diphtheria, ,dysentery (amoebic or bacillary), food poisoning, leprosy, leptospirosis, malaria, measles, meningitis, meningococcal septicaemia (without meningitis), mumps, ophthalmia neonatorum, plague, paratyphoid fever, relapsing fever, rabies, rubella, smallpox, scarlet fever, typhus, tetanus, tuberculosis, typhoid fever, viral haemorrhagic fevers, viral hepatitis, whooping cough and yellow fever.

Employers also have a responsibility to ensure that their staff are immunised against infectious disease; that they receive ongoing training in the prevention and control of infection; and that their personal development plan shows what

training they have completed and what they need to do.

Infection Control Guidance for Care Homes, DH, 2006

Time to reflect

 1.2 Immunisation

What diseases are you immunised against? Are your immunisations up to date? What could happen if you failed to be immunised properly?

Evidence activity

 1.2 Employers' roles and responsibilities regarding infection prevention and control

This activity gives you the opportunity to demonstrate your understanding of your employer's roles and responsibilities in relation to the prevention and control of infection.

What are your employer's responsibilities in relation to infection prevention and control? Why is it important that your employer fulfils these responsibilities?

LO2 Legislation and policies relating to prevention and control of infections

2.1 Current legislation and regulatory body standards that are relevant to the prevention and control of infection

Table 11.1 Legislation relevant to infection prevention and control

Legislation	Purpose of the legislation
Health and Safety at Work *etc.* Act (HASWA) 1974	Ensures the health and safety of everyone who may be affected by work activities.
Management of Health and Safety at Work Regulations (MHSWR) 1999	Require employers and managers to carry out risk assessments to eliminate or minimise risks to health and safety, including from pathogens.

Legislation	Purpose of the legislation
Personal Protective Equipment at Work Regulations (PPE) 1992	Minimise the risks to health and safety associated with **cross-infection**.
The Health Act 2006	Aims to prevent and control healthcare-associated infections (HCAIs).
The Health and Social Care Act 2008	Aims to protect public health by preventing and controlling the spread of infectious diseases.
Reporting of Injuries, Diseases and Dangerous Occurrences Regulations (RIDDOR) 1995.	Require that certain work-related injuries, diseases and dangerous occurrences are reported to the HSE or local authority.
Public Health (Control of Disease) Act 1984 and The Public Health (Infectious Diseases) Regulations 1988	Require that outbreaks of infection, changes in resistance to antibiotics and notifiable diseases are reported to the HPU so that they can be managed to prevent their spread.
Food Safety Act 1990 and the Food Hygiene Regulations 2006	Minimise the risks to health and safety associated with food handling.
Control of Substances Hazardous to Health Regulations (COSHH) 2002	Minimise the risks to health and safety from the use of hazardous substances, including pathogens.
Hazardous Waste Regulations 2005	Require that waste is dealt with so as to avoid putting health at risk.
Environmental Protection (Duty of Care) Regulations 1991	Require that waste, including contaminated waste, is properly stored and adequately packaged while awaiting removal from the premises.

Key term

Cross-infection is the spread of pathogens from one person, object, place or part of the body to another.

Regulatory bodies are organisations set up by the Government to establish national standards for qualifications and best practice and to ensure that the standards are consistently observed. They include:

■ The Care Quality Commission in England, which regulates health and social care provided by the NHS, local authorities, private companies and voluntary organisations. Its standards of quality and care state that people can expect to be cared for in a clean environment where they are protected from infection.

www.cqc.org.uk

■ The General Social Care Council in England, Care Council for Wales, Scottish Care Council and Northern Ireland Social Care Council. Their codes of practice dictate the standards of practice and conduct that social care workers and employers should meet, which includes protecting individuals from danger or harm.

www.gscc.org.uk; www.ccwales.org.uk; www.sssc.uk.com; www.niscc.info

■ The GMC (General Medical Council), whose guides and strategies for improvement shape the role of healthcare professionals with regard to infection prevention and control.

http://www.gmc-uk.org

■ The Nursing and Midwifery Council (NMC), whose code or 'Standards of conduct, performance and ethics for nurses and midwives' is a key tool in protecting and promoting health and well-being, requiring nurses and midwives to manage risks, including risk of infection.

www.nmc-uk.org

■ The Health Professions Council (HPC), whose 'Standards of Conduct, Performance & Ethics' require **allied health professionals** to deal safely with risk of infection by taking precautions to protect everyone, including themselves, from cross-infection.

www.hpc-uk.org

Key term

Allied health professionals are clinical healthcare professionals as distinct from medicine, dentistry and nursing, who work in a healthcare team to make the healthcare system function.

Competence is to do with having knowledge, understanding and capability.

■ The Office for Standards in Education, Children's Services and Skills (Ofsted), which regulates and inspects care service provision for children and young people. For a care provider to meet Ofsted's standards and regulations, it has to demonstrate that children and young people are not at risk from cross-infection because of low standards of hygiene.

www.ofsted.gov.uk

Some occupations are not covered by regulatory standards or codes of practice, for example health care assistants in England and Wales. Instead, national occupational standards (NOS) set out the **competences** that apply to their job roles and level of experience. NOS for workers in the health and social care sectors are written by the Children's Workforce Development Council (CWDC), Skills for Health and Skills for Care.

www.cwdcouncil.org.uk;
www.skillsforhealth.org.uk;
www.skillsforcare.org.uk

Evidence activity

(2.1) Legislation and regulatory body standards

This activity gives you the opportunity to demonstrate your knowledge of current legislation and regulatory body standards that are relevant to the prevention and control of infection.

Summarise the Acts and Regulations, regulatory body standards and national occupational standards that are relevant to your responsibilities in relation to infection prevention and control.

(2.2) Local and organisational policies relevant to the prevention and control of infection

You read earlier that policies set out the arrangements an organisation has for complying with legislation. Infection prevention and control policies describe the measures that organisations take to comply with the legislation listed in Table 11.1.

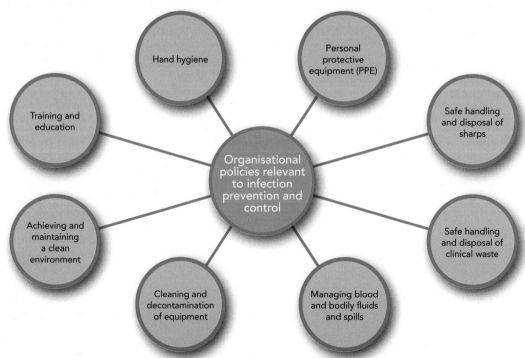

Figure 11.2 Organisational policies relevant to infection prevention and control

Local authorities and health trusts produce **evidence-based policies** that guide health and social care settings within their districts and regions to comply with legislation while taking account of local needs. National initiatives and campaigns also help shape how local health and social care providers can minimise and prevent the spread of infection. For example, the RCN 'Wipe it out' campaign is aimed at reducing the **prevalence** of HCAIs, as are its booklets 'Good practice in infection prevention' and 'Guidance on Uniforms and Work Wear'.

Key terms

Evidence-based policies are policies that have been proved to work.
Prevalence is the proportion of individuals in a population having a disease.

The Department of Health has produced a number of documents addressing infection prevention and control at a local level, such as:

■ 'Essential Steps to Safe Clean Care: Reducing Healthcare Associated Infections', which guides local health and social care providers in the use of best practice to prevent and manage the spread of infections

■ 'A Matron's Charter: An Action Plan for Cleaner Hospitals', which explains how staff, patients and visitors can make their local hospital a cleaner, safer place

■ 'Infection Control Guidance for Care Homes', which describes how everyone involved in providing residential care can protect residents and staff from acquiring infections.

The Health Protection Agency provides support and advice to, for example, local authorities and health and emergency services. Its 'Guidance on infection control in schools and other childcare settings' describes the importance of immunisation, personal hygiene and a clean environment.

Evidence activity

(2.2) Local and organisational policies

This activity gives you the opportunity to demonstrate your knowledge of local and organisational policies relevant to the prevention and control of infection.

1. Describe infection prevention and control policies written for your workplace. What is the purpose of each?

2. Describe infection prevention and control policies written for health and social care organisations in your locality. Which organisations produced them? Why was it necessary for them to be produced?

LO3 Systems and procedures relating to the prevention and control of infections

(3.1) Procedures and systems relevant to the prevention and control of infection

While policies set out the arrangements an organisation has in place for complying with legislation, procedures describe the activities or practices that need to be carried out for policies to be implemented. Figure 11.3 introduced you to a range of policies that are relevant to infection prevention and control. You will read more about hand hygiene and PPE shortly, but the following checklist summarises routine safe practices or **standard precautions** that protect not only the individuals you work with but also you and your colleagues. Note that the checklists are not a substitute for your workplace's procedures.

Key term

Standard precautions are based upon a set of principles designed to minimise exposure to and transmission of a wide variety of micro-organisms.

Safe handling and disposal of sharps, for example needles, scalpels, stitch cutters and glass ampoules

■ Do not attempt to handle or dispose of sharps until you have had the appropriate training.

■ Keep handling to a minimum and do not pass directly from hand to hand.

■ Never re-sheath needles and do not use needles that are broken or bent.

■ Do not dismantle syringes or needles – dispose of them as a single unit.

■ Dispose of sharps in the designated container at the point of use, i.e. where you are working.

■ Do not fill containers more than two-thirds full and store them in an area away from the public.

Safe handling and disposal of clinical waste

Clinical waste is any waste that poses a threat of infection, for example, body fluids, such as blood; body waste, such as urine, faeces, vomit; soiled swabs, dressings, clothing and bed linen; sharps. Safe handling and disposal of clinical waste requires that you:

■ have had the appropriate training

■ wear appropriate PPE and maintain good hand hygiene

■ dispose of body fluids and waste down the sluice, or bag as follows:

■ yellow bag – infected waste and used swabs and dressings, to be incinerated

■ clear alginate bag inside a red plastic bag – soiled and infected clothing and linen, to be laundered

■ report any dangerous handling and disposal of clinical waste to your manager.

Managing blood, body fluids and spills

Do not attempt to clean up spills or collect and handle specimens until you have had the appropriate training.

Spills

■ Wear appropriate PPE.

■ Clean up as soon as you can, using cleaning materials and disinfectants that are appropriate to the type of spill and the surface that has been spilled on.

Collecting and handling specimens

■ Wear appropriate PPE.

■ Make sure containers are suitable, sterile and leak-proof.

■ Label containers with relevant information and complete any accompanying forms.

■ Send specimens to the lab as soon as possible – never leave them lying around.

■ Enter test results into patient records as soon as you receive them and highlight any abnormal results to the appropriate person.

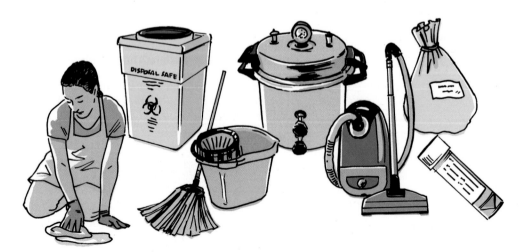

Figure 11.3 Standard precautions

Decontamination of equipment

Do not attempt to use decontamination techniques and equipment until you have had the appropriate training. Always follow manufacturer's instructions and do not use any equipment if you are not confident that it has been installed and maintained properly.

Single-use equipment, for example nebulisers and disposable catheters, should not be decontaminated and re-used. Dispose of them as appropriate. Re-usable equipment, such as bed pans and surgical instruments, must be decontaminated before re-use through a process of cleaning and disinfection or cleaning and sterilisation.

Key term

Single-use equipment is items that can only be used once.

■ Cleaning, using hot water and detergent, removes visible contamination but may not destroy pathogens. It is suitable for environmental cleaning.

■ Disinfection uses chemicals or heat and reduces the number of **viable** pathogens. Washer-disinfectors and ultrasonic baths use very high temperatures to disinfect equipment that would be damaged by chemicals. Chemicals, such as formaldehyde and peroxide, are used when heat is insufficient.

■ Sterilisation ensures that an object is totally free from pathogens. You may have access to a sterile services department (SSD), or you could use a bench-top vacuum steam steriliser.

Key terms

Mucous membranes are mucous-secreting membranes lining the body cavities and canals that connect with the external air, such as the alimentary canal and respiratory tract. Viable means alive and able to reproduce.

Achieving and maintaining a clean environment

A dirty environment holds a risk of infection. Dust and dirt, body fluids and waste, and household waste such as leftover food, provide conditions that support the growth and reproduction of a variety of pathogens. Health and social care settings should therefore have:

■ fixed schedules for thorough cleaning of all areas, using properly maintained cleaning equipment that is appropriate to the surface being cleaned

■ appropriate and clean facilities for the disposal of non-clinical, household waste.

Time to reflect

 3.1 Training

What training have you had in relation to infection prevention and control? How does training- or the lack of it, impact on your work?

Training

All health and social care professionals should be trained in infection prevention and control, as part of their induction and on an ongoing basis to maintain and update their knowledge and skills. Training should cover the principles of infection prevention and control, including:

■ relevant legislation

■ policies and procedures, including standard precautions

■ roles and responsibilities

■ risk assessment

■ use of PPE

■ environmental and personal hygiene, including hand washing and skin care.

Evidence activity

 3.1 Procedures and systems for the prevention and control of infection

This activity gives you the opportunity to demonstrate your knowledge of procedures and systems relevant to the prevention and control of infection.

Describe infection prevention and control procedures or standard precautions that:

■ you are required to follow in your work

■ a colleague, who has a different job role from you, has to follow in their work.

3.2 The potential impact of an outbreak of infection on the individual and the organisation

Minor outbreaks of infection are characterised by close neighbours, for example in a ward, classroom or adjacent rooms in a residential care home, developing similar signs and symptoms over a period of days or weeks. They are usually easily managed. A serious outbreak is characterised by 20 or more people throughout a health or social care setting developing signs and symptoms within 24 hours. Serious outbreaks are dealt with using serious outbreak procedures.

It is important to recognise potential outbreaks promptly so that prevention and control measures can be put in place as soon as possible. You read about the characteristics of a possible outbreak earlier. It is also important to report suspicions of or an actual outbreak without delay to the individual who has responsibility for managing infection control.

When a suspected outbreak has been reported, the individual or team responsible for managing infection will assess the situation and decide what action to take. This could include:

■ isolating the individual or group of people, including staff, who are infected and restricting staff movement in order to minimise exposure to the source of infection

■ ensuring that staff who are exposed to the infection use appropriate PPE and have a sufficient supply of alcohol gel

■ ensuring that appropriate antibiotics are available

■ restricting visiting or closing the affected ward, department or setting

■ informing the local HPU if the infection is a notifiable disease

■ keeping relatives and friends informed

■ employing additional staff, as cover for those who are sick or whose time is devoted to isolation nursing.

When the outbreak has been controlled, the environment and any equipment used during the outbreak should be thoroughly decontaminated and an audit carried out to check:

■ the effectiveness of infection prevention and control procedures

■ whether staff are following procedures to the letter

■ whether there are any barriers to following procedures, for example time constraints, staff shortages and lack of resources

■ the need for further training.

It is also important to assess how patients felt the situation was dealt with. Isolation nursing and the removal of familiar objects and routines can create feelings of isolation, loneliness, depression and boredom; and disruption to routine can be stressful. There can be a stigma attached to having an infectious disease, for example, the fervent use of infection control measures can make people feel dirty or 'unclean' and that their disease will affect the attitudes of staff. And having a diagnosis sign on the door compromises their confidentiality, even though staff have a duty of care to protect others from exposure to the infection.

Patients need to be encouraged to talk about their experiences of being in isolation so that strategies can be put into place for the future. And they and their relatives, who are understandably anxious, need to be given information to help them to understand the need for the measures that are being taken.

The impact of an outbreak of infection on an organisation can also be significant. For example:

■ Hospital-based infections such as *C. difficile* and MRSA are the focus of huge amounts of attention from the media, impacting on the reputation of the hospitals concerned and the morale of staff.

■ Having to buy in additional resources, such as staff, impacts on finances.

■ Discontinuity of care due to using agency staff affects the emotional well-being of patients.

■ Additional work involved in dealing with an outbreak of infection is time consuming and can jeopardise job satisfaction and the day-to-day running of the organisation.

Evidence activity

3.2 Potential impact of an outbreak of infection

This activity gives you the opportunity to demonstrate your understanding of the potential impact of an outbreak of infection on the individual and the organisation.

Talk with your manager about an outbreak of infection at your workplace. How was the outbreak dealt with? How did it affect people and the organisation? Why did it have those effects? What steps were taken subsequent to the outbreak? Has there been a further outbreak of the same infection? If so, why?

LO4 The importance of risk assessment in relation to the prevention and control of infections

 ## What is meant by 'risk'?

A hazard is anything with the potential to cause harm, and a risk is the likelihood that a **hazard** will cause harm. For example, a broken paving stone is a hazard – it has the potential to cause someone to trip, fall and break a leg. But the likelihood or risk of this happening depends on factors such as age and ability. An able-bodied child is less likely to fall and break a bone than a frail older person or an adult with visual impairment.

The expression 'at-risk group' is used to describe a group of people who have a higher-than-average risk of being harmed by hazards, for example because of their age, lifestyle, existing health status and genetic inheritance.

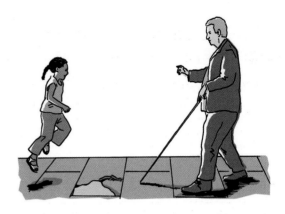

Figure 11.4 Hazards and degree of risk

Evidence activity

 ### Define the term risk

This activity gives you the opportunity to demonstrate your knowledge of the definition of 'risk'.

In your own words, explain what is meant by the term 'risk'.

Case Study

 ### Care in the community?

Cum-a-Cropper Community Centre is situated on a busy main road. It is an old house on three floors and the front door opens straight onto the pavement. Its ground floor kitchen/dining room, which is open plan and freely accessible, is much in need of a makeover, as are the two toilets, both on the second floor, neither of which has adequate disabled facilities. There is a lounge on the first floor and a TV and games room on the second floor. The garden is grassed.

The community centre is used by groups of children, young people, mothers and toddlers, elderly people, and people with learning and physical difficulties, including sensory impairments.

What hazards can you identify at Cum-a-Cropper Community Centre? How does the risk to health and safety vary within the different groups of people using the centre?

 ## The potential risks of infection within the workplace

Infection can occur anywhere where pathogens are present. Failure to prevent pathogens being brought into health and social care settings, for example by patients, staff and visitors, and to control outbreaks of infection once they have established, can have dire effects on vulnerable, at-risk groups.

HCAIs

HCAIs are infections acquired in hospital or brought into hospital by people already infected. They include:

■ MRSA (Meticillin-resistant *Staphylococcus aureus*), a bacterium that is resistant to the antibiotic meticillin. Many of us carry *Staph aureus* (SA) on our skin without developing an infection, but if it enters the body, it can cause blood poisoning and infections such as boils, abscesses and impetigo. It is spread by direct contact with infected patients and also indirectly, by touching contaminated sheets, towels, clothes and dressings. At-risk groups include people who take frequent courses of

Table 11.2 Routes of the spread of infection

Main route of spread of infection	Examples of pathogenic infections
Skin. Direct contact is skin-to-skin contact between two people. Indirect contact is touching things that another person has used and contaminated.	Bacterial infections such as MRSA and *C. difficile*; infestations such as lice; and fungal infections such as ringworm.
Airways (inhalation).	Bacterial and viral infections such as influenza, pneumonia, bronchitis and tetanus.
Digestive tract, when consuming food and drink.	Bacterial and viral infections such as *E. coli*, Salmonella, rotavirus and norovirus.
Use of health care instruments, such as sharps.	Viral infections such as HIV AIDS and Hepatitis B.

antibiotics, are already in poor health, have an open wound or skin condition such as psoriasis, or have an in-dwelling device such as a **catheter** or intravenous drip.

> ## Key term
>
> A catheter is a plastic tube inserted into the body to drain fluid.

■ *Clostridium difficile* (*C. difficile*), a bacteria present in the large bowel that does not usually cause problems in healthy people. It is spread in the same way as MRSA, but contaminated surfaces are more likely to be bedpans and toilets. Symptoms include stomach ache, diarrhoea, inflammation and bleeding of the bowel, blood poisoning and fever. It can also be fatal. At-risk groups include elderly people and people in hospital, particularly if they are taking antibiotics, which destroy the bacteria that prevent *C. difficile* causing problems.

Head lice

The head louse is a tiny, wingless parasitic insect that lives among human hairs and feeds on blood from the scalp. They are very common and their bites cause the scalp to itch, which, if scratched, can become infected. While they cannot fly or jump, lice have claws that allow them to cling firmly to hair. They spread mainly through head-to-head contact, but also indirectly when clothing and hair equipment are shared. At-risk groups are people who have close contact, especially children.

Ringworm

Ringworm is caused by the dermatophyte fungus that lives on dead skin, hair and nails. When it affects the skin between the toes, it is known as athlete's foot, and appears as red, scaly patches. Ringworm of the scalp starts as a small sore that becomes scaly, causing hair to fall out or break into stubbles. Ringworm of the nails causes them to become thick, discoloured and brittle. It is spread directly and indirectly, for example from damp clothing and wet floors and surfaces. At-risk groups include people who use changing room facilities and swimming pools, and people in hospitals and residential care who share bathrooms.

Influenza

Influenza is a highly infectious illness caused by a flu virus. It infects the respiratory system, causing fever, aches and pains, a dry cough, nausea and loss of appetite. Like the common cold, it is spread by inhaling small droplets of virus-containing saliva that are coughed or sneezed into the air by an infected person. It is also spread by indirect contact, for example when an infected person touches surfaces, such as door handles, with unwashed hands. At-risk groups include elderly people and people with weak immune systems, such as cancer and AIDS patients.

Time to reflect

 Infections

Think about the infections you have had from time to time. What caused them? Why do you think you caught them? How did they affect you? How could you avoid catching them again?

Pneumonia and bronchitis

Pneumonia is a bacterial or viral infection of the lung tissue, and bronchitis is a bacterial infection of the **bronchi**. They are spread in the same way as influenza and can occur together as broncho-pneumonia. Symptoms include aches and pains, fever, chest pain, cough, breathlessness, and yellow/green, sometimes bloodstained sputum. At-risk groups include people who are frail and elderly and already in poor health, for example with a chest disease. Pneumonia is a common cause of death in people who are already in poor health, for example, people in the late or terminal stages of a cancer.

> ### Key term
>
> Bronchi are the large airways that carry air from the trachea into the lungs.

Tetanus

Tetanus is caused by the bacterium *Clostridium tetani*, which is found in soil and animal manure. If the bacterial **spores** get into a wound they release a toxin that attacks the nervous system and causes problems such as muscle spasm, as in lockjaw. At-risk groups include people who work with soil and animal manure, children playing outdoors, and people in health and social care settings where cleanliness is not maintained.

> ### Key term
>
> A spore is a temporary, dormant structure into which a bacterium changes when conditions for its survival become hazardous.

Food poisoning

Food poisoning is caused by poor standards of personal hygiene, poor hygiene in food storage, preparation and eating areas, and incorrect storage and cooking temperatures. Food poisoning bacteria include *Escherichia coli* (*E. coli*) and Salmonella, and viruses such as rotavirus and norovirus. In addition to growing and reproducing in food, they are carried by people on their bodies and clothes; by animals in their urine and faeces; and on kitchen surfaces and equipment. Signs and symptoms include nausea, stomach ache, diarrhoea and vomiting, and at-risk groups include babies, children, elderly people and people with pre-existing health problems.

Hepatitis B

Hepatitis B is a highly infectious virus that damages the liver. It is 50 to 100 times more infectious than HIV (Human Immunodeficiency Virus) and, like HIV, is carried in body fluids such as blood, saliva, semen and vaginal fluid. At-risk groups are drug users who use contaminated needles, patients exposed to contaminated equipment and blood, for example during transfusions, and people who have unprotected sex. Hep B is also an important complication of accidental **needle stick injuries** and therefore a risk factor for unvaccinated healthcare and body art workers.

www.patient.co.uk; www.nhs.uk; http://kidshealth.org; www.bupa.co.uk; www.bbc.co.uk

> ### Key term
>
> A needle stick injury is a skin puncture by a hypodermic needle or other sharp object.

Evidence activity

 Potential risks of infection within the workplace

This activity gives you the opportunity to demonstrate your knowledge of the potential risks of infection within your workplace.

Bearing in mind the type of setting in which you work, the care that is provided and the characteristics of the people you support, for example their age, lifestyle and existing health status, outline potential risks of infection within your workplace.

 ## Carrying out a risk assessment

The Management of Health and Safety at Work Regulations (MHSWR) 1999 require your employer to carry out risk assessments to eliminate or minimise any risks associated with infection. And because you have a responsibility to cooperate with your employer's or manager's efforts to improve health and safety, you should be thinking 'risk assessment' as you carry out each and every activity.

Time to reflect

(4.3) Risk assess or risk averse?

Do you think 'risk assessment' as you carry out your activities? Or are you blind to things that could go wrong? Can you see the benefit of being on the alert for potential hazards and associated risks?

According to the HSE, there are five steps to a risk assessment. In relation to the prevention and control of infections:

Step 1: Identify hazards

■ Inspect the cleanliness and hygiene of people, equipment and the working environment.

■ Check that facilities for maintaining cleanliness and hygiene are in good repair.

■ Check that infection prevention and control procedures are understood and followed to the letter.

■ Check that systems are in place for monitoring the use of procedures, educating everyone concerned about the importance of following procedures and supervising them to ensure that they put their learning into practice.

■ Review records relating to infectious outbreaks to check that they are appropriately dealt with.

Step 2: Decide who might be harmed and how

Harm in this scenario is exposure to and the consequences of infection; and the people who might be harmed are the people you support, you, your colleagues and any visitors.

Step 3: Assess or evaluate the risks

Assess or evaluate the risks arising from the hazards and decide whether the existing precautions are adequate or if more should be done. If something needs to be done, take steps to eliminate or control the risks.

As you know, a hazard is anything with the potential to cause harm, but the risk that it will cause harm depends on a variety of factors, including age, ability, health status and so on. However, because of the vulnerability of the people you support, the physical proximity that you share with them and the fact that the setting where you work is accessed by the visiting public, the chances are that all the hazards you

identify could have dire consequences for the health of everyone concerned.

Are existing precautions adequate? Can you eliminate the hazards? Can you control associated risks?

Step 4: Record the findings and say how the risks can be controlled to prevent harm

Inform everyone about the outcome of the risk assessment, as everyone will be involved in controlling the risk.

It is very important to let everyone know the upshot of your risk assessment. Risks will remain unless you let people know how they must adapt their work practices.

Step 5: Review the assessment from time to time and revise it if necessary

Review is similarly important. Unless you review the effect of changes to work practices, you won't know if they are working! Also, you may have been asked to use new equipment, materials and procedures, which could lead to new hazards. So do not be afraid to suggest further changes if necessary. While you do not want to continually re-invent the wheel, there is an argument for never standing still, that things can only get better!

www.hse.gov.uk

Evidence activity

(4.3) Carrying out a risk assessment

This activity gives you the opportunity to demonstrate your knowledge of the process of carrying out a risk assessment.

1. Identify an infection hazard, for example, that colleagues aren't washing their hands as often as they should.

2. Who might be harmed and how?

3. What are the risks to health caused by the hazard? What can be done to eliminate or control these risks?

4. How could you make people aware of changes that need to be made to eliminate or control the risks?

5. When do you think you should review the effectiveness of the changes?

The importance of carrying out a risk assessment

Managing the risk of infection by carrying out a risk assessment helps to maintain your health and that of the people you support, your colleagues and members of the public. Because ill health harms lives, you have a moral obligation to help manage risk. It also harms the reputation and financial standing of an organisation, which in turn would affect your employment status. In addition, there is a legal requirement to carry out risk assessments.

A risk assessment should also alert you to your standard of work practice, and whether you are enacting your duty of care to the health of everyone affected by your actions, including yourself.

www.hse.gov.uk

 Evidence activity

(4.4) Explain the importance of carrying out a risk assessment

This activity gives you the opportunity to demonstrate your understanding of the importance of carrying out a risk assessment.

Identify a couple of activities that you carry out and that have been risk assessed, for example, preparing food and helping someone use the toilet. Why do you think these activities have been risk assessed? Why is it important that you follow procedures for these activities to the letter?

LO5 The importance of using personal protective equipment (PPE) in the prevention and control of infections

(5.1) Demonstrate correct use of PPE

PPE is equipment that is intended for use by workers to protect them against risks to their health or safety. It must be used wherever there are risks to health and safety that cannot be adequately controlled in other ways. It must come with instructions on how to use it safely, and people who use it must be trained in its use and supervised to make sure they use it correctly.

Section 5.7 describes the correct practice in putting on and taking off PPE; and Section 5.8 describes the correct procedure for its disposal.

 Practice activity

(5.1) Correct use of PPE

This activity gives you the opportunity to practise using PPE correctly.

Ask an experienced colleague to observe you using PPE, including putting it on, taking it off and its disposal. Are you both confident that you use it correctly?

(5.2) & (5.3) Different types of PPE & The reasons for using PPE

There are different types of PPE, each helping prevent the spread of pathogens from one person, object, place or part of the body to another.

Body protection

Some procedures involve contact with blood, body fluids and waste. If there is a risk of extensive splashing to your skin and clothing, you should wear a full-body fluid-repellent gown. If splashing would be restricted to your trunk area, or you are carrying out procedures that involve contact with skin lesions and mucous membranes, a disposable, single-use apron is more suitable.

You should also wear a disposable apron if you are handling food, cleaning, making beds, disposing of waste and decontaminating equipment. Do not wear an apron all the time, 'just in case', but do wear one where there is a possibility of risk, not just to protect you against any potential infection but also to protect others against any pathogens you may be harbouring in your clothes.

Face protection

Some cleaning materials cause breathing problems, such as asthma. Dirt and dust, which may contain bacterial spores, can be inhaled during cleaning. And, as you know, some infections are caught by inhaling the small droplets coughed or sneezed into the air by an infected person. To protect your airways and lungs against inhalation hazards, use PPE that covers your nose and mouth, such as a face mask or disposable filtering face piece.

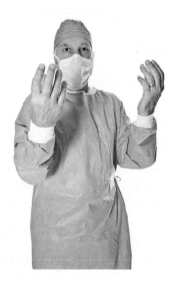

Figure 11.6 PPE

Eye protection

Activities that require you to work with chemicals, body fluids and waste are splash hazards. Wear PPE, such as visors and safety goggles, to protect your eyes.

Gloves

Single-use, disposable gloves are absolutely vital for protecting you and the people you work with against infection. You should use them for all procedures that involve contact with:

■ people suspected or known to have an infection

■ anything that may have been touched or used by someone who has an infection

■ body fluids and waste, including soiled linen and clothing

■ skin lesions and mucous membranes

■ sterile instruments

■ hazardous chemicals.

  Evidence activity

5.2 & 5.3 Different types of PPE and the reasons for their use

This activity gives you the opportunity to demonstrate your knowledge and understanding of types and use of PPE.

Complete the following table to show that you know when to use PPE, what PPE to use and why you should use it.

Items of PPE	When I wear it	Why I must wear it

5.4 & 5.6 Current regulations and legislation relevant to PPE & Your employers' responsibilities regarding the use of PPE

Relevant legislation and regulations	Responsibilities of your employer
Personal Protective Equipment at Work Regulations (PPE) 1992	To provide you with PPE that: • is appropriate and suitable • is maintained and stored properly • has instructions on how to use it safely • you can use correctly.
Health and Safety at Work, etc. Act (HASWA) 1974	To write health and safety policies and procedures regarding the use of PPE and make you aware of them.
Management of Health and Safety at Work Regulations 1999	To carry out risk assessments to eliminate or reduce risks to health and safety, including using PPE, and provide you with clear information, supervision and training in how to use PPE.
Provision and Use of Work Equipment Regulations (PUWER) 1998	To make sure suitable replacement PPE is always readily available and that it is well looked after and properly stored when not being used, for example in a dry, clean cupboard, or its box or case.
Control of Substances Hazardous to Health Regulations (COSHH) 2002	To carry out risk assessments on activities that involve exposure to hazardous substances and write procedures for their correct and safe use, including using PPE.
Health and Social Care Act (2008)	To make sure PPE is clean and fit for purpose, to minimise the risk of HCAIs.
Department of Health (2004) Standards for better health (England only)	To maintain the safety of patients, staff and visitors by having systems that ensure a reduced risk of infection for patients, including using PPE.
Food Safety Act 1990 and the Food Hygiene Regulations 2006.	To make sure that food safety hazards are controlled, including using PPE.
Hazardous Waste Regulations 2005	To make sure that hazardous waste, including used PPE, is dealt with so as to avoid putting health at risk.
Environmental Protection (Duty of Care) Regulations 1991.	To make sure that waste, including used PPE, is properly stored and adequately packaged while awaiting removal from the premises.

Evidence activity

5.4 & 5.6 Regulations and legislation relevant to PPE and employers' responsibilities

This activity gives you the opportunity to demonstrate your knowledge of current regulations and legislation relevant to PPE and of your employer's responsibilities regarding the use of PPE.

Make a list of the Regulations and Acts of Parliament that are relevant to your work with regard to infection prevention and control, and describe how this legislation affects your employer's responsibilities regarding the use of PPE.

5.5 Your responsibilities regarding the use of PPE

The Health and Safety at Work, *etc.* Act 1974 states that it is your duty while at work to take reasonable care of yourself and anyone else who may be affected by your actions. In relation to prevention and control of infection, this means knowing:

■ what PPE to use, when and how to use it and why

■ the correct procedures for putting it on and taking it off

■ appropriate decontamination and disposal methods.

You also have a responsibility to cooperate with your employer in relation to health and safety issues. This means:

■ following procedures and complying with requests to use PPE – in some jobs, failure to use PPE properly can be grounds for disciplinary action, even dismissal; however, you can refuse to wear PPE if it puts your safety at risk, for example if it is the wrong size or you might be at risk because of poor fit

■ making sure you get proper training regarding the use of PPE

■ raising concerns when you feel that PPE isn't being used appropriately

■ suggesting changes in its use that you think would be beneficial.

www.direct.gov.uk

'A Short Guide to the Personal Protective Equipment at Work Regulations 1992', HSE 2005

 Research & investigate

5.5 Responsibilities

Find out what could happen if you failed to:

- comply with requests to wear PPE
- attend training in the use of PPE
- raise concerns that PPE wasn't being used appropriately.

 Evidence activity

5.5 Your responsibilities regarding the use of PPE

This activity gives you the opportunity to demonstrate your knowledge of your responsibilities regarding the use of PPE.

Describe your responsibilities with regard to the use of PPE.

5.7 Correct practice in the application and removal of PPE

It is important that you know the correct procedure for putting on and removing a range of PPE.

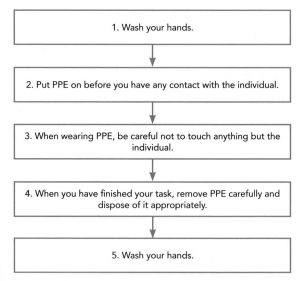

Figure 11.7 Five key points about the use of PPE

If you need to wear a gown, put that on first. Choose the appropriate gown for the task and the right size for you. The opening should be at the back and it should be secured at the neck and waist.

Face protection goes on next. Some masks are fastened with ties, others with elastic. If yours has ties, place it over your mouth, nose and chin and tie the upper set at the back of your head and the lower set at the base of your head/top of your neck. If it has elastic head bands, separate the two bands, hold the mask over your nose, mouth and chin, then stretch the lower band round the base of your head/top of your neck and the upper band round the upper back of your head. Adjust to fit.

Eye protection is third to go on. Position goggles or a visor over your eyes and secure them to your head using the ear pieces or head band. Adjust to fit.

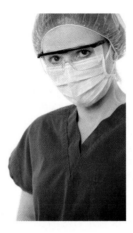

Figure 11.8 Face and eye protection

Gloves are last to go on. Choose the type needed for the task in the size that fits you best. Insert your hands and adjust for comfort and so that you do not feel restricted. If you are wearing a gown, tuck the cuffs under each glove to provide a continuous barrier protection for your skin.

When wearing PPE, safe work practice dictates that you:

■ do not touch or adjust your PPE while working

■ do not touch anything with contaminated gloves

■ take your gloves off if they get torn, and wash your hands before putting on a new pair.

At the end of an activity, the outside of anything on your front and arms is considered to be contaminated. Clean areas are inside the gloves and gown, the back of the gown and apron, and the ties and elastic of face and eye protection.

As gloves are the most contaminated items of PPE, they are taken off first. Using a gloved hand, grasp the outside of the opposite glove near the wrist and peel the glove away from the hand so that it is inside out. Hold the removed glove in the other, gloved hand, slide one or two fingers of the ungloved hand under the wrist of the remaining glove and peel it off from the inside, creating a bag for both gloves. Dispose of as appropriate.

Eye protection comes off next. Grasp the 'clean' ear or head pieces and lift away from your face. Dispose of as appropriate

Body protection is third to come off. Untie your apron, roll up so only the 'clean' part is visible and dispose of appropriately. Remove a gown by:

■ slipping your hands inside at the neck and shoulder and peeling away from the shoulders

■ slipping the fingers of one hand under the cuff of the opposite arm and pulling your hand into the sleeve, grasping the gown from inside

■ pushing the sleeve off the opposite arm.

Fold or roll into a bundle with only the 'clean' part visible and drop into the appropriate container.

Finally but most importantly, wash your hands. You will read about good hand washing technique shortly.

www.cdc.gov

Evidence activity

 Correct practice in the application and removal of PPE

This activity gives you the opportunity to demonstrate your knowledge of how to apply and remove PPE.

Produce a poster to be displayed in your staff room that tells colleagues how they should put on and take off PPE. Check out websites and PPE catalogues for diagrams to illustrate your poster.

 The correct procedure for disposal of used PPE

Clinical waste includes all items contaminated by body fluids and waste that are or could be infectious.

Single use PPE, for example white or clear plastic aprons and disposable gloves, masks and eye protection, should be used for just one procedure or **episode of care**. If it becomes contaminated by body fluids and waste, it must be disposed of as clinical waste in a yellow bag or container for collection and incineration by trained personnel. If it is not contaminated it should be double bagged and disposed of as domestic waste.

Key term

An episode of care is one of a series of care tasks in the course of a continuous care activity.

Reusable PPE should be decontaminated according to the manufacturer's instructions.

Blue disposable plastic aprons should be used for food handling only and disposed of in domestic waste bins. Domestic household gloves should be washed with detergent and hot water and left to dry after each use to remove visible soil. If they are worn frequently, are torn or becoming stained, they should be disposed of in domestic waste bins and replaced.

Time to reflect

5.8 Disposal of PPE

Think about the PPE you use. Which of it is disposable and which can you re-use?
How do you dispose of single-use items?
What do you do with reusable items?
Do you need to make changes to your methods of disposal?

Waste bins should be lidded, foot-operated and kept clean, and the bags within them should never be filled more than two-thirds full. Waste bags awaiting collection must be secured to prevent leakage and labelled to show the place of origin. They should be stored in a designated area that is kept clean and locked, to prevent access by the public, animals and vermin.

Evidence activity

5.8 Correct procedure for disposal of used PPE

This activity gives you the opportunity to demonstrate your knowledge of the correct procedure for disposal of used PPE.

Produce a set of coloured, illustrated memory cards to remind your colleagues how they should dispose of used PPE.

LO6 The importance of good personal hygiene in the prevention and control of infections

6.1 The key principles of good personal hygiene

Infection prevention and control is based on the use of practices and procedures that reduce the likelihood of infection being spread from one person, object, place or part of the body to another. High standards of personal hygiene are key to infection prevention and control, not least because much of health and social care requires being in very close proximity with individuals.

Ten top tips for maintaining good personal hygiene

1. Keep your hands clean. This is top of the list in controlling the spread of infections such as those that cause diarrhoea and vomiting and respiratory disease. You will read about good hand washing technique in the next section.

2. Shower or bath daily. Perspiration and dirt provide the perfect environment for many bacteria, fungi and viruses to live and reproduce, and stale sweat is not pleasant to smell. Use a good-quality, unperfumed antiperspirant.

3. Keep your hair clean and tidy and cover or tie it back if it is longer than collar length, especially when handling and serving food and drink. By paying regular attention to your hair, you will look and smell fresh and also be aware of any infestations.

4. Keep your nails short and clean. Bitten nails look unpleasant, and dirt under nails harbours a range of **micro-organisms**. False nails are also a health and safety hazard and should not be worn at work.

5. Keep your feet clean and covered up. Dirty, sweaty feet also look unpleasant and are a **reservoir** for micro-organisms.

Key terms

Micro-organisms are organisms such as bacteria, parasites and fungi that can only be seen with the use of a microscope.
A reservoir is an environment in which a micro-organism can live and reproduce.

6. Keep your clothes clean. Parasites such as fleas and pubic lice can live in clothing, and dirty clothing smells, particularly if you smoke. Do not wear sleeves that go below your elbows at work, so that you can wash your hands and forearms effectively.

7. Keep your teeth clean. Nothing looks worse than dirty, stained teeth, and an unclean mouth provides living conditions for the bacteria that cause bad breath.

8. Do not wear jewellery or body piercings, apart from a plain ring, metal ear studs and a fob watch. Jewellery can carry micro-organisms, and piercings can be infected, especially when new.

9. Cover wounds with a coloured plaster and check what you can and can't do while wearing the plaster, especially if you work with food.

10. Either shave regularly or keep facial hair clean and tidy. Your organisation may have requirements with regard to beards and moustaches.

1. Wet hands and forearms and apply soap.

2. Rub palm to palm.

3. Rub with fingers interlaced.

4. Massage between fingers, right palm over back of left hand, left palm over back of right hand.

5. Scrub with fingers locked, including fingertips.

6. Rub in a circular movement, with thumbs locked.

7. Rinse thoroughly.

8. Dry palms and backs of hands using a paper towel.

9. Work towel between fingers.

10. Dry around and under nails.

'Good practice in infection prevention and control', RCN, 2005

Note: Alcohol gel should be applied using the hand washing technique described above.

 Evidence activity

 6.1 The key principles of good personal hygiene

This activity gives you the opportunity to demonstrate your knowledge of the key principles of good personal hygiene.

How do you maintain good personal hygiene? In what ways could you improve your personal hygiene? Why is it so important for a health or social care worker to maintain good personal hygiene?

 Practice activity

6.2 Demonstrate good handwashing technique

This activity gives you the opportunity to develop a good handwashing technique.

Using the information above, practice.

6.2 & 6.3 Good hand washing technique & Correct sequence for hand washing

Hand hygiene involves washing with soap and water to ensure that all areas are decontaminated. It is a standard precaution against the spread of infection and should be carried out prior to any activity with an individual, whether the hands are visibly dirty or not.

Evidence activity

(6.3) The correct sequence for hand washing

This activity gives you the opportunity to demonstrate your knowledge of the correct sequence for hand washing.

Role-play washing your hands to a colleague, to show that you know the correct sequence for washing your hands effectively.

(6.4) When and why hand washing should be carried out

Hands are top of the list when it comes to the spread of infection, and hand hygiene contributes significantly to reducing the risks of cross-infection. In fact, it is known to be the single most important thing we can do to reduce the spread of disease.

Time to reflect

(6.4) Now wash your hands

When do you wash your hands at work? Do you think you wash them often enough? If not, what prevents you from washing them? Shortage of time? The condition of your skin? The soap isn't very nice? There are never enough towels?

Hand washing should be carried out before:

■ having direct contact with a patient, such as giving personal care and carrying out first aid or healthcare procedures, for example catheter care, PEG feeding and collecting specimens

■ administering medication

■ using PPE

■ handling food.

It should be carried out after:

■ having direct contact with a patient, as above

■ removing PPE, including gloves

■ using the toilet, coughing, sneezing and touching personal clothing, hair etc

■ domestic activities such as handling raw and waste food, cleaning and making beds.

Evidence activity

(6.4) When and why hand washing should be carried out

This activity gives you the opportunity to demonstrate your understanding of when and why hand washing should be carried out.

Think of five or six activities that you carry out in your day-to-day work. For which of these activities would you need to wash your hands? When would you wash them: before the activity, after the activity, or before and after? Why would you wash your hands as you have described for these activities?

(6.5) The types of products that should be used for hand washing

You have a duty of care to the people you work with, their family and friends, your colleagues and yourself to help prevent cross-infection. For this reason, you should raise the alarm if hand washing facilities and products aren't available for everyone to use.

Key terms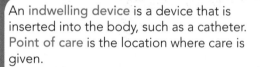

An **indwelling device** is a device that is inserted into the body, such as a catheter. **Point of care** is the location where care is given.

Evidence activity

(6.5) Types of products that should be used for hand washing

This activity gives you the opportunity to demonstrate your knowledge of the types of products that should be used for hand washing.

Survey your workplace for hand washing products and facilities. Does it score well? Or are there any shortfalls in provision? Who should you report shortfalls to? Why is it important that hand washing products and facilities are in good supply?

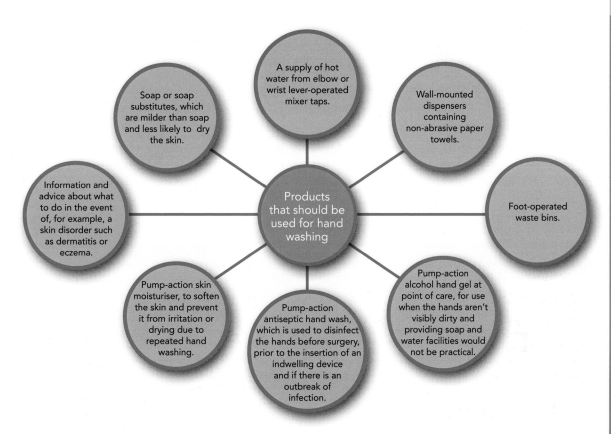

Figure 11.10 Products that should be used for hand washing

6.6 Correct procedures that relate to skincare

Healthy, intact skin provides an effective barrier against cross-infection. Cover any breaks in your skin with an impermeable waterproof dressing and check the dressing regularly, replacing it if necessary. And keep your hands in good condition by using a good-quality **barrier hand cream**.

Key term

A barrier hand cream helps reduce the effects of skin contact with harmful substances.

Occupational skin diseases are caused by irritants and allergies. Soap, water and alcohol gel used for hand hygiene can cause irritation, such as irritant contact dermatitis; and latex rubber gloves can cause allergies, such as allergic contact dermatitis. Signs of occupational skin disease include dryness, redness, itching, inflammation and vesicles. The skin may eventually become cracked, scaly and thickened. In addition, existing skin disorders such as eczema can be made worse by frequent hand washing. If, as a result of wearing gloves and washing your hands, you develop signs of an occupational skin disease or your existing condition gets worse, seek medical advice from an appropriate person, for example your GP or Occupational Health Officer.

Gloves protect against risk of infection, but wearing them can cause skin problems, for example when they are inappropriate to the task, are too large or small, or are damaged. Sensible precautionary measures help to reduce skin problems:

■ Never wear gloves for more than one hour at a time, particularly single-use gloves.

■ Never use lubricants such as powder to help put on gloves.

■ Never use barrier cream when wearing gloves.

■ After taking gloves off, wash and dry your hands, using a mild soap and a non-abrasive paper towel, and apply a quality moisturiser to return lost oils to the skin.

'Hand protection and skin care management', MRC, 2006

6.6 Correct procedures relating to skincare

This activity gives you the opportunity to demonstrate your knowledge of the correct procedures relating to skincare.

Keep a record of how you care for your hands at work. Are you happy that you are looking after them sufficiently well? How can you improve your skin care regime? Why is it important to look after your hands as well as you can? Who can you speak to if you have any concerns about the condition of your hands?

Assessment summary

Your reading of this chapter and completion of the activities will have prepared you to demonstrate your learning and understanding of the role of the health and social care. To achieve the unit, your assessor will require you to:

Learning outcomes	Assessment Criteria
Learning outcome **1**: Understand roles and responsibilities in the prevention and control of infections by:	**1.1** explaining employees' roles and responsibilities in relation to the prevention and control of infection See Evidence activity 1.1, p. 204
	1.2 explaining employers' responsibilities in relation to the prevention and control of infection See Evidence activity 1.2, p. 206
Learning outcome **2**: Understand legislation and policies relating to prevention and control of infections by:	**2.1** outlining current legislation and regulatory body standards that are relevant to the prevention and control of infection See Evidence activity 2.1, p. 208
	2.2 describing local and organisational policies relevant to the prevention and control of infection See Evidence activity 2.2, p. 209
Learning outcome **3**: Understand systems and procedures relating to the prevention and control of infections by:	**3.1** describing procedures and systems relevant to the prevention and control of infection See Evidence activity 3.1, p. 211

Learning outcomes	Assessment Criteria
Learning outcome **3**: Understand systems and procedures relating to the prevention and control of infections by:	(3.2) explaining the potential impact of an outbreak of infection on the individual and the organisation See Evidence activity 3.2, p. 212
Learning outcome **4**: Understand the importance of risk assessment in relation to the prevention and control of infections by:	(4.1) defining the term risk See Evidence activity 4.1, p. 213
	(4.2) outlining potential risks of infection within the workplace See Evidence activity 4.2, p. 215
	(4.3) describing the process of carrying out a risk assessment See Evidence activity 4.3, p. 216
	(4.4) explaining the importance of carrying out a risk assessment See Evidence activity 4.4, p. 217
Learning outcome **5**: Understand the importance of using Personal Protective Equipment (PPE) in the prevention and control of infections by:	(5.1) demonstrating correct use of PPE See Practice activity 5.1, p. 217
	(5.2) describing different types of PPE See Evidence activity 5.2 & 5.3, p. 218
	(5.3) explaining the reasons for use of PPE See Evidence activity 5.2 & 5.3, p. 218
	(5.4) stating current relevant regulations and legislation relating to PPE See Evidence activity 5.4 & 5.6, p. 219
	(5.5) describing employees' responsibilities regarding the use of PPE See Evidence activity 5.5, p. 220

Learning outcomes	Assessment Criteria
Learning outcome **5**: Understand the importance of using Personal Protective Equipment (PPE) in the prevention and control of infections by:	(5.6) describing employers' responsibilities regarding the use of PPE See Evidence activity 5.4 & 5.6, p. 219
	(5.7) describing the correct practice in the application and removal of PPE See Evidence activity 5.7, p. 221
	(5.8) describing the correct procedure for disposal of used PPE See Evidence activity 5.8, p. 222
Learning outcome **6**: Understand the importance of good personal hygiene in the prevention and control of infections by:	(6.1) describing the key principles of good personal hygiene See Evidence activity 6.1, p. 223
	(6.2) demonstrating good hand washing technique See Practice activity 6.2, p. 223
	(6.3) describing the correct sequence for hand washing See Evidence activity 6.3, p. 224
	(6.4) explaining when and why hand washing should be carried out See Evidence activity 6.4, p. 224
	(6.5) describing the types of products that should be used for hand washing See Evidence activity 6.5, p. 225
	(6.6) describing correct procedures that relate to skincare See Evidence activity 6.6, p. 226

Good luck!

Weblinks

Royal College of Nursing	www.rcn.org.uk
Healthcare Republic, a website for healthcare professionals	www.healthcarerepublic.com
Health Protection Agency	www.hpa.org.uk
Daily Mail newspaper	www.dailymail.co.uk
Chartered Institute of Environmental Health	www.cieh.org
Care Quality Commission	www.cqc.org.uk
General Social Care Council in England	www.gscc.org.uk
Care Council for Wales	www.ccwales.org.uk
Scottish Care Council	www.sssc.uk.com
Northern Ireland Social Care Council	www.niscc.info
General Medical Council	www.gmc-uk.org
Nursing and Midwifery Council (NMC)	www.nmc-uk.org
Health Professions Council (HPC)	www.hpc-uk.org
Office for Standards in Education, Children's Services and Skills (Ofsted)	www.ofsted.gov.uk
Children's Workforce Development Council (CWDC)	www.cwdcouncil.org.uk
Skills for Health	www.skillsforhealth.org.uk
Skills for Care	www.skillsforcare.org.uk
Health information for patients	www.patient.co.uk
NHS website	www.nhs.uk
Children's health information	http://kidshealth.org
Health information from BUPA	www.bupa.co.uk
BBC website	www.bbc.co.uk
Government website about public services	www.direct.gov.uk
Centre for Disease Prevention and Control	www.cdc.gov

12 Move and position individuals in accordance with their plan of care

For Unit HSC 2028

What are you finding out?

For a number of reasons, many of the individuals who use health and social care services need help and support to move and change position. Incorrect moving and handling techniques, whether **manual** or with the help of equipment, can cause injury, to both the person being moved and the person helping them make the move. Legislation seeks to protect the health and safety of everyone involved in moving and handling activities, through policies, guidelines and risk assessments, and through procedures and agreed ways of working that are written into individual care plans.

The reading and activities in this chapter will help you to:

■ Understand anatomy and physiology in relation to moving and positioning individuals

■ Understand current legislation and agreed ways of working when moving and positioning individuals

■ Be able to minimise risk before moving and positioning individuals

■ Be able to prepare individuals before moving and positioning

■ Be able to move and position an individual

■ Know when to seek advice from and/or involve others when moving and positioning an individual.

> ### Key term
> Manual involves using human effort, skill, power, energy.

> ### Key terms
> A ligament is a band of tissue that connects bones, typically to support a joint.
> A tendon is a band of tissue that connects a muscle with a bone.

LO1 Anatomy and physiology in relation to moving and positioning

1.1 The anatomy and physiology of the human body in relation to the importance of correct moving and positioning of individuals

The musculoskeletal system is the system of muscles, **tendons**, bones, joints and **ligaments**. Its purpose is to move the body and maintain its form.

Muscles

There are three types of muscle, cardiac (heart), smooth and skeletal, and each is made up of cells or fibres that can contract (shorten). Skeletal (also known as striped or striated) muscle is attached to tendons, which attach to bones. When the fibres of a skeletal muscle contract, the muscle shortens, pulling the tendon, which pulls on the bone to which it is attached. For example, when the biceps muscle contracts, it pulls on the distal biceps tendon, which pulls on the radius, a bone in the forearm. This causes the arm to bend. When the triceps contracts, the triceps tendon pulls on the ulna, the other bone in the forearm. This causes the arm to straighten.

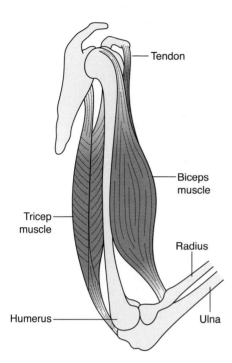

Figure 12.1 The interplay between muscles and bones to bring about movement

A strain can occur when a muscle or tendon is over-stretched or torn, for example by pulling or jerking someone roughly during a manual handling activity; or during an activity that involves pushing, when the muscle or tendon is forced to contract too strongly.

Bones

There are two types of bone. Cortical or compact bone forms the dense outer layer of bones and is thickest in places that bear the greatest load. Cancellous or spongy bone forms the less dense, softer and weaker inner layer but is also found at the ends of the long bones (in the limbs), next to joints and within the vertebrae of the backbone. Spongy bone contains red bone marrow in which blood cells are produced.

Although it can mend, a **fractured** bone is extremely painful.

Key term

Fractured means broken.

1. The most common type of fracture is the simple fracture, when a bone breaks cleanly. In some instances, a simple

fracture can be caused by the slightest of pressure, such as a gentle grip or clasp when helping someone move, or by standing for just a very short period, for example while repositioning from wheelchair to chair.

2. An impacted fracture happens when the ends of two bones are forced into one another, for example when someone extends their arms to stop themselves falling.

3. A jagged, spiral fracture happens as a result of a sharp sudden twist of a bone, such as when someone is twisted when being repositioned.

4. A compression fracture, where a bone breaks into fragments, can result from being crushed, for example by falling equipment.

Research & investigate

(1.1) The causes of broken bones

Check out the incidence of broken bones where you work.

1. What proportion of these breaks were simple, impacted, jagged or due to compression?

2. What caused the breaks?

3. How do you think the breaks could have been avoided?

Joints

A joint is the connection between two bones. There are three types of joint:

1. fixed, such as in the skull, where no movement can take place

2. cartilaginous, in which the bones are firmly joined together by cartilage, for example between the ribs and the vertebrae of the spinal column or back bone, allowing only slight movement

3. synovial, in which the bones are held in place by muscles and ligaments and there is extensive movement, due to the presence of cartilage, which lines the bones forming a smooth, slippery surface, and synovial fluid, which acts as a lubricant. There are four types of synovial joint (see Table 12.1).

The spinal column

The spinal column is made up of 24 individual bones called vertebrae, which are stacked on top of each other in a natural curved 'S' shape that provides the body with strength and flexibility. Between the vertebrae are discs or circular pads of cartilage. They have a tough outer layer and a jelly-like centre, allowing them to squeeze or stretch as the vertebrae move, cushioning the vertebrae and acting as shock absorbers.

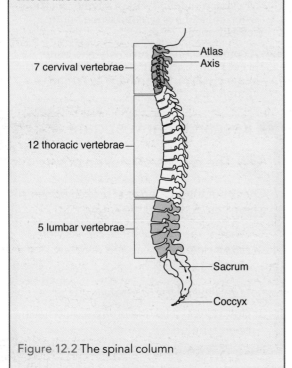

Figure 12.2 The spinal column

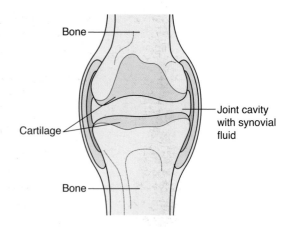

Figure 12.3 A synovial joint

Forcing a joint beyond its normal range of movement can sprain the ligaments holding the bones together. For example, the ligaments on the outside of the ankle can be sprained when the ankle turns over, forcing the sole of the foot to face inward. Sprains also occur when someone is forced into a position, for example when a dragging movement causes twisting or stretching of a joint.

Table 12.1 The four types of synovial joint

Type of joint	Type of movement	Example of joint
Ball and socket	Rotation, allowing movement in nearly all directions	Hip and shoulder
Hinge	Rather like a door hinge, allowing movement in one plane only	Jaw, knee and elbow
Gliding	Bones slide over each other	Wrist and ankle
Pivot	One bone rotates alongside another	The joint between the atlas and axis vertebrae in the neck, allowing the head to turn from side to side

Evidence activity

1.1 The importance of correct moving and positioning of individuals

This activity enables you to demonstrate your knowledge of anatomy and physiology in relation to correct moving and positioning of individuals.

Complete the following table to show your understanding of how incorrect moving and positioning can affect the musculoskeletal system and cause injury.

Moving and positioning technique	Possible effect on the musculoskeletal system
Pulling, jerking	
Pushing	
Gripping, clasping	.
Twisting	
Any technique that requires a weakened individual to bear their own weight, for example standing	
Any technique that carries a risk of a fall	
Any technique that uses equipment	
Any activity that prevents the body assuming its natural 'S'-shaped curve	
Any technique that forces a joint beyond its normal range of movement	

1.2 The impact of specific conditions on the correct movement and positioning of an individual

Many individuals who use health and social care services need help and support to move and change position. A range of moving and positioning activities are shown in Table 12.2, and organisations that provide support in this way are obliged to have in place procedures and agreed ways of working that describe exactly how each manoeuvre must be carried out.

Table 12.2 Moving and positioning activities

Aim of activity	Objectives of activity
Support an individual to sit, stand and walk	• Move forward and backwards in a chair. • Move from sitting in a chair to standing, and vice versa. • Move from sitting on the edge of a bed to standing, and vice versa. • Walk. • Prevent from falling and raise from a fall.

Aim of activity	Objectives of activity	
Support an individual to move in bed	•	Get in and out of bed and turn in bed.
	•	Lie at an angle.
	•	Sit up from lying and onto the edge of the bed.
	•	Slide up and down when lying and sitting.
	•	Maintain the correct posture and appropriate position.
Support an individual to move laterally (side to side)	•	From bed to trolley, and vice versa.
	•	Standing and seated transfers from bed to chair, and vice versa.
	•	Transfer from chair to chair.
	•	Transfer from chair to commode or toilet, and vice versa.
Hoisting	•	Fitting a sling with the individual in bed or in a chair.
	•	Fitting a sling with the individual in bed or in a chair using glide sheets.
	•	Hoisting from bed to chair, and vice versa.
	•	Hoisting from the floor.
	•	Transferring to the toilet or bath using sling-lifting or a stand aid hoist.

Many people have conditions that impact on their mobility and on the support they need to move and reposition. For this reason, procedures must be adapted and agreed ways of working put in place that meet their specific needs.

Specifically tailored moving and repositioning activities must be devised for people who have:

■ a history of falls due, for example, to low blood pressure, vertigo, problems with balance, the side effects of medication, alcohol abuse or low **haemoglobin** levels that bring on fainting

■ bone and joint conditions, such as rheumatoid arthritis, in which the joints become inflamed and painful; osteoarthritis, in which the cartilage of the joints becomes worn, stiff and painful; and osteoporosis, in which the density of the bones is much reduced, increasing the risk of fracture

■ a physical disability that affects movement and mobility, such as amputation, muscular dystrophy, multiple sclerosis, stroke, Parkinson's disease, Huntington's disease, cerebral palsy and epilepsy

■ a sensory impairment, such as impaired sight or hearing, which limit ability to hear how to help in a manoeuvre or see where to move to

■ a health care attachment, such as a PEG feeding tube, catheter, oxygen therapy

■ variations in capabilities during the day and night, for example, an individual may be able to move themselves during the day but not at all at night

■ reduced tissue viability. Tissue viability is to do with the ability of the skin to remain intact and healthy; reduced tissue viability manifests as skin breakdown and pressure ulcers. Skin breakdown is caused by failure to care for skin exposed to moisture from urine, sweat and **exudate**; and pressure ulcers are due to pressure (of the body on the bed or chair), shear (pressure created by pushing and pulling in a lateral direction) and friction (created by two surfaces moving over each other)

Key term

Exudate is fluid that seeps out of injured tissues.
Haemoglobin is the protein in red blood cells that carries the oxygen needed by the body to create energy.
Comatose means unable to exhibit any voluntary movement or behaviour and unable to understand what is happening.

They must also be devised for people who are:

■ paralysed and unable to move

■ unconscious – someone who is **comatose** is unable to comprehend how to help in manoeuvres

■ emotionally disturbed or distressed, aggressive or confused or who have diminished understanding, such as a learning difficulty or dementia. Conditions like these can manifest in challenging and unexpected behaviour, which add to the risks of moving and repositioning.

Evidence activity

1.2 Specific conditions affecting movement and positioning

Check out your workplace's safe moving and handling procedures for three individuals with different needs. How do they compare? In what ways are they different? Why are they different?

LO2 Current legislation and agreed ways of working when moving and positioning individuals

 2.1 Current legislation and agreed ways of working that affect working practices related to moving and positioning individuals

The purpose of health and safety legislation is to protect health, safety and well-being. Health and safety policies set out the arrangements that an organisation has for complying with legislation, and health and safety procedures and agreed ways of working describe how work activities must be carried out for policies to be implemented and the law obeyed.

Time to reflect

2.1 Laying down the law

● What health and safety legislation affects the way that you carry out moving and positioning activities?

● What policies does your employer have in place to ensure that you comply with the law when carrying out moving and positioning activities?

● Where are moving and positioning procedures stored in your workplace? When did you last look at them, to make sure that your work practice is accurate?

There are a number of pieces of legislation that aim to protect everyone involved in moving and repositioning activities. If your job requires you to help someone move or reposition, whether manually or with the help of equipment, you should familiarise yourself with the legislation and your workplace's policies, and ensure that you follow to the letter procedures and agreed ways of working.

The Health and Safety at Work etc. Act 1974 does not specifically cover moving and repositioning activities. However, it requires employers to:

■ write health and safety policies and procedures, including ones that relate to moving and positioning activities, and make employees aware of them

■ ensure everyone's health, safety and welfare, as far as is reasonably practicable.

In addition it requires you to:

■ take reasonable care of yourself and anyone else who may be affected by your activities

■ cooperate with your employer in relation to health and safety issues, including those related to moving and repositioning

■ not interfere with or misuse anything provided in the interest of health and safety, for example equipment used for moving and repositioning.

The Manual Handling Operations Regulations 1992 (amended 2002) apply to a wide range of manual moving and repositioning activities, including lifting, lowering, pushing and pulling.

Table 12.3 Responsibilities under the Manual Handling Operations Regulations 1992

Responsibilities of employers	Your responsibilities
• Avoid the need for hazardous manual handling, so far as is reasonably practicable. • Assess the risk of injury from any hazardous manual handling that can't be avoided. • Reduce the risk of injury from hazardous manual handling, so far as is reasonably practicable.	• Follow work practices that are in place for your safety. • Use properly any equipment that is provided for your safety. • Cooperate with your employer on health and safety matters. • Inform your employer if you identify hazardous handling activities. • Take care to ensure that your activities do not put others at risk.

Getting to grips with manual handling. A short guide. HSE 2006

The Management of Health and Safety at Work Regulations 1999 aim to minimise risks to health and safety through the process of risk assessment. Risk assessment requires employers to:

■ assess the risks associated with moving and repositioning activities

■ take sensible measures to tackle them

■ ensure that you are competent to carry out moving and repositioning activities, through training and supervision.

The Workplace (Health, Safety and Welfare) Regulations 1992 aim to minimise risks to health and safety associated with working conditions. Employers must therefore ensure that minimum standards are met with regard to:

■ moving and repositioning equipment

■ the environment within which moving and repositioning activities take place, for example the space available, lighting and temperature.

A number of moving and repositioning activities require the use of equipment. *The Provision and Use of Work Equipment Regulations (PUWER) 1998* aim to minimise the risks to health and safety associated with its use. Employers have a responsibility to ensure that:

■ equipment is safe, well maintained and appropriate for the job

■ employees use equipment safely and correctly, through training and supervision.

The Lifting Operations and Lifting Equipment Regulations (LOLER) 1998 aim to reduce health and safety risks due to using lifting equipment. Employers are required to ensure that lifting

equipment used for moving and repositioning activities is:

■ strong, stable and marked to indicate safe working loads

■ safely positioned and installed to minimise any risks

■ used safely and appropriately by trained and supervised employees

■ maintained and inspected by competent people.

■ Research & investigate

 Well equiped?

What equipment is available at your workplace for carrying out moving and positioning activities? What specific activities is it used for? How and by whom is it maintained? How would you know it was safe to use?

The Personal Protective Equipment at Work Regulations (PPE) 1992 aim to minimise the risks to health and safety associated with cross-infection. Employers have a responsibility to minimise the risk of cross-infection during moving and repositioning activities by:

■ providing employees with appropriate personal protective equipment (PPE)

■ ensuring that employees use and dispose of PPE safely and correctly, through training and supervision.

The Reporting of Injuries, Diseases and Dangerous Occurrence Regulations (RIDDOR)

1995 require that certain work-related injuries, diseases and dangerous occurrences are reported to the HSE or local authority. Employers have a responsibility to train employees in how to report injuries and dangerous occurrences associated with moving and repositioning activities.

Evidence activity

2.1 Legislation related to moving and positioning individuals

This activity enables you to demonstrate your knowledge of how current legislation and agreed ways of working affect working practices related to moving and positioning individuals.

Think about three different moving and positioning activities in which you participate. For each, describe:

- the relevant legislation
- workplace policies that ensure compliance with the legislation
- your responsibilities in implementing the policies and ensuring best practice.

2.2 **Health and safety factors that need to be taken into account when moving and positioning individuals and using equipment**

Moving and repositioning activities, whether manual or using equipment, are health and safety hazards for everyone concerned. This section looks at the health and safety hazards or risk factors that need to be taken into account when moving and repositioning individuals.

The activity

■ Musculoskeletal injuries or disorders (MSDs) are the most common occupational illness in Great Britain. They include back and joint injury, sprains and strains. If the activity requires manual effort, does it involve any of the movements known to cause MSDs? (See Figure 12.4.)

■ If the activity requires the use of equipment, is it appropriate, safe and well maintained, and do you know how to use it properly? If the answer to any of these questions is no, then equipment carries a risk of accident and injury.

■ Is the activity appropriate for the individual concerned, or would an alternative activity meet their needs? You read earlier about conditions that impact on an individual's ability to move and reposition. Individuals with these conditions require specifically tailored support; anything else would put their health and safety at risk.

■ Are you trained to carry out the activity and are you confident to carry it out safely? Never perform any activity for which you haven't been trained and always ask for help if you have any concerns.

The load

Before attempting to help an individual move or reposition, be aware of factors such as their:

■ weight – would moving them manually put your health at risk? Does the equipment you intend to use indicate that it can carry their weight safely?

■ size – does their size or shape affect your ability to get hold of them safely and securely?

■ behaviour – do you anticipate any unexpected movement that would put health and safety at risk?

Time to reflect

2.2 Been there, got the T-shirt …

Have you ever hurt yourself as a result of carrying a heavy, awkward load? Did the experience impact on your ability to carry on as usual? How long were you out of action? What would you say to someone else who appeared to be struggling with an unwieldy, bulky load?

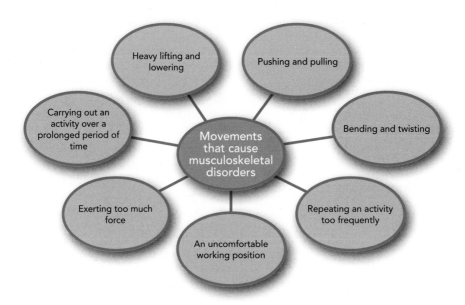

Figure 12.4 Movements that cause musculoskeletal disorders

The working environment

■ Does the environment or space in which you work constrain your posture? For example, do obstructions or a lack of space restrict your movements or make movement uncomfortable? Postural constraint is a further cause of MSD.

■ Is the floor level and free from slip and trip hazards?

■ Can you see what you are doing, or is lighting dazzling or insufficient?

■ Can you hear, or is background noise distracting, preventing you from hearing instructions accurately?

■ Is there a comfortable working temperature, neither too hot nor too cold?

■ Is ventilation comfortable, not too drafty or humid?

■ Is the environment clean and fresh smelling?

Your capabilities and those of the others in your team

■ Are you trained and confident in your ability to do the activity safely?

■ Are your clothing and footwear appropriate, or do they restrict movement?

■ Are you fit and strong enough?

■ Do you have a disability that prevents you carrying out certain activities?

■ Does your health status affect your ability, for example, are you pregnant or do you have an MSD?

■ Are you able to give the activity the time it requires, or do high job demands, time constraints, fatigue and stress tempt you to cut corners?

Other factors

■ Do you need to take precautions against the risk of cross infection, for example by using PPE?

■ Are you trained and confident in your ability to report and record any accidents and injuries?

 Research & investigate

(2.2) How safe is your workplace?

Carry out a brief survey of the environment in which you work. On a scale of 1 = excellent to 5 = poor, how does it score with regard to enabling safe moving and positioning?

Evidence activity

(2.2) Health and safety factors

This activity enables you to demonstrate your knowledge of the health and safety factors that need to be taken into account when moving and positioning individuals and using equipment.

Think about two individuals you help to move and position, one of whom requires the use of equipment. For each individual, make a list of the health and safety factors you need to consider when helping them move and position, including those that relate to the equipment that is used.

LO3 Minimising risks before moving and positioning individuals

(3.1) Accessing up-to-date copies of risk assessment documentation

Health and safety legislation that relates to moving and positioning requires that every manual or equipment-aided moving and positioning activity is assessed for risks, and that steps are taken to eliminate or minimise any risks. The results of risk assessments must be recorded, manually and/or electronically, and everyone involved made aware of the health and safety procedures they contain.

Risk assessment records should be stored in filing cabinets or electronic storage systems in a clearly known and accessible location, for example a staff room or office, so that everyone can keep themselves familiar with their content. Anyone who carries out an activity must follow to the letter the procedures described in the risk assessment.

Risk assessments need to be routinely reviewed and updated, to take account of, for example, changes in legislation and developments in moving and handling techniques and equipment. Good practice dictates that you keep up to date with the law and the latest moving and handling procedures.

 Practice activity

(3.1) Access up-to-date copies of risk assessment documentation

This activity gives you an opportunity to demonstrate that you can access up-to-date copies of risk assessment documentation

- Where are moving and handling risk assessments stored at your workplace?
- How do you access them?
- Why is it necessary to review them?
- How do you know that the risk assessments you access are up-to-date?

(3.2) Preparatory checks using care plans and moving and handling risk assessments

Moving and handling risk assessments record procedures for carrying out activities such as those listed in Table 12.2. Care plans contain information about an individual's abilities and needs, including instructions for moving and handling activities that are specific to them.

Before helping anybody to move or reposition, make a preparatory check of their care plan. This serves to remind you of any special requirements for the activity and also whether the requirements have been updated since you last carried out the activity. If there are no special requirements, check and follow the moving and handling risk assessment for the manoeuvre. Failure to follow procedures laid out in care plans and risk assessments flies in the face of best practice and puts everyone involved at risk.

Practice activity

3.2 Preparatory checks

This activity gives you an opportunity to demonstrate that you can carry out preparatory checks using an individual's care plan and the moving and handling risk assessment.

Think about three people that you help to move and position.

■ What documentation describes the moving and handling activities in which they need support?

■ Where is this documentation stored?

■ Why is it important to follow the procedures described in this documentation?

3.3 Identify any immediate risks to the individual

Don't follow procedures blindly. Before you initiate any move, be on the alert for risks that could affect the individual's health and safety.

Questions you should ask yourself prior to carrying out any moving and handling activity

1. Is the activity appropriate? Changes in an individual's physical health, for example, their weight, mobility, balance, tendency to fall, sight, hearing and tissue viability can put health and safety at risk. Similarly, changes in their mood and mental health, such as level of dependency, understanding, behaviour and ability to help in the manoeuvre can also affect health and safety.

2. Is the working environment free from obstruction and noise, and is it well lit?

3. Is the equipment you are going to use appropriate, and are you confident and competent in its use?

4. Is there evidence to show that equipment is safe and well maintained?

5. Are you and any others involved in the manoeuvre appropriately trained, fit and healthy, sufficiently strong and appropriately dressed?

6. Is there any possibility of cross-infection? Infection is a major cause of illness and hospitalisation among people living in residential care homes, and healthcare-associated infections (HCAIs) may be serious, even life threatening.

Evidence activity

3.3 Identify any immediate risks to the individual

Produce a set of reminder cards to alert your colleagues to any risks to individuals prior to carrying out moving and handling activities. Use the categories 'Activity', 'Load', 'Working environment', 'Workers' capabilities' and 'Other factors'.

3.4 Actions to take in relation to identified risks

It is very difficult to completely eliminate risks. The aim of risk assessment is to create procedures to reduce risks 'to the lowest level reasonably practicable'.

Table 12.4 Minimising risks associated with moving and positioning

Risk factor	Action to take to minimise the risks
Activity	Don't carry out any activity unless you have been trained.
	Don't carry out any activity unless you are sufficiently strong, fit and healthy.
	If an activity puts great pressure on you, request the support of a team.
	If a manual activity poses a risk, consider using equipment instead.
	Don't use equipment unless you have been trained.

Risk factor	Action to take to minimise the risks
Activity	Use equipment that is appropriate to the activity and the needs of the individual.
	Inspect equipment before use to make sure it is safe and well maintained.
	Follow procedures within care plans and risk assessments.
	Report any concerns.
Load	Prior to the activity, assess individuals for changes in their physical and emotional condition that could affect the manoeuvre.
	Know what can affect their behaviour so you can plan for unexpected movements.
	Know their weight in order to decide whether you are strong enough to help in the manoeuvre and that any equipment you intend to use can carry them safely.
	Take their size and shape into account when planning how to grasp or support them.
	Report any changes in the individual that impact on moving and positioning.
	Report any concerns.
Working environment	Don't carry out any activity if there isn't sufficient space for you to move in comfort.
	Don't carry out any activity if there isn't sufficient space to use equipment properly.
	Don't carry out any activity if the light, noise, ventilation and temperature could compromise comfort and safety.
	Report any concerns.
Capabilities	Ensure that you are trained in moving and handling, including using equipment.
	If you work in a team, know your responsibilities and commit to developing teamwork skills.
	Ask for supervision to check that you are competent and work safely.
	Wear appropriate clothing, including PPE if necessary.
	Stay fit and healthy and let your employer know if you are pregnant or if a manoeuvre causes you pain or discomfort.
	Report concerns related to high job demands, time constraints, fatigue and stress that you think could interfere with your ability to work safely.
Other factors	Follow procedures for working with people who are infected.
	Follow procedures if you think that you may have an infectious disease.
	Follow procedures for reporting accidents and injuries related to moving and handling.

Evidence activity

(3.4) Describe actions to take in relation to identified risks

Think about three moving and handling manoeuvres that you carry out on a day-to-day basis.

■ What risks are associated with each in terms of the activity itself, the load, the working environment, workers' capabilities and other factors, such as risk of infection?

■ How would you deal with each risk?

(3.5) Action to take if an individual's wishes conflict with their care plan in relation to health and safety and their risk assessment

The individuals who use health and social care services have a right to lead their lives independently, without unreasonable demands, and to make personal choices about the provision and timing of their care. For this reason, you should consult with the people you support to find out how they wish to be cared for and when. Where decisions about care are made on behalf of an individual, they should take into account any known wishes and beliefs. Providing care and support in ways not agreed with an individual can bring accusations of neglect and abuse.

Conflict can arise when individuals decline to be cared for according to their care plan or a risk assessment and make decisions that carry an element of risk. For example, they may elect to exercise their independence and move without your help; they may choose to be uninvolved in a manoeuvre, even though their **active participation** would help and protect you; or they may decide they don't want to move at all, even though to do so is in their best interests. Although you might see these decisions as eccentric or unwise, everyone has a right to make decisions that carry an element of risk to themselves, and you have a responsibility to support individuals in exercising their right to take risks.

Key term

Active participation is when a person takes an active rather than a passive role in their own care and support.

However, you also have a responsibility to protect their health and safety as well as your own and any colleagues' involved. In the event of a seemingly unwise decision, discuss the safety implications for everyone concerned and point out your duty to follow safe procedures and comply with health and safety law. Make every attempt to convince the person of the importance of following their care plan or the relevant risk assessment, while at the same time indicating your wish to respect and promote their rights.

If, having discussed the possible consequences of their decision, you cannot steer someone away from an ill-advised decision, support them according to their wishes and choices and record the incident. If their decision is likely to endanger your health and safety, seek help.

Evidence activity

(3.5) What to do if there are conflicting interests

This activity gives you an opportunity to demonstrate your knowledge of what to do in the event that an individual's wishes conflict with their care plan in relation to health and safety and their risk assessment.

Check out your workplace's policy for accommodating individuals when their wishes conflict with the health and safety procedures you are required to follow. Use your findings to produce an information sheet or poster for colleagues who you feel need support in dealing with situations that could become difficult.

(3.6) Preparing the immediate environment for moving and repositioning activities

You read earlier that the Workplace (Health, Safety and Welfare) Regulations 1992 require employers to minimise risks to health and safety associated with the working environment. Factors within the working environment, which can be someone's own home, that can jeopardise the safety of moving and positioning activities include a lack of space and obstructions, such as general clutter and **fixtures** and **fittings**.

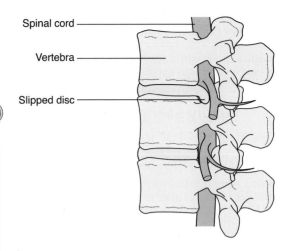

Figure 12.5 A slipped disc

Key terms

A fitting is any item that is free standing or hung by a nail or hook.

A fixture is any item that is bolted to the floor or walls.

A slipped disc occurs when one of the discs of the spine is ruptured and the jelly-like substance inside leaks out, putting pressure on the spinal cord. It causes intense back pain as well as pain in other areas of the body.

Adequate, accessible space is vital for a normal range of joint and muscle movements. Working in cramped, cluttered conditions uses awkward movements such as twisting, leaning sideways, stooping, overreaching, and turning and balancing in a small area. Awkward movements force the spinal column out of its natural curved 'S' shape, overstretching muscles and joints and causing MSDs, for example, a **slipped disc**, joint injury, sprains and strains. MSDs are very debilitating. Apart from long periods of reduced mobility and pain that can affect everyday activities and the ability to sleep, they can also affect your job prospects.

Working in cramped conditions increases the risk of accidents, for everyone concerned. According to the Health and Safety at Work etc. Act 1974, you have a responsibility to take reasonable care of yourself and anyone else who may be affected by your activities. So before carrying out any moving

and positioning activities, make sure that everyone involved has enough space to move freely and comfortably and that there is enough space to use equipment properly. Assess the area for obstructions that could restrict movement, such as furniture, wheelchairs, televisions, shelving, cupboards, even curtains and curtain rails, and deal with them to make the space as tidy and free from clutter as possible. If you are working in a team, coordinate your tasks such that you don't restrict each other.

Other hazards that can jeopardise the safety of moving and handling procedures include:

■ slip and trip hazards, for example slippery floors, worn carpets, missing tiles; changes in floor levels, such as slopes, steps and stairs; clutter and other trip hazards

■ lighting that is uncomfortable and not user-friendly, for example bulbs that provide insufficient light, creating dark areas, lighting that dazzles or glares, and badly designed light fittings

Practice activity

(3.6) Preparing the immediate environment

Complete the following table to show how you ensure that the environment in which you carry out three moving and handling activities is as free from risk as possible.

Description of moving and handling activity	How I ensure that there is adequate space for the move	Details of other hazards that I remove
1.		
2.		
3.		

■ distracting **ambient** conditions, such as startling or repetitive noise; uncomfortable temperatures – too hot or too cold; high humidity; poor ventilation, including cold drafts; dirt and bad smells.

(3.7) Apply standard precautions for infection prevention and control

Helping someone to move or reposition requires close body contact and, on occasion, contact with blood and body fluids. Standard precautions are the practices adopted by health and social care workers when there is a chance that they may come into contact with blood or body fluids. They are a set of principles designed to minimise exposure to and transmission of a wide variety of **pathogens**.

> ### Key term
> Ambient means in the surrounding environment.

Before carrying out any moving and positioning activities, remove or reduce the risks associated with these hazards 'to the lowest level reasonably practicable'.

Practice activity

(3.7) Apply standard precautions for infection prevention and control

This activity gives you an opportunity to demonstrate that you apply standard precautions for infection prevention and control.

Think of 3 moving and handling activities you carry out in which there is a risk of contact with blood or body fluids. For each one, describe the precautions you take to prevent the spread of infection.

> ### Key term
> A pathogen is a disease-producing bacterium, fungus, virus, infestation or prion.

See Chapter 11, 'The principles of infection prevention and control'.

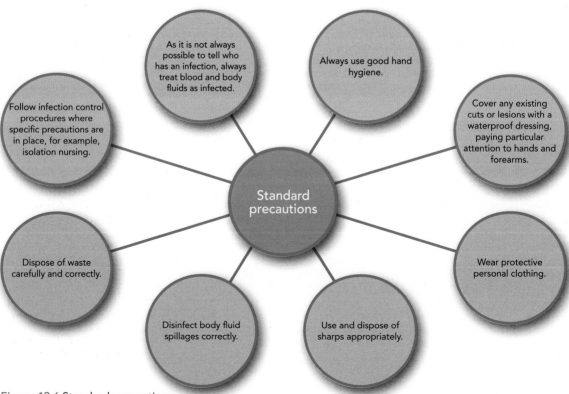

Figure 12.6 Standard precautions

LO4 Preparing individuals before moving and positioning

 Communicate effectively with individuals to ensure they understand the details and reasons for the action/activity being undertaken and agree the level of support they require

There are countless actions and activities carried out in health and social care, and unless an individual understands what is happening and why they can feel very frightened. They can also lose their dignity and feel that things are being 'done' to them without their having any choice. Imagine the fear associated with having to have, for example, a CT scan or an endoscopy; not knowing why certain things are being done; finding the experience distressing or painful; worrying about how long the procedure will last; and being terrified about the eventual diagnosis. It is essential, therefore, that you reassure the people you work with by describing in full any activity you need to carry out, why it needs to be carried out and how you will carry it out.

You also need to reach an agreement with them about the level of support they require. Human nature is such that we want to stay as independent as possible for as long as we can. Taking away someone's independence takes away their control, prevents them from doing what they want to do when they want to do it, and destroys any feelings of self-worth. Reassure the individuals you work with that you don't intend to 'take over'; that you want to work with them, in a partnership; that you respect what they can do; and that you value their active participation, especially since that makes your job easier and more enjoyable!

Many people find it difficult to admit to needing help and support, especially with everyday activities. Asking for help and support can be embarrassing and can challenge their pride and status. Talk with them about what they can do and what they would like to do. Read between the lines and watch their body language for clues as to where support would be appreciated. It may be as simple as helping them to get up from a chair or clean themselves after using the toilet. It may be that they need help to walk or reposition, because of **vertigo** or pain. Or it may be that movement is tiring, they can't see where they are going, or they are afraid of falling.

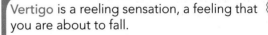

Key term

Vertigo is a reeling sensation, a feeling that you are about to fall.

 Time to reflect

4.1a Do you care?

Does it ever occur to you that the individuals for whom you provide care and support may be frightened, feel they have lost independence and control, and that what they have to undergo takes away their pride and self-respect? If you were in their shoes, how would you like to be treated?

 Time to reflect

4.1b Can you help?

Think about the people you work with who find it difficult to admit to needing help and support. How do they show their feelings? Are they on the defensive, embarrassed, apologetic? How do you reassure them that it is OK to receive help and support? Why do you think it is important to give this reassurance?

Chapter 1 describes communication techniques that help people understand each other. You need to develop and put effective communication skills into practice to ensure that the individuals you support understand the details and reasons for your activities with them.

Agreeing the level of support you give maintains independence and dignity. It promotes partnership working and people's right to be cared for in a way that meets their needs and takes account of their choices. The following sections look at how you can give that support, including the use of moving and handling aids and equipment.

Practice activity

(4.1) Communicating effectively with the individual

This activity gives you an opportunity to demonstrate that you communicate effectively with individuals to ensure that they understand the details and reasons for the action/activity being undertaken and agree the level of support they require.

Talk to two or three of the individuals you work with. Ask them for feedback on and how you can improve your ability to:

■ communicate to them the details and reasons for your work with them

■ agree with them the level of support they need.

They are the experts in their care. Listen to them and act on what they tell you!

(4.2) Obtaining valid consent for the planned activity

Individuals in receipt of care and support have a right to be cared for in a way that meets their needs and takes account of their choices. To impose care on people without respecting their wishes is not only **unethical**, it is also illegal.

Key terms

Unethical behaviour is behaviour that is not right, moral or honourable.

Before carrying out a caring activity or procedure for a competent adult or child, including helping them to move or reposition, you must obtain their consent. Competence means being able to understand and weigh up the information needed to make a decision. Always assume the people you support are competent unless they demonstrate otherwise. But remember:

■ An unexpected decision or one with which you don't agree does not prove they are incompetent. It might just indicate that they need further information or a more simple explanation.

■ They can change their minds and withdraw consent at any time. Always check that consent remains to your caring for them as previously agreed.

UK country definitions of valid consent

England and Northern Ireland

For consent to be valid, it must be given voluntarily by an appropriately informed person (the patient or, where relevant, someone with parental responsibility for a patient under the age of 18) who has the capacity to consent to the intervention in question. Acquiescence where the person does not know what the intervention entails is not 'consent'.

Wales

For consent to be valid, it must be given voluntarily by an appropriately informed person who has the capacity to consent to the intervention in question. The informed person may either be the patient, someone with parental responsibility or a person who has authority under a Power of Attorney. Consent will not be legally valid if the patient has not been given adequate information or where they are under the undue influence of another. Acquiescence where the person does not know what the intervention entails is not 'consent'. Where a patient does not have capacity to give consent, then treatment may be given providing it is given in accordance with the Mental Capacity Act 2005.

Scotland

In order for valid consent to treatment to exist, the patient must have been given, and been able to understand, a certain degree of information about the nature, purpose and possible outcomes of the proposed treatment. The case law in Scotland and England broadly suggests that, for the purpose of avoiding civil liability for treatment without consent, a doctor must provide such information as would be provided by a responsible body of medical opinion.

Some people are competent to make some decisions but not competent to make others. Advocacy services and a variety of different communication methods can help people with learning or communication difficulties to understand any proposed care and treatment. Younger children who fully understand what is involved in a procedure can give consent, but when they don't or can't understand, or when they won't give consent, someone with parental responsibility can be asked to do so on their behalf.

Consent must be given voluntarily. Neither you, your colleagues, an individual's family or friends are allowed to influence or put pressure on them to consent to care or treatment. In fact, a competent adult is fully entitled to refuse care, even where it would clearly be of benefit. And if an incompetent person indicated in the past, while competent, that they would refuse treatment in certain circumstances (an 'advance refusal'), and those circumstances arise, you must abide by that refusal. However, people can be treated without their consent when:

■ the treatment is for a mental disorder and the person is detained under the Mental Health Act 1983

■ they are suffering from a notifiable disease (Public Health (Control of Disease) Act 1984).

Consent should be given using a form of communication with which the individual is most comfortable, for example it may be spoken or written, or be non-verbal, such as British Sign Language or **Makaton**. However, a signature on its own is not sufficient – a consent form must record the decision and discussions that took place in order that the decision could be reached.

Key term

Makaton uses signs and symbols to enable people with communication and learning difficulties to communicate.

Practice activity

 Obtain valid consent for the planned activity

This activity gives you an opportunity to demonstrate that you obtain valid consent for any moving and handling activity you plan to carry out.

Build on your work for Practice activity 4.1 by checking with the individuals that you do indeed gain there consent for any help and support you plan to give them.

LO5 Be able to move and position an individual

 Follow care plans to ensure that individuals are positioned using agreed techniques and in a way that avoids causing undue pain or discomfort

Moving can be painful and uncomfortable. Bone and joint conditions, strains, sprains and pressure ulcers can make even the slightest movement distressing. Everyone needing help and support to move should be risk assessed to identify techniques that either eliminate the risk of pain and discomfort or reduce it to an absolute minimum. And once those techniques have been agreed or consented to by the individual concerned, they must be written into their care plan and routinely reviewed.

You must follow to the letter the instructions within an individual's care plan, but remember, only carry out moving and handling activities for which you have been trained and in which you are competent.

Time to reflect

Training

● What moving and handling activities have you been trained to carry out?

● Do you ever participate in moves for which you have had no formal training?

● Imagine that you help an individual to move using a technique for which you haven't received training and either they or you get injured. What might be the outcome for you?

Ten top tips for moving and positioning individuals

To ensure that individuals are moved and positioned using agreed techniques and in a way that will avoid causing undue pain or discomfort, before starting the activity:

1. Check the care plan, the moving and handling risk assessment, that equipment is clean, safe and well maintained, and that you have valid consent to carry out the activity.

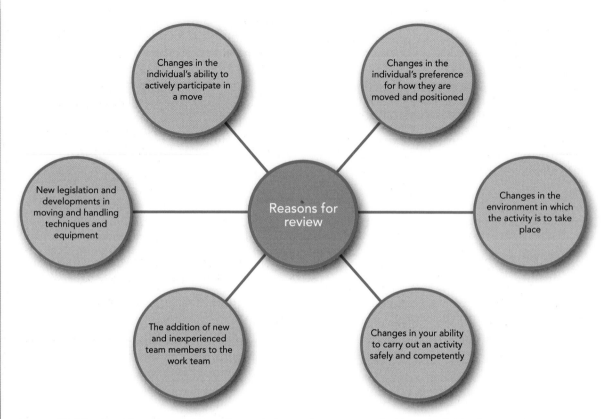

Figure 12.7 Review of moving and handling techniques that are recorded in an individual's care plan

2. Assess any immediate risks to everyone concerned and get help where you think there is a risk you can't deal with.

3. Tell the individual what you need to do, why they are to be moved and handled in a particular way, and help them understand how they can actively participate.

4. Prepare the immediate environment – remove any potential hazards and make sure there is enough space for the move to take place.

5. If appropriate, get help.

While carrying out the activity:

6. Use the correct technique and the correct equipment.

7. Observe the individual throughout, and if they show any adverse reaction, such as pain and distress, stop and get help.

8. If you run into difficulties, get help.

9. Use appropriate equipment to maintain the individual in the required position.

When the activity is finished:

10. Use appropriate documentation to record what you have done, any difficulties you encountered, any pain or discomfort

experienced by the individual, your suggestions for changes to the activity, and note when the next positioning manoeuvre is due.

Practice activity

 5.1 Following the care plan

This activity gives you an opportunity to demonstrate that you follow care plans to ensure that individuals are positioned using agreed techniques and in a way that avoids causing undue pain or discomfort.

Ask your colleagues or a supervisor to observe you as you carry out moving and positioning activities as described in care plans. Act on their feedback to ensure that you use techniques competently and confidently.

Check with the individuals themselves that the help you give them maintains their comfort. Act on their feedback to ensure you support them in such a way that you avoid causing them any pain or discomfort.

5.2 Effective communication with others involved in the manoeuvre

Many moving and positioning activities require teamwork, particularly when the individual concerned is heavy or requires a high level of care. Effective teamwork protects the health and safety of everyone involved.

Ideally team members should be similar in height and strength in order to:

■ avoid awkward movements, such as overreaching – you read earlier that awkward movements can cause MSDs

■ ensure that the individual's weight is evenly shared – being overloaded and unbalanced can also cause an MSD

■ keep the move as smooth and comfortable as possible for everyone concerned.

An effective team needs a good leader whose experience is worthy of respect and in whom the rest of the team has confidence. Apart from setting a good example by carrying out moving and positioning activities according to agreed techniques, a leader must be able to communicate effectively when:

■ ensuring everyone involved, including the individual concerned, understands the reason for the manoeuvre and their specific role in enabling it to take place safely

■ working with everyone to agree commands, such as 'Ready, steady, pull!'

■ issuing commands during the manoeuvre

■ evaluating the manoeuvre and how it could be improved.

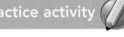

Practice activity

 5.2 Demonstrate effective communication with any others involved in the manoeuvre

This activity gives you an opportunity to demonstrate that you can communicate effectively with others involved in a manoeuvre.

Keep a log of moving and positioning activities for which you have to allocate and explain roles, agree and issue commands, and evaluate manoeuvres. Reflect on your communication skills. Are they effective? Is there room for improvement? what do the others think about your communication skills? Act on their feedback.

5.3 Aids and equipment used for moving and positioning

There is a plethora of aids and equipment that can be used to help individuals move, reposition and retain a comfortable posture. They include:

■ mobility scooters and wheelchairs

■ walking frames, trolleys and sticks

■ manual and electric mobile hoists, which are used to move people from, for example, bed to chair, wheelchair to car

■ wall and ceiling track hoists, which consist of a rail or track fixed to the wall or ceiling, along which a seat or sling is moved

■ sling lifts and bath hoists, which are fixed to the floor and have either a sling or a chair seat to lower and raise people into and out of the bath

■ stand aids, to help a person from sitting to standing and to transfer a short distance

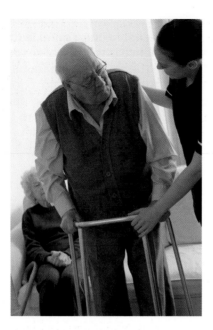

Figure 12.8 Aids and equipment

■ slide sheets, for repositioning a person in bed or moving them from bed to trolley – their low friction surface prevents the shearing that can lead to pressure ulcers. Some slide sheets have a non-slip area that allows the person to get a heel grip and turn themselves over

■ monkey poles and bed ladders, to help a person move from lying down to sitting up

■ inflatable lifting cushions and backrests, to enable people to stand up from a chair and sit up in bed respectively

■ swivel aids, turntables and turn disks, for transferring people from one sitting or standing position to another

■ transfer boards, for lateral transfer, for example, bed to chair, chair to wheelchair, wheelchair to car

■ handling belts, for gripping a person prior to a move, often used in conjunction with swivel aids, transfer boards and slide sheets

■ leg lifters.

Evidence activity

(5.3) **Aids and equipment used for moving and positioning**

Complete the table below.

Aids and equipment used in moving and positioning activities at my workplace	Function

---

(5.4) ## Equipment that maintains the individual in the appropriate position

Because some individuals are unable to maintain a stable posture, they require frequent repositioning, aided or unaided. This can be tiring and uncomfortable, disrupt their concentration, affect their quality of life, compromise their dignity and cause pressure ulcers.

Research & investigate

(5.4) Reposition for repose

What equipment is available at your workplace to help individuals maintain a stable, comfortable posture?

Frequent repositioning can be avoided by using equipment that maintains the appropriate position, for example:

■ support chairs, standing frames and wheeled walkers that have head, arm, knee and foot supports and straps; chest and hip pads, all of which can be adjusted for comfort and safety

■ positioning wedges, such as those used to prop someone into position when in bed

■ orthopaedic supports, braces and immobilising slings

■ slide sheets that allow movement in one direction only, helping people who tend to slide forwards or to the side to stay upright.

 Evidence activity

 5.4 Equipment used to maintain the appropriate position

Make a list of the individuals you work with who are unable to maintain a stable posture. Describe how you help them to do so. Remember to maintain their confidentiality.

5.5 Encouraging individuals to actively participate in manoeuvres

You read earlier that active participation is a way of working in which people using health and social care services are regarded as active partners in their care or support, as opposed to being passive recipients. There are many ways in which you can encourage individuals to cooperate in manoeuvres, and it is important that you do so, for two main reasons:

1. to ensure they stay as independent as possible for as long as possible

2. to help protect your health and safety – a problem shared is a problem halved!

Before you carry out a moving and positioning activity, ask the individual how they think they can help and what help they think they would like. Answers will vary on a day-to-day basis, depending on mood, motivation, level of confidence, fear of falling, fear of pain, physical health status and so on. Remind them that you are there to provide support and that you want them to be in control.

Sometimes you may be asked to help in a way that is not within your job scope, in which you haven't been trained, or that you know could risk health and safety. Some moving and handling manoeuvres are so risky that they have been condemned. Be sensitive when explaining why you can't accommodate their request, and reach a compromise that will enable you to work within health and safety guidelines while at the same time meeting their needs.

Condemned moving and handling manoeuvres

- Drag lift
- Australian or shoulder lift
- Orthodox or cradle lift
- Any manoeuvres involving the individual's hands being placed around the handler's neck or body
- Any manoeuvres involving the lifting of most of or the entire body weight of an individual without the use of a mechanical lifting aid

 Evidence activity

 5.5 Encouraging individuals' active participation

Think about three moving and positioning activities in which you encourage individuals to actively participate. In what ways do they help in the move? Why is it useful for them to contribute like this?

5.6 Monitoring the individual throughout the activity so that the procedure can be stopped if there is any adverse reaction

You read earlier that it is important to observe an individual throughout a manoeuvre and that you should stop and get help if they show any adverse reaction. Adverse reactions include:

■ distress due to fear, pain, discomfort, a lack of confidence in the handler and anxiety about relying on equipment

■ a failure to follow instructions, due to difficulty in hearing or understanding, or a change in the ability or desire to cooperate

■ a change in **muscle tone**, unexpected movement, loss of balance

■ sprained joints, trapped fingers and limbs, and dislodged health care attachments, due to poor positioning

■ changes in medical status, for example a drop in blood pressure, loss of consciousness, restricted ability to breathe

■ fatigue.

Key term

Muscle tone is the tension or resistance to movement in a muscle that enables us to keep our bodies in a certain position.

Be on the alert for adverse reactions throughout every manoeuvre you perform. If you detect any risks to health and safety, stop what you are doing and get help without delay.

Evidence activity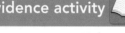

5.6 Monitor the individual throughout the activity

This activity gives you an opportunity to demonstrate that you monitor individuals when helping them to move or reposition so that you can stop the procedure in the event of an adverse reaction.

Think about three moving and positioning activities that you stopped because of an adverse reaction. What caused the individual involved to react in these ways? What have you learnt from these experiences?

5.7 Report and record the activity, including when the next positioning manoeuvre is due

It is extremely important that you follow your workplace's procedures for reporting and recording any moving and positioning manoeuvres you undertake, including accidents, incidents and near misses. Verbal reports should be made to the relevant person, and written records should be made in care plans and on appropriate accident/incident report forms.

Research & investigate

5.7 Record keeping

What does your workplace's policy require of you with regard to reporting and recording:

● moving and handling activities?

● the timing of moving and handling activities?

Report and record any adverse reactions during a manoeuvre. This will trigger a review of the manoeuvre to ensure that the situation does not recur. And use care plans to record details of every manoeuvre that is carried out and when the next is due. Failure to reposition someone, in bed or in a chair, to transfer them when necessary to the toilet or bath, and to generally help them keep moving as much as possible, amounts to neglect. As you read earlier, skin breaks down after a prolonged period of exposure to urine, sweat and exudate, and pressure ulcers can develop after lengthy periods of sitting or lying in the same position. So it is important that you and your colleagues know when to reposition the people you work with.

Any hazards you identify with the manoeuvre, the individual concerned, aids and equipment and the working environment must be reported and recorded without delay. Similarly, any accidents, incidents and near misses must be reported and recorded. Unless hazards, accidents, incidents and near misses are reported, their cause can't be investigated and they will continue to put health and safety at risk.

Finally, make sure your colleagues and line manager know about any personal factors such as MSDs, illness or pregnancy that might affect your ability to carry out manoeuvres in the future.

Evidence activity

(5.7) Reporting and recording

This activity gives you an opportunity to demonstrate that you know how to report and record moving and positioning activities, including when the next positioning manoeuvre is due.

Produce an information sheet for use in a training session that tells your colleagues how to report and record any moving and positioning activities they undertake, and the importance of noting when the next positioning manoeuvre is due.

LO6 Knowing when to seek advice from and/or involve others when moving and positioning an individual

(6.1) Seeking advice and/or assistance to move or handle an individual safely

Time to reflect

(6.1) Help!

- In what circumstances do you currently get help or advice to carry out moving and handling activities?

- Why might you not seek help?

- What might be the outcome if you carried out an activity for which you didn't feel 100% confident or competent?

If you are pregnant, feel yourself coming down with an infection, have an MSD or are concerned that you are not physically big or strong enough to participate in a particular manoeuvre, get advice from your manager about whether or not you should carry it out.

If you are asked to participate in a manoeuvre in which you haven't been trained, politely refuse but get help – apply for training! Health and care work depends on people being able to pull together – if you can't do a job due to lack of training, you're not much good to anyone.

You may be asked to help in a manoeuvre:

- which is outside the confines of the care plan

- which is not within the scope of your job role

- that you know could cause injury.

Get help when you cannot reach a compromise that will enable you to work within health and safety guidelines.

If, despite being trained, you are not confident in being able to carry out a manoeuvre competently, seek advice from an experienced colleague. Ask them to supervise you and help where necessary until you can demonstrate the required level of competence.

If you have concerns that a manoeuvre is no longer appropriate for the individual, for example, because of a change in their health or ability to understand instructions, get help. The manoeuvre may have to be reviewed and adapted.

If you have concerns that any aids or equipment are not sufficiently clean or well maintained, get help. Don't put health and safety at risk by using unsafe equipment.

Evidence activity

(6.1) Describe when advice and/or assistance should be sought to move or handle an individual safely

This activity gives you an opportunity to demonstrate that you know when to seek advice regarding safe moving or handling.

Make a list of the occasions when, because of fears for safety with regard to moving or handling an individual, you have sought advice or assistance.

(6.2) Sources of information about moving and positioning individuals

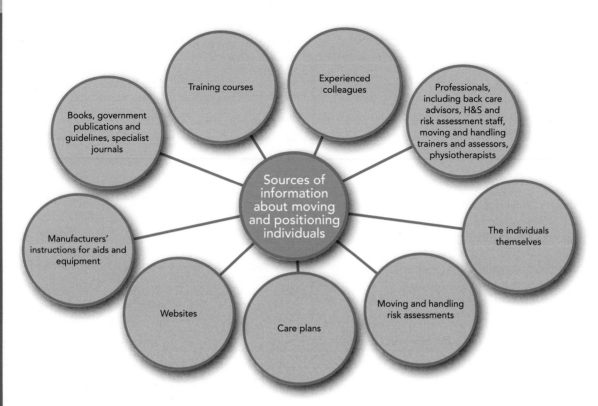

Figure 12.9 Sources of information about moving and positioning individuals

Evidence activity

(6.2) Sources of information about moving and positioning

Produce a list of sources of information about moving and positioning individuals, which can be retained within care plans and risk assessment records.

Assessment summary

Your reading of this chapter and completion of the activities will have prepared you to be able to engage in personal development in health, social care or children's and young people's settings.

To achieve the unit, your assessor will require you to:

Learning outcomes	Assessment Criteria
Learning outcome **1**: Understand anatomy and physiology in relation to moving and positioning individuals by:	(1.1) outlining the anatomy and physiology of the human body in relation to the importance of correct moving and positioning of individuals See Evidence activity 1.1, p. 233

Learning outcomes	Assessment Criteria
Learning outcome 1: Understand anatomy and physiology in relation to moving and positioning individuals by:	1.2 describing the impact of specific conditions on the correct movement and positioning of an individual See Evidence activity 1.2, p. 235
Learning outcome 2: Understand current legislation and agreed ways of working when moving and positioning individuals by:	2.1 describing how current legislation and agreed ways of working affect working practices related to moving and positioning individuals See Evidence activity 2.1, p. 237
	2.2 what health and safety factors need to be taken into account when moving and positioning individuals and any equipment used to do this See Evidence activity 2.2, p. 239
Learning outcome 3: Be able to minimise risk before moving and positioning individuals by:	3.1 accessing up-to-date copies of risk assessment documentation See Practice activity 3.1, p. 239
	3.2 carrying out preparatory checks using: • the individual's care plan • the moving and handling risk assessment See Practice activity 3.2, p. 240
	3.3 identifying any immediate risks to the individual See Evidence activity 3.3, p. 240
	3.4 describing actions to take in relation to identified risks See Evidence activity 3.4, p. 242

Learning outcomes	Assessment Criteria
Learning outcome **3**: Be able to minimise risk before moving and positioning individuals by:	(3.5) describing what action should be taken if the individual's wishes conflict with their plan of care in relation to health and safety and their risk assessment See Evidence activity 3.5, p. 242
	(3.6) preparing the immediate environment, ensuring: • adequate space for the move in agreement with all concerned • that potential hazards are removed See Practice activity 3.6, p. 243
	(3.7) applying standard precautions for infection prevention and control See Practice activity 3.7, p. 244
Learning outcome **4**: Be able to prepare individuals before moving and positioning by:	(4.1) demonstrating effective communication with the individual to ensure that they: • understand the details and reasons for the action/activity being undertaken • agree the level of support required See Practice activity 4.1, p. 246
	(4.2) obtaining valid consent for the planned activity See Practice activity 4.2, p. 247
Learning outcome **5**: Be able to move and position an individual by:	(5.1) following the care plan to ensure that the individual is positioned: • using the agreed technique • in a way that will avoid causing undue pain or discomfort See Practice activity 5.1, p. 248
	(5.2) demonstrating effective communication with any others involved in the manoeuvre See Practice activity 5.2, p. 249

Learning outcomes	Assessment Criteria
Learning outcome 5: Be able to move and position an individual by:	**5.3** describing the aids and equipment that may be used for moving and positioning See Evidence activity 5.3, p. 250
	5.4 using equipment to maintain the individual in the appropriate position See Evidence activity 5.4, p. 251
	5.5 encouraging the individual's active participation in the manoeuvre See Evidence activity 5.5, p. 251
	5.6 monitoring the individual throughout the activity so that the procedure can be stopped if there is any adverse reaction See Evidence activity 5.6, p. 252
	5.7 demonstrating how to report and record the activity noting when the next positioning manoeuvre is due See Evidence activity, 5.7 p. 253
Learning outcome 6: Know when to seek advice from and/or involve others when moving and positioning an individual by:	**6.1** describing when advice and/or assistance should be sought to move or handle an individual safely See Evidence activity 6.1, p. 253
	6.2 describing what sources of information are available about moving and positioning individuals See Evidence activity 6.2, p. 254

Good luck!

Web links

Health and Safety Executive   www.hse.gov.uk
Royal College of Nursing   www.rcn.org.uk

Various websites promoting moving and handling aids and equipment.

For Unit HSC 3020

In care, it is vital that people have the right care to meet their needs. It is therefore important that procedures are followed to ensure that needs are met. Further, it is vital that individuals are at the centre of this process so they feel that they are actively involved in their own care. Good, effective care planning can ensure all these criteria are met. Care packages should never be made for the ease or convenience of care workers.

The reading and activities in this chapter will help you to:

■ Understand the principles of person-centred assessment and care planning

■ Be able to facilitate person-centred assessment

■ Be able to contribute to the planning of care and support

■ Be able to support the implementation of care plans

■ Be able to monitor a care plan

■ Be able to facilitate a review of care plans and their implementation

LO1 Understand the principles of person-centred assessment and care planning

 1.1 **Explain the importance of a holistic approach to assessment and planning of care or support**

Individuals may need care at various times in their life. Figure 13.1 shows some of the reasons why this could be.

Because there is such a range of individuals, it follows that there is a range of needs. To meet these needs, care planning is vital.

Holistic health means seeing the whole person, not just their physical health, but also their emotional, sexual, social, intellectual, mental and spiritual health. When we care for someone, we need to consider all these needs, which can be interlinked.

Key term

Holistic means acknowledging the 'whole'.

Time to reflect

1.1 Who is 'healthy'?

Consider an 18-year-old wheelchair user who attends college, hopes to go to university, regularly sees his friends, has close relationships with his family and has a long-term girlfriend. Would it be considered that this person had poor health? Compare this with an 18 year old who is physically healthy but is neither at college nor has a job, he lost all contact with his family two years ago, he has nobody he can refer to as his friends and as of yet, has not had a partner. Which of these two teenage boys do you feel has the best health?

Traditionally, health has been seen as mostly physical but, increasingly, it is the norm and good practice to consider an individual's holistic health. Only concentrating on physical aspects of care could miss key needs. A consequence could be that as well as not caring for that aspect of their health, the physical side of their health may worsen too.

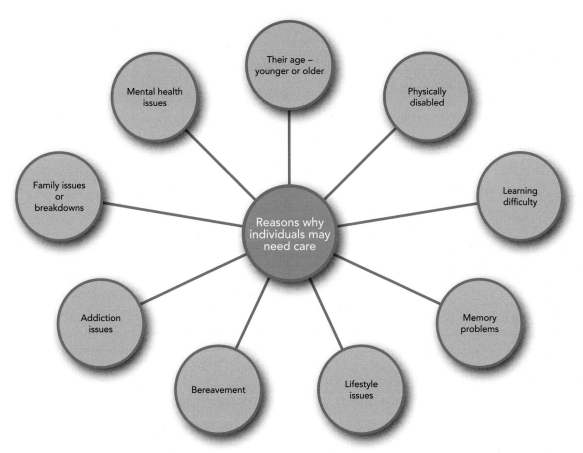

Figure 13.1 Why individuals may need care

Case Study

 Jean

Jean (76) is continually being admitted to hospital after falling. She is given pain relief, has her wounds dressed and has any broken bones cast. Her physical care needs are assessed and supported and, between them, her carers 'fix' her.

Jean is, however, unhappy, lonely and depressed. She always falls at the same place, getting in and out of her house. As she explains, 'That step will kill me one winter!' Because of this, she now avoids going out as much as possible. She rarely goes to the shops, and when she does, she stocks up on freezable, processed foods. She has stopped going to the library and the day care centre completely. She rarely sees her friends. She is also now putting on weight.

1. In what ways are assessments of Jean failing?

2. What are the consequences of this on her holistic health?

3. What simple action could improve Jean's life significantly?

It is important that an individual is looked at holistically, acknowledging all their facets, otherwise important aspects of that person will not be recognised. An individual needing care is more than a 'service user'; they are a person, with a history, a life and an identity. Ignoring this could be detrimental to the quality of care delivered.

Being person centred is about listening to and learning about what people want from their lives, and helping people to think about what they want now and in the future. Family, friends, professionals and services work together with the individual to make this happen. The case study of Robert shows how detrimental ignoring an individual's holistic needs could be.

Case Study

 1.1b Robert

Robert is an elderly man whose dog is his only company, and sometimes his only reason to get up in the morning. When he was assessed, his carer didn't take his dog into account, or what would happen to it if Robert wasn't around. When Robert went into hospital after having a stroke, his carers referred to his notes, but as there was no mention of a dog, nothing was arranged. When Robert returned from hospital, he found that his dog had died. Robert was devastated. In the six months that followed, Robert's health deteriorated very quickly.

Explain the consequences of not being person centred and assessing Robert holistically.

Evidence activity

1.1 The importance of holistic assessment and planning

Consider an individual you know and, with their permission, describe their needs holistically.

1.2 ## Describe ways of supporting the individual to lead the assessment and planning process

The role of clients in their care planning is recognised in legislation such as the Children Act (1989), NHS & Community Care Act (1990) and The Carer (Recognition) Act (1995), which prioritised it as best practice and marked a way

forward for all future care planning. Since then the idea has evolved that individuals requiring care should be involved in every stage of the planning process.

Research & investigate

 1.2 Key legislation

The Children Act (1989), NHS & Community Care Act (1990) and The Carer (Recognition) Act (1995) are key pieces of legislation in health and social care. For each, find out about:

- its purpose
- its key features.

Consider the reasons why people need care, as show in Figure 13.1. Such a range of reasons results in a wide range of needs. To meet all these individual and specific needs, care planning is vital. Usually the planning process involves the stages outlined in Figure 13.3. This process needs to be a continuous cycle, as needs can change. A care plan which is meeting needs when implemented, may not be meeting them six months later.

When assessing and planning, it is vital that the individual leads the process. This may sound obvious, but it is surprising how often this is overlooked and care professionals may think they 'know what's best'. Care professionals must remember that the individual is at the foundation of care planning; it is their body, their discomfort, their life and fundamentally, their care. Care planning which is not person centred is meaningless. It is not acceptable to 'go through the motions', care workers must value an individual's role in this process – that is best practice. It is essential to **empowering** people in their own care.

Key term

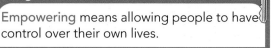

Empowering means allowing people to have control over their own lives.

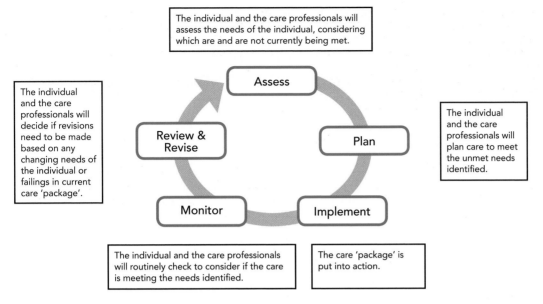

Figure 13.2 The care planning process

Top tips to support an individual to lead assessment and planning

■ Ask the individual what they want and what they consider their needs to be. Leading questions should be avoided, e.g. 'Your current hygiene arrangements are fully meeting all your needs, aren't they?' This may lead to agreement when it may not actually be the case. Also, **open questions** are preferred to **closed questions** so, instead of asking 'Are you happy?' try, 'Tell me about how you feel at the moment.'

■ Care workers should meet with individuals face to face. Assessment is not done best over the telephone or email. Individuals need to feel valued enough to be met in person.

■ Care workers should make clear that everything will be kept **confidential**. This will reassure the individual that it is okay to divulge necessary information.

■ Discussions should be in a simple format. Bamboozling individuals with **acronyms**, jargon and technical terminology will not help them to lead the assessment. However, care workers should avoid patronising individuals by using language that is too simplistic. A balance of detailed information that is clear and simple is important.

■ Employ **empathy** throughout. It is vital that care workers consider how the individual feels, which will help strengthen the care worker/individual relationship.

■ If anything needs repeating, it should be done patiently and clearly. At the end, care workers should clarify and summarise to ensure that everything is understood and to minimise mistakes. Any terminology should be clarified, as an individual's interpretation of 'priority', for example, may differ from yours or from another organisations'.

■ Give copies of documents to everyone. Allow time for individuals to read them and ask questions, and ensure that documents are signed. This is an opportunity for any mistakes or disagreements to be highlighted, and is a record for any future queries.

Key terms

Acronyms are words formed from the initial letters of several words, e.g. NHS.
Closed questions result is set answers, e.g. yes/no, true/false.
Confidential means private, only allowing people with authority to access the information.
Empathy the ability to view a situation from another individual's perspective.
Open questions can, in theory, result in any answer and can be better for getting people's opinions than closed questions.

Not every individual is in a position to lead fully in the process (due to age, communication difficulties, sensory impairments, mental health problems, learning difficulties) and so the use of an advocate may be needed. An advocate is someone who represents another. Advocates will not make decisions on an individual's behalf, but will seek information, ask questions, present the information to the individual in an unbiased way, allowing the individual to be informed and hence make decisions. Advocates ensure that individuals' rights and interests are supported.

The website Action for Advocacy is an excellent source on advocacy. In their words, 'Advocacy is taking action to help people say what they want, secure their rights, represent their interests and obtain services they need.'

Carers should aim to allow active participation when assessing and planning care. This not only leads to better care, but will also aid ownership of any care packages and further, help with an individual's self esteem and feeling valued and respected.

 1.3 **Describe ways the assessment and planning process or documentation can be adapted to maximise an individual's ownership and control of it**

There is little point involving individuals if they cannot access the process or documents. If individuals have issues affecting their abilities, they will feel little or no ownership over the process.

Key term

Active participation recognises an individual's right to participate as independently as possibly; the individual is regarded as an active partner in their own care, rather than a passive recipient.

Key term

Makaton is a system using gestures in combination with pictures and symbols to communicate messages. Information can be found on the Makaton website.

Evidence activity

 1.2 **The importance of supporting an individual to lead assessment and planning**

Produce a report on the ways you would support the individual you described in Evidence activity 1.1 to lead their assessment and planning process.

Research & investigate

 1.3 Active listening

Find out about active listening. In particular, find out about Egan's steps to active listening, and the use of the SOLER strategy.

Research & investigate

 1.3 Self advocacy

Find out about self advocacy. What is it? What is its purpose?

Time to reflect

 1.2 Barriers to communication

An individual is meeting with a care worker. They have a desk between them. The care worker is looking at the form he is completing and does not raise their head or make eye contact. There is a computer screen facing the care worker, which has the individual's details on, but the individual cannot see it.

1. How do you think the individual is feeling in this situation?

2. What suggestions would you make?

Care workers need to consider the logistics of meetings. Meetings should be arranged in a suitable location. If an individual has to travel long distances, possibly at cost to themselves, they may feel they are not a priority. Arrange meetings at times that are convenient, showing flexibility and openness. Make sure all are comfortable; ensure that chairs, tables, refreshments, etc. are available. If the individual has any disabilities, make sure that facilities meet these needs, for example, wheelchair access, disabled parking and toilets. Ideally, arrange meetings in the client's own home, fully working the process around them.

Care workers should employ effective verbal communication skills. Language should be appropriate to the age, ability and understanding of the individual. Being confused or embarrassed because they do not understand is to a positive outcome. If the person speaks a language other than English, ensure that interpreters are available, respecting the right of the individual to fully participate.

Effective non-verbal communication skills will make individuals feel more comfortable. Care professionals need to consider their facial expressions, eye contact, posture (whether sitting or standing), gestures, etc. A smiling, friendly face, nodding when an individual is talking, shows that the care worker is respecting what the individual has to say. A scowling, slouching care worker may not make an individual feel that what they are saying is important. One strategy to use is active listening.

Communication aids can be used to assist discussions. For individuals with visual impairments, Braille and the spoken word could be used. For individuals with hearing impairments, hearing aids, sign language, a signer, lip reading and the written word could be used. For those with emotional difficulties or behavioural issues, **Makaton**, picture aids, photographs, visits, plans, flash cards, etc. could be used to help. These are effective at ensuring inclusiveness and allowing individuals to fully participate in all stages of care planning.

Figure 13.3 Actions to help individuals take ownership of the care planning process

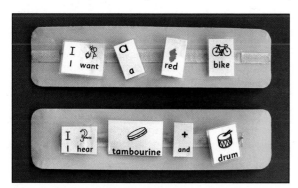

Figure 13.4 Using images to assist communication

Evidence activity

1.3 Adapting planning and documents

Produce a detailed list of 'Top tips' for a new care worker on the ways assessing and planning documents can be adapted to maximise an individual's ownership and control.

LO2 Be able to facilitate person-centred assessment

2.1 Establish with the individual a partnership approach to the assessment process

Alongside the individual, there are many people who can be involved in assessment, all able to give their opinion and professional expertise. A partnership approach is effective when professionals from different disciplines work together. It can be most effective where there is a key worker (sometimes referred to as care coordinator, facilitator, care manager or similar) who can assist individuals in managing their care planning process. It is important that they coordinate assessment, request written reports and professional opinions, or invite others to case meetings.

It is vital that the key worker explains the process of a partnership approach to the individual, outlines the benefits to them and reassures them of any confidentiality issues, etc. It is imperative that the individual is comfortable with a partnership approach and does not feel intimidated or that everyone is 'ganging up on them'.

Evidence activity

2.1 How to establish a partnership approach

You need to explain a partnership approach to an individual. Produce a statement of what you would say.

2.2 Establish with the individual how the process should be carried out and who else should be involved in the process

The individual and the key worker should consider who may be involved in the process. This could potentially be an exhaustive list as the needs are unique and complex.

The individual needs to consider how the process should develop, depending on the urgency or complexity of care needs. Whichever method is chosen, best practice is assessment through a Single Assessment Process, which is where people's needs are assessed, but without procedures being needlessly duplicated by different agencies, with information shared appropriately. Then, with an individual's permission, the information will be shared with other professionals who will be involved in provision. Decisions should be made as to the format in terms of weight of opinion, time allocated, themes, care setting, etc.

Evidence activity

2.2 The process and who else should be involved

Choose an individual whom you know, someone from a 'soap', or an individual in the media. (This individual will be used for various Evidence activities in this unit, so try to choose an individual with a variety of needs.)

Describe all the people who may be able to help this individual, and a process of assessment that may be beneficial.

2.3 Agree with the individual and others the intended outcomes of the assessment process and care plan

Outcomes are the desired results or consequences of actions. First, outcomes must to be identified; a **care plan** without them is not as effective. Second, ensure that outcomes are agreed throughout the partnership. It would be ineffective to have a partnership approach to assessment and then have separate intended outcomes. The individual and others such as carers, friends, relatives and professionals can all have useful input into what intended outcomes are appropriate.

Key term

A care plan may be know by other names, such as a support plan, individual plan or care delivery plan. It is the document in which day-to-day requirements and preferences for care and support are detailed.

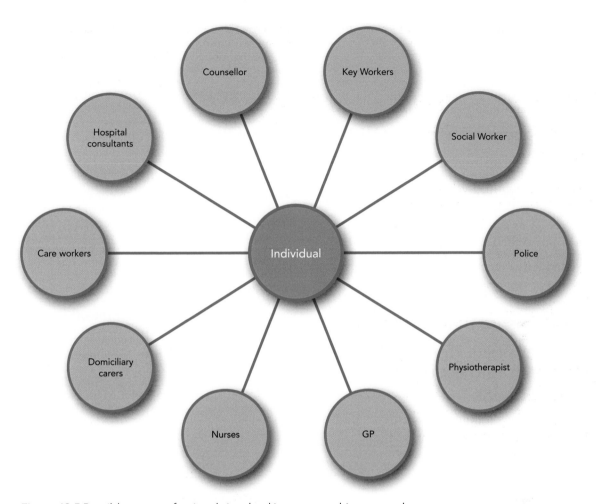

Figure 13.5 Possible care professionals involved in a partnership approach

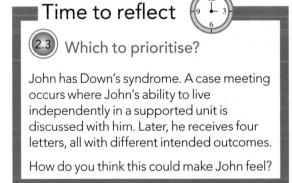

Time to reflect

(2.3) Which to prioritise?

John has Down's syndrome. A case meeting occurs where John's ability to live independently in a supported unit is discussed with him. Later, he receives four letters, all with different intended outcomes.

How do you think this could make John feel?

In their research 'Introducing an outcome focus into care management and user surveys', the Social Policy Research Unit at York University state that there are three types of outcomes.

The Outcomes Framework

■ Maintenance of quality of life – e.g. maintaining acceptable levels of personal comfort and safety, social contact, meaningful activity, participation in normally accepted social roles, control over daily life and routines.

■ Change – e.g. improving confidence, or accessibility of the environment, reducing risk, improving means of communication, or regaining self care skills.

■ Impacts of Service Process – e.g. whether people feel treated as an individual, valued and respected, or whether services fit well with other sources of assistance, or the users' preferences and priority outcomes.

To make these outcomes as useful as possible, all intended outcomes are SMART:

Specific

Measurable

Achievable

Realistic

Time related

SMART targets ensure that there is less confusion, and they can then be measured as to whether they have been met or not. Intended outcomes must be formally written into care plans, so success at meeting them can be judged. It may be useful to prioritise intended outcomes or to break them down into more manageable, attainable results.

 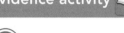 **Evidence activity**

2.3 **How to agree intended outcomes**

Using the same individual as for Evidence activity 2.2, use SMART targets to establish intended outcomes for the individual.

2.4 **Ensure that assessment takes account of the individual's strengths and aspirations as well as needs**

The aim of any assessment is to ensure that the individual has the best quality of life and

optimum health and well-being. This does not just mean helping an individual to *not be* ill, *not be* in pain, *not be* disadvantaged; it is about them being the best they can be.

Key term

The optimum is the best or most favourable point, degree or amount – the ideal.

One way to describe this is to consider positive and negative definitions of health. Negative definitions are when we are seen as healthy because we *don't* have a condition, an illness or impairment. A positive definition of health is when something is achieved or gained; being as fit and healthy as you can be, having the best health, wanting to add life to years and years to life. It focuses more on well-being than just health for the sake of 'getting by'. The World Health Organisation's definition of health takes a more positive view of health as 'Health as a state of complete physical, mental and social well-being and not merely the absence of disease or infirmity' (WHO, 1946). This also includes mental and social well-being, so is a more holistic definition of health.

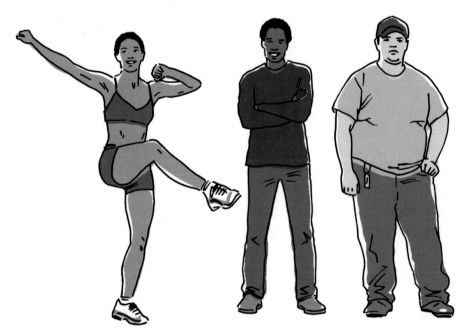

Figure 13.6 Positive and negative definitions of health

This principle is just the same for meeting an individual's needs. It is not enough to deal with all the areas where they are in need. It is about their well-being being as good as possible; allowing people to do what they can do (their

strengths), and what they'd like to do (aspirations). Ensuring that individuals remain independent and autonomous is essential for their self-esteem and feelings of worth.

Case Study

 2.4 Becky

Becky is an able woman who is a wheelchair user. Her carer is assessing her. He asks Becky about all the things she cannot do. Becky explains that she struggles with certain personal hygiene matters, washing clothing, housework (e.g. vacuuming, sweeping), transport, etc. These are noted. Becky is never given the opportunity to say the things she can do, e.g. ironing, doing her own hair and makeup, dusting and polishing her house. Becky also loves dancing and watching dance programmes like *Strictly Come Dancing*; she would love to be in a dance group or to go to watch dance acts.

All the services Becky requires to meet her unmet needs, e.g. personal hygiene matters, washing clothing, housework transport, etc. are put into place.

1. How might Becky feel when **domiciliary carers** iron her clothes for her, dust and polish her house or do her hair?

2. Becky never goes to any dance classes or to see any dance shows. How could this affect her health and well-being?

Key term

Domiciliary carers, sometimes referred to as 'home carers', are carers who provide support in an individual's own home.

Research & investigate

2.4 Positive and Negative definitions of health

Find out about positive and negative definitions of health.

Find definitions and the advantages and disadvantages of each.

Evidence activity

2.4 Taking account of individuals' strengths and aspirations as well as needs

Using the same individual as for Evidence activity 2.2, design a set of questions which would allow identification of the individual's strengths and aspirations.

2.5 Work with the individual and others to identify support requirements and preferences

It is imperative that individuals are able to highlight their support requirements and preferences. A good written template for this will be best practice, ensuring that:

■ all assessments are standardised, limiting variations between individuals

■ nothing is missed out by any assessor.

Many examples of care assessment documentation can be found online. It is important to ensure that set templates allow room for individualised commentary, otherwise it is not person centred.

Research & investigate

2.5 Care planning documentation

Use the internet to find a variety of documents used by care professionals to assess an individual.

Consider the criteria covered in each document. Are there similarities?

The document should be worked through, remembering any issues discussed earlier in 1.2 and 1.3. It is often a good idea to allow the individual to consider their assessment beforehand, instead of it being 'sprung upon them'. Ideally, offer the individual a document beforehand, to record any reflections on their own needs. Doing this means that they can really consider their care needs beforehand, so the process can be more person centred.

When individuals and others are assessing, they may do this at two levels, general and specialist. The general level may deal with everyday aspects, such as day-to-day needs. Specialist assessment would be through an appropriate specialist, such as a nurse, GP, occupational therapist, psychologist or physiotherapist. Specialists will assess specific needs, as they have the expert knowledge and opinion. All assessments will be facilitated and collated by the key worker. However, although getting specialist assessment is vital, the individual's opinions or judgements should not be disregarded or seen as 'supplementary'.

Evidence activity

Identifying support requirements and preferences

Using the same individual as for Evidence activity 2.2, assess your individual using a form similar to the one in Figure 13.8 (or any other you have found).

LO3 Be able to contribute to the planning of care or support

3.1 Take account of factors that may influence the type and level of care or support to be provided

Once the individual has been assessed, the next stage is to decide what care and support is required to meet these needs. Many factors will influence this.

Feasibility of aspirations

If something is feasible, it is possible. Sometimes, with the best will in the world, certain aspirations are not achievable. This may be because of:

- Time – there may not be enough time to organise certain care or support, or by the time it has been organised it may be too late.

- Money – resources in health and social care are not **infinite**, and sometimes individuals can not have what they would like or, unfortunately, what they need. Care organisations that are funded by the government have budgets and have to prioritise how they spend their money. Equally, charities have limited funds and are dependent on donations from government and individuals. On occasions, individuals themselves may have to fund services and obviously, if they cannot, then they may not be able to access that support.

Key term

Infinite means never ending, without a limit.

- Staffing – certain care may need a certain quantity and quality of staff. As with money, there may not always be the staff to meet the needs of the individual and, clearly, staff need paying too.

- Health/ability of individual – there may be times when the individual's health or abilities may make any of their preferences or aspirations difficult, and it may be that as a result of this, these cannot be met.

The individual's beliefs, values and preferences

Belief, values and preferences have to be taken into account when planning to meet an individual's needs. This could be something simple, such as preparing food a certain way, for example, an individual may prefer grilled bacon with the fat cut off. If bacon was then fried, with the fat left on, with extra lard used in the pan, the individual may not eat it, and hence miss a meal. Therefore the need would be unmet.

	Fully independent	Independent with support	Completely dependent
Physical Health Needs			
Mobility	☐	☐	☐
Breathing	☐	☐	☐
Pain	☐	☐	☐
Skin	☐	☐	☐
Sexual needs	☐	☐	☐
Foot care	☐	☐	☐
Eating, drinking and swallowing	☐	☐	☐
Lifestyle changes desired(diet/alcohol/smoking etc)	☐	☐	☐
Medications	☐	☐	☐
Personal Care			
Getting in/out of bed	☐	☐	☐
Washing	☐	☐	☐
Bathing/showering	☐	☐	☐
Toileting	☐	☐	☐
Hair care/personal hygiene	☐	☐	☐
Dressing	☐	☐	☐
Oral health	☐	☐	☐
Cooking/food preparation	☐	☐	☐
Housework/laundry	☐	☐	☐
Shopping	☐	☐	☐
Worship	☐	☐	☐
Emotional Well-being			
Sleeping	☐	☐	☐
Confidence and disorientation	☐	☐	☐
Memory	☐	☐	☐
Depression	☐	☐	☐
Bereavement or loss	☐	☐	☐
Social Well-being			
You, your family, and friends	☐	☐	☐
Carer support	☐	☐	☐
Pets	☐	☐	☐
Social contacts	☐	☐	☐
Childcare/parenting/other caring responsibility	☐	☐	☐
Accommodation			
Location	☐	☐	☐
Accommodation	☐	☐	☐
Warmth	☐	☐	☐
Access to and around the accommodation	☐	☐	☐
Amenities of the accommodation	☐	☐	☐
Security & safety	☐	☐	☐
Education & Employment			
Help finding work or training	☐	☐	☐
Studying or qualifications	☐	☐	☐
Your leisure activities (pastimes and hobbies)	☐	☐	☐
Financial Well-being			
Benefits	☐	☐	☐
Management of personal finances	☐	☐	☐
Help with debt	☐	☐	☐
Miscellaneous			
Use this space here to tell us of any issues or problems or questions you have	☐	☐	☐

Figure 13.7 An example of a simple assessment form

Case Study

(3.1) Margaret

Margaret is living in a nursing home. She has trouble communicating. Every time the care worker helps Margaret to wash, she runs a bath even though Margaret prefers a shower. Her carer also 'gives Margaret a little treat' by putting bath salts in, but Margaret hates these as she thinks they scratch her legs and bottom as they don't dissolve properly. She would prefer bath oils. The care worker then washes Margaret's hair in a supermarket's own brand shampoo and doesn't use a conditioner; she rinses her hair with bath water, not clean water. This upsets Margaret, as she loved having nice, shiny hair.

Consider how something as simple as this washing practice is not respecting Margaret's values and preferences.

As well as preferences in day-to-day activities, it is vital the religions spiritual or lifestyle beliefs of an individual are also respected and promoted. An individual's religion will affect the day-to-day care a person receives – their diet, their dress, their washing rituals, their prayer routines, etc. A carer not actively promoting any beliefs in the planning of care would not be ensuring that rights to equality and diversity are being met; indeed, the care plan could even be discriminatory. All aspects of care planning need to be anti-discriminatory – the language used, the resources available, the staff employed, the locations, etc.

Risks associated with achieving outcomes

Occasionally there may be risks involved in achieving outcomes, and this may affect the ability to provide the type and level of care to be provided. These could be general health and safety risks, or specific risks to the individual's well-being. For example, if an individual desired an outcome where they were able to live independently, without support, this may not be possible if carers, their family and friends and others believe that they may be at risk. Service providers have a duty of care to ensure that all individuals are safe and free from harm. If anything were to happen to an individual, they may be deemed responsible for poor-quality care and mismanagement of the situation. It may

be that a long-term target could be established for a desired outcome, but short-term targets may need to be in place to judge how risk-free or how feasible the intended outcome would be in the future.

However, this needs to be balanced with the rights individuals have to the life they choose. This can sometimes be an ethical dilemma for care workers.

Research & investigate

(3.1) Ethics

1. Research ethics and ethical dilemas.

Try to find out about ethical dilemas which care workers may be faced within health and social care.

Availability of services and other support options

If a service isn't available, it is clearly not possible for an individual to access it. Often, services are not spread out equally across the nation, and an excellent service which someone has accessed in one place may not be available elsewhere. Plus, even if it is available, there may be travel involved, or opening hours may not match the times when an individual needs them.

Evidence activity

(3.1) Factors that may influence the type and level of care

Using the same individual as for Evidence activity 2.2, describe any factors that may influence the type or level of care or support provided for the individual.

(3.2) Work with the individual and others to explore options and resources for delivery of the plan

All options for delivery need to be explored with the individuals and others involved, to consider the most effective and efficient ways to deliver the plan. Working together, sharing ideas, considering all the benefits and disadvantages of options, and generally considering the **logistics** of a plan's delivery is ideal. This will involve the person in their care and hence continue to be person centred, and will also highlight any potential downfalls before they occur.

Key term

Logistics refers to the full management of a task or procedure, from beginning to end.

Once options are decided, the specific details need to be established, i.e. the frequency, times, duration and staffing. Sometimes, the full original plan is referred to as the macro-plan, whereas the day-to-day, more specific care plan is often called the micro-plan. It is essential that all are clear on the details, as the misunderstanding of minutiae could lead to problems.

Care could be provided from the following options and resources:

■ Informal support – unpaid non-professionals, often spouses, parents or siblings.

■ Formal support – paid, qualified staff whose job it is to provide care.

■ Care or support services – the range of services available from health and social care.

■ Community facilities – communities often have a wealth of services for individuals. Libraries, day centres, town halls, community centres, etc. all have facilities which could have a positive effect on an individual.

■ Financial resources – some services are offered by private organisations at a cost. Some individuals have to use these services because they are only available privately; others may choose a private service in the belief that it provides better choice and quality. This would obviously draw on an individual's finances.

■ Individuals' personal networks – individuals may be part of teams, clubs, societies or religious groups that could impact positively on their lives.

A good care plan would draw on all of these to provide the right 'package' of care designed by, and right for, the individual.

Time to reflect

 The unlikeliest places!

Harold goes to his local Working men's Club three times a week. He has a pint (or two!) and watches sport on the television. He has some good friends there; they'd miss him if he wasn't around. At Christmas, the club provides a meal for the senior club members and a gift from the club funds. In the summer, there is a trip to the coast, which Harold never misses. He often assists with the club bingo, selling tickets, etc.

1. What benefits are there from the personal network Harold has?

2. Why would it be bad practice if a care plan did not acknowledge this?

Evidence activity

 Exploring options and resources for delivery of the plan

Using the same individual as for Evidence activity 2.2, describe any options and resources the individual may have to support delivery of any plans.

 ## Contribute to agreement on how component parts of a plan will be delivered and by whom

If it is not agreed at the outset what will be delivered and by whom, problems could occur.

1. Duplication – if it is not stated who is responsible for a task, more than one person could assume that they were, and so it could be delivered more than is needed. This is clearly inefficient and a waste of resources, as well as potentially being intrusive in someone's life.

2. Omissions – a potentially worse situation would be if it is not stated who is responsible for a task and everyone assumes it is not their responsibility, so no one delivers. This evidently means that the individual doesn't receive the care they need.

The need to agree and formalise how components of the plan will be delivered is even more important when single assessment and working in partnerships is being practised. If it is made clear who is responsible for what, it also highlights who is accountable for any failings in the care plan or provisions, so no one can claim later that 'I didn't know!'

What?	• What services exactly will be delivered?
Where?	• Which particular care setting will the care be delivered in, and which room?
When?	• When will delivery take place, and how often, and what time?
How?	• How will the delivery take place?
By Whom?	• What staff, expertise is needed and how much?

Figure 13.8 Care delivery details

Case Study

 3.3 Susan

As scheduled, Susan's bandages were changed yesterday by the district nurse. Today, a domiciliary care worker arrives to help with some cleaning and hygiene care. The domiciliary carer starts to take the bandages off. Susan complains, explaining that the district nurse told her to keep them on until her visit next week. The domiciliary carer tells her to stop getting confused and let her do her job. Susan gets very upset, as she knows she is right and doesn't like the tone the care worker takes with her.

What aspects of care do you believe the domiciliary care worker is doing wrong here?

Evidence activity

3.3 Contributing to agreement on who delivers which components of a plan

Using the same individual as for Evidence activity 2.2, describe some suggested plan components and whom they could be delivered by.

3.4 Record the plan in a suitable format

Similar to when assessing, considerations may need to be made for needs and preferences when planning. The plan may be on paper and, for some individuals, this may be the most appropriate format. However, for some groups of individuals, other formats may be of use.

■ For people with learning difficulties, simpler language and avoidance of technical language may beneficial. Symbols or signs, such as Makaton, could be used. Equally, the organisation Photosymbols provides a full gallery of images which could be used. In their words, 'Photosymbols are a collection of pictures for making easy-read information. They are designed to be placed alongside words to make information easier to understand.'

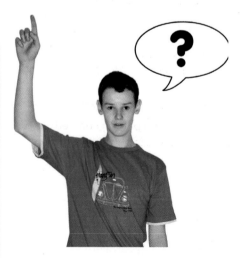

Figure 13.9 Using images to make communication easier

■ For the visually impaired, Braille, the use of large font or Makaton symbols can all be helpful. Or the care plan could be presented in an audio format.

■ For the hearing impaired, the use of sign language, a signer or lip reading may help when explaining the plan or when the individual has questions. The individual may also benefit from a hearing aid.

Present the plan in a way that is appropriate to the age, needs, ability and preferences of the individual and, if in doubt, ask them! It is not offensive to ask someone how they would like the documents to be presented; it is offensive to not ask. Whatever format is chosen however, it must be clear, with good standards of English or whichever language the document is in and easy to follow.

Practice activity

(3.4) **Recording the plan in a suitable format**

While at your real work environment, record any plans you have in a suitable format for the individual in question.

LO4 Be able to support the implementation of care plans

(4.1) **Carry out assigned aspects of a care plan**

Often, this can be seen as the simplest part of the planning process and, if good assessment and planning has taken place, it can be. Quite simply, this is where the care plan is put into effect.

Success at this stage is more likely if:

■ assessment has been person centred

■ examination of needs and preferences was holistic

■ planning of delivery has been person centred

■ a partnership approach has been applied

■ there have been opportunities for it to be checked and amended.

If this has occurred, implementation *should* be fairly straightforward. However, this is not guaranteed and communication still needs to happen to ensure that any issues are highlighted immediately.

This is a key stage, when the care workers who are appointed to deliver particular aspects are deployed and, in theory, the needs of the individual start to be met. This could be an emotional time. On one hand, the individual and others around them may be anxious about how the care plan will work, whether it will be successful and whether or not needs will indeed be met. However, the individual and others around them may be excited and pleased about positive changes to their lives which they have been waiting for. Hence, sensitivity and patience may be needed with the individual to ensure that they cope with this transition.

Practice activity

(4.1) **Carry out assigned aspects of the plan**

While at your real work environment, carry out assigned aspects of the plan. Collate witness statements and any documentation as evidence.

(4.2) **Support others to carry out aspects of a care plan for which they are responsible**

As a potential key worker, one essential role is to oversee implementation of the care plan and support others in their roles. Key workers will often be the first port of call for any questions, not just from the individual but also from any of the partnerships involved in provision and delivery of the care plan.

It is important that key workers deal with any issues quickly, patiently and in a way that is supportive. If a key worker is unapproachable, reprimanding or judgemental, anyone involved in the delivery of the care plan, including the individual, may not feel confident to seek clarification, request guidance or ask for assistance.

However, if those responsible for the care delivery are not performing, then the key worker must ensure that they are challenged. This must be dealt with in a professional, supportive way. But equally, if someone is not providing the care that they should be, key workers need to have the authority and the ability to report this and deal with it. If necessary, disciplinary action needs to be taken. Everyone needs to be accountable for their role.

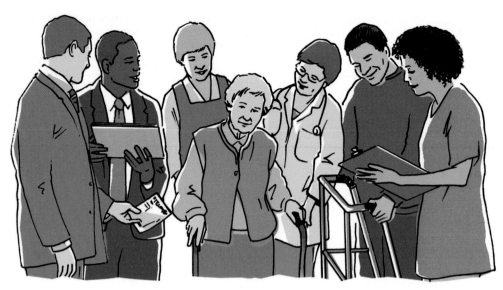

Figure 13.10 And… action!

Time to reflect

4.2 Could you?

What characteristics would make a good, supportive key worker?

Research & investigate

4.2 Accounting

Define accountability.

Why do you think accountability is important in health and social care?

Practice activity

4.2 Supporting others to carry out aspects of a care plan

While at your real work environment, support others to carry out aspects of the plan for which they are responsible. Collate witness statements and any documentation as evidence.

4.3 Adjust the plan in response to changing needs or circumstances

At the outset it may be noted that the plan needs immediate changes, before the scheduled review date. In this case, the plan needs adapting to take account of this. Clearly, this needs to be done immediately.

Reasons the plan needs changing could be due to:

■ a need was missed

■ the individual's needs alter

■ the individual changes accommodation, possibly even geographical area (which may result in a different local authority or service providers being responsible for their care)

■ the informal care supplied changes

■ services open, close or opening hours change

■ care worker problems, e.g. staff sickness, industrial action or redundancies.

Case Study

4.3 Harpreet and Avaninder

Harpreet has mobility problems due to a recent hip and knee replacement. The main care giver is his wife, Avaninder, who assists with all his dietary, hygiene and toileting

contd.

Case Study

contd.

needs. Harpreet has a care plan in place which details services provided by others, e.g. transport, physiotherapy, medical care. When returning home from shopping one day, Avaninder slips and damages her back. An ambulance is called and, after a short period in hospital, she is sent home to rest in bed for approximately a week to allow her bruised and tender back to heal.

1. Why will the current care plan no longer be effective?

2. Imagine you are the key worker for this household. What adjustments to the care plan would you make?

Practice activity

4.3 **Adjusting the plan in response to changing needs or circumstances**

While at your real work environment, adjust a care plan in response to changing needs or circumstances. Collate witness statements and any documentation as evidence.

LO5 Be able to monitor care plans

5.1 **Agree methods for monitoring the way a care plan is delivered**

Once the care plan is being implemented, everyone needs to be aware of how the care plan will be monitored (checked). Methods for monitoring need to be agreed with the individual and the care team.

■ **How often?** This may depend on the severity of the needs of the individual, as well as the level of changes being made. The more severe the needs or the greater the level of change, the greater the need for more frequent monitoring. Monitoring may be at set, frequent

points, or the care delivered may be so simple that there only needs to be monitoring if an issue arises.

■ **How?** What method should be used to feed back on whether the care plan is effective or not? This could be in person if it is decided that it is most suitable, and case meetings may be needed. However, it may be judged that face-to-face feedback isn't required and written reports would be sufficient. Under all circumstances, verbal feedback on its own should be avoided, as there is no recording of this.

■ **Who will feed back?** Clearly, the more care workers, family and friends feeding back, as well as the individual, the more evidence there will be on the effectiveness of the delivery. However, this has to be balanced with information overload. A line may need to be drawn at people on the **periphery** of the care delivery.

Key term

Being on the periphery means on the edge, or having minor involvement in something.

Whatever is decided, it must be after discussions with the individual and using the methods they desire and feel are suitable.

Evidence activity

5.1 **Agreeing methods for monitoring the delivery of a care plan**

Using the same individual as for Evidence activity 2.2, produce a poster describing methods which could be used for monitoring the way a care plan is delivered.

5.2 **Collate monitoring information from agreed sources**

It is the key worker's role to collate (collect) all the information from the agreed sources, allowing an overview of all the expert perspectives of those involved. The key worker needs to ensure that the information they collate from the agreed sources follows essential guidelines, which will ensure that monitoring is as effective as possible.

Rule 1 – Accuracy . When care workers report their observations, they should ensure they are as accurate as possible. This ensures there is little doubt over the meaning of what they are saying. Information could be used to alter a care plan and the care an individual gets, it could be used in any investigations or tribunal and could also be read by any of the parties involved, including the individual themselves, so every statement needs to be accurate and true.

Rule 2 – Objectivity. Although it can sometimes be difficult to not put one's own viewpoint or opinion on what one sees, hears or thinks, it is vital this is avoided. When reporting on an individual's care all elements of subjectivity need to be removed. Avoid 'I think' and 'I believe'. Waffle should also be avoided as this could cloud judgements.

Rule 3 – Facts. It is more effective to comment on a *measured* difference. Instead of reporting 'It looks like Hilda has lost weight since she has moved into the residential home', it might be more beneficial, to say 'In the two weeks since Hilda has moved into the residential home, her weight has reduced by 7lbs'. Comments making clear how many meals eaten, hours spent sleeping, fluids consumed, and exercise done etc will lead to a better monitoring.

Figure 13.11 Rules for collating information

 Practice activity

(5.2) Collating monitoring information from agreed sources

While at your real work environment, collate monitoring information from agreed sources. Provide documentation as evidence.

 (5.3) Record changes that affect the delivery of the care plan

Whatever changes are made as a result of any monitoring, these changes need to be recorded in as much detail as the initial plans were, to ensure that all parties are in full support and knowledge of what the changes are.

It is also important to remember that changes can be exceptionally subtle. Not all changes are obvious, and may not even be acknowledged by the individual. Changes such as increasing feelings of depression, feelings of isolation or lower self-esteem may not be so apparent, and could easily be rectified by adapting somebody's pain relief for example. Good care workers will not only make a conscious effort to monitor these changes, but will also record them.

Information needs to be stored in one place, and kept easily accessible. Changes need to be recorded immediately and information should be shared with the individual and others, so they are kept up to date.

 Time to reflect

(5.3) Singing from the same hymm sheet?

Consider what would happen if changes were made to a care plan but not recorded or stored?

 Practice activity

(5.3) Recording changes that affect the delivery of the care plan

While at your real work environment, record changes that affect the delivery of the care plan. Provide documentation as evidence.

LO6 Be able to facilitate a review of care plans and their implementation

 (6.1) Seek agreement with the individual and others about who should be involved in the review process and criteria to judge effectiveness of the care plan

When the care plan is ready to be reviewed at the scheduled time, the individual should discuss the success of the plan from their perspective. Individuals should be given the opportunity to reflect on how they feel their care plan has met their needs before any meeting, so they can consider, articulate and prepare for any discussions. This again is making the process person centred, not just the assessment and planning, but throughout.

Once a review is in place, individuals and others involved should be asked about who should be involved in the review process. A balance needs to be made between the range of information received and relevance. One course of action is to speak with the individual about whom they would like to be involved in the review process.

■ Many of the people involved in the assessment stage may be called upon, as they may be able to provide feedback which can be more comparative, i.e. before and after the care plan.

■ The individual may have different friends or family around them whom they believe can provide useful feedback.

■ The individual may have care workers to whom they have become particularly close, or spent significant amounts of time with and feel they would like them to be consulted about their progress.

■ There may be care workers with whom relationships have been poor and the individual may not respect or trust any comments from them.

Clearly, the key worker needs to bear any of these reservations in mind, but they also have to balance an individual's personal feelings with getting the most accurate picture of whether the care plan has been successful.

In theory, the criteria to judge the effectiveness of the care plan should have been decided with the individual at the outset, as one could argue that the goalposts have been moved if these are put into place at the end of the plan. However, if significant changes have occurred, new criteria need to be established with the individual to judge the success of the care plan, which takes these changes into account.

1. If another care plan is designed, it will continue with the same inappropriate care.

2. The care plan may continue when it is not needed any more.

3. The care plan may end when it is still needed.

Care workers may believe that only small 'tweaks' to the care plan may be needed, e.g. more frequent trips to the dentist to assist with denture care. On the other hand, more significant changes may be reported, e.g. a belief that a move from living in the individual's own home to nursing care would be more suitable. Whatever the feedback, it is vital that it is recorded and shared.

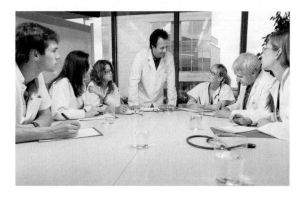

Figure 13.12 Gathering feedback

Evidence activity

(6.1) The review process

Using the same individual as for Evidence activity 2.2, provide suggestions for who should be involved in the review process and the criteria to judge the effectiveness of the care plan.

Practice activity

(6.2) Feeding back about how the plan is working

While at your real work environment, seek feedback from the individual and others about how the plan is working. Provide witness statements and documentation as evidence.

(6.2) Seek feedback from the individual and others about how the plan is working

As with monitoring, it is vital that the individual and everyone involved in their care is able to comment on how the plan has worked, whether it has been successful and where there may be room for improvement.

If the individual or care workers do not highlight successes or failures, then there are three possible problems:

(6.3) Use feedback and monitoring/other information to evaluate whether the plan has achieved its objectives

At the 'end' of a care plan, it is good practice to consider whether the plan has met its objectives. The worst situation would be if the plan were just to 'fizzle out' with no reflection, discussion, review or agreement. It will not be possible to make any revisions to the plan if this stage were not considered.

Case Study

 (6.3) Mark

Mark is a 9-year-old child with a combination of visual and hearing impairments. Mark and his parents want him to move to a mainstream school. His care plan for the last year has targeted how he could cope with the move. When his care plan is due for review, there are a variety of reports and monitoring to be consulted.

- The report from Mark's teacher at his current school for visually impaired children includes details of his educational achievements that year, and whether he could cope with studying a Key Stage 2 curriculum at the local Primary School. She feels he can, with appropriate support, e.g. signers and larger-print books. There is also commentary on his improved social skills, how he is now interacting with the other children more and becoming increasingly able to both make and keep friends.

- The report from his Educational Welfare Officer has details about Mark's improved confidence and self-esteem, and how Mark is now developing more in accordance with the developmental norms of a boy his age. There are also more detailed studies of his cognitive abilities, which show significant improvements in all areas.

- Mark's social worker reports on how Mark has coped with the travel to his current school and the logistics of him moving to a local state school. Whereas in past years, he has been upset going to school, now the driver reports that he is happy and far more independent.

- A report from the Local Education Authority Admissions Officer outlines the application procedures for the schools in his catchment areas, including the move to high school and the issues around a move to any of the schools, in particular for a child with special needs.

Case Study

- The feedback from his parents details how Mark has gained in confidence in the last year, how at times he reports feeling bored at the school and wants to take part in more challenging activities. They say he misses his old friends and is a bright boy; they feel he would be better suited to and challenged by a mainstream school.

- Most importantly, a review from Mark explains that he loves his current school, but sometimes finds the work easy and he misses his friends from his street whom he socialises with at evenings and weekends. He knows going to the local primary school will be tough, but he says he is determined and wants to give it a shot. He really wants to go to the local high school at the same time as his friends do and sit as many GCSEs as possible.

1. Why is it useful to have all these reviews and feedback?

2. What would be the problem if all of the monitoring was requested *apart from* Mark's?

3. Do you think Mark's objective of transferring to his local mainstream primary school is possible?

Practice activity

(6.3) Using feedback and monitoring to evaluate the success of the plan

While at your real work environment, use feedback and monitoring/other information to evaluate whether the plan has achieved its objectives. Provide witness statements and documentation as evidence.

6.4 Work with the individual and others to agree any revisions to the plan

Once feedback has been received and examined thoroughly, the next stage is for the individual and others to decide on any revisions to the plan. There are five outcomes that could be agreed upon.

1. **Closing the plan if all objectives have been met**. Some people may only need care provision for a set period of time; maybe their condition wasn't chronic (e.g. they had broken a bone), or they have recovered from an illness. In such cases, the care plan may come to a natural end if the individual becomes independent and no longer has any unmet needs.

2. **Reducing the level of support to reflect increased independence** – if an individual is improving, or is able to take on more tasks for themselves, then it may be possible to reduce the care delivered.

3. **Increasing the level of support to address unmet needs** – sometimes, an individual's care needs increase; they may have become more ill, weaker, or the level of informal care available may have decreased, in which case the revised care plan will need to reflect this and the level of care delivered will need to increase. It may be that as they have aged, future needs have become more apparent, e.g. a woman showing signs of the menopause may now need support in this area.

4. **Changing the type of support** – an individual may have become more independent in one area but more dependent in another, or the support originally offered wasn't in the right style. In these cases, the type of care may need to be altered.

5. **Changing the method of delivering the support** – a service provider may not be deemed the most appropriate for the needs of the individual; it may be too far, not suitable, or a more suitable service may have become available. It may be that the same support is delivered in a different setting. For example, if care was required when an individual was in hospital, the same care may need to be arranged at the individual's home on their discharge or if they are admitted to another care setting.

It is worth noting that for some individuals, care plans may never actually finish – an individual may have a care plan all of their life, so it will always need to be monitored, reviewed and adapted. The key principle here is that care plans are not only reviewed and amended as necessary but that, at each stage, the individual is central to this.

Evidence activity

6.4 How to support an individual to lead assessment and planning

Produce a report on the ways you would support the individual you described in Evidence activity 1.1 to lead their assessment and planning process.

6.5 Document the review process and revisions as required

Due to the importance of the care planning process, it is vital that all revisions are documented appropriately and that any revisions are clear. It may be best to have a complete new copy, dated so there is no confusion as to which care plan everyone is working to. Copies of the new care plan need to be circulated to the appropriate people.

It is vital that the individual's or anybody else's opinions on revisions are noted. If anybody has any reservations or disagreements about any changes, these need to be recorded.

The storage and access of documents also needs to be considered:

■ **Storage** – all care plans should be stored securely. Paper documents and electronic documents need to be organised, tidily and chronologically, in a way which means they can be found easily if they need to be referred to. Both written and electronic data needs to be stored in line with the Data Protection Act 1998.

■ **Confidentiality** – when documents are stored, confidentiality must be paramount. Only those with authority to access the information can do so. This will ensure that the individual trusts service providers. Care workers need to ensure that individuals understand that confidentiality will be upheld. Written documents need to be in a place which is secure, restricted or locked and not left where anybody else could view them. Electronic documents need to be stored in places which are password protected, on personal user areas (shared areas should be avoided) and not on removable storage (e.g. USB memory sticks) as these could be lost.

Key term

Chronologically means in order of time or occurrence.

Research & investigate

(6.5) Data Protection Act 1998

Find out as much as you can about the Data Protection Act, its purpose, principles, etc.

Evidence activity

(6.5) The importance of supporting an individual to lead assessment and planning

Produce a report on the ways you would support the individual you described in Evidence activity 1.1 to lead their assessment and planning process.

Having excellent documents and exemplary recording and storage of notes is clearly the best way to give quality care to the service user. However, it will also support care workers, especially if there are any questions, complaints or investigations into the quality of care. Good documentation will:

- ■ protect those care workers who are doing their work properly

- ■ highlight any care workers who are not doing their work properly.

Case Study

(6.5) Shanice

Shanice is an elderly woman who has no known conditions or impairments other than what would be expected for a woman of her age. Her children are very concerned about the care she has received over the last 15 years, for example, she has had unmet needs and been left for days at a time without scheduled visits. She first moved into a residential home to assist with her social and emotional needs 4 years ago, but since then she has had to move twice; once because it was too far away from her home town, friends and family, and again because the care home closed. In the new care home, her children are very concerned about the standard of personal care. Shanice's clothes are sometimes dirty, especially her underwear, although there is no evidence to prove that Shanice has any issue with bowel or bladder control. She has lost weight, become increasingly anxious and at times seems nervous. She has aged faster than would be expected from her developmental norms.

Her children have reported Shanice's care to the Care Quality Commission and it is being investigated. Her files, case notes and care plans since she first started receiving care are being requested.

1. Why is it important to look at all the documents relating to Shanice's care over the last 15 years?

2. Draw your conclusions about some possible negative findings.

3. Are there any possible positives that may come to light here?

Assessment summary

Your reading of this chapter and completion of the activities will have prepared you to be able to engage in personal development in health, social care or children's and young people's settings.

To achieve the unit, your assessor will require you to:

Learning outcomes	Assessment Criteria
Learning outcome 1: Understand the principles of person centred assessment and care planning by:	1.1 explaining the importance of a holistic approach to assessment and planning of care or support See Evidence activity 1.1, p. 260
	1.2 describing ways of supporting the individual to lead the assessment and planning process See Evidence activity 1.2, p. 262
	1.3 describing ways the assessment and planning process or documentation can be adapted to maximise an individual's ownership and control of it See Evidence activity 1.3, p. 263
Learning outcome 2: Be able to facilitate person centred assessment by:	2.1 establishing with the individual a partnership approach to the assessment process See Evidence activity 2.1, p. 264
	2.2 establishing with the individual how the process should be carried out and who else should be involved in the process See Evidence activity 2.2, p. 264
	2.3 agreeing with the individual and others the intended outcomes of the assessment process and care plan See Evidence activity 2.3, p. 266
	2.4 ensuring that assessment takes account of the individual's strengths and aspirations as well as needs See Evidence activity 2.4, p. 267

Learning outcomes	Assessment Criteria
Learning outcome 2: Be able to facilitate person centred assessment by:	(2.5) working with the individual and others to identify support requirements and preferences See Evidence activity 2.5, p. 268
Learning outcome 3: Be able to contribute to the planning of care or support by:	(3.1) taking account of factors that may influence the type and level of care or support to be provided See Evidence activity 3.1, p. 270
	(3.2) working with the individual and others to explore options and resources for delivery of the plan. See Evidence activity 3.2, p. 271
	(3.3) contributing to agreement on how component parts of a plan will be delivered and by whom See Evidence activity 3.3 on p. 272
	(3.4) recording the plan in a suitable format See Practice activity 3.4, p. 273
Learning outcome 4: Be able to support the implementation of care plans by:	(4.1) carrying out assigned aspects of a care plan See Practice activity 4.1, p. 273
	(4.2) supporting others to carry out aspects of a care plan for which they are responsible See Practice activity 4.2, p. 274
	(4.3) adjusting the plan in response to changing needs or circumstances See Practice activity 4.3, p. 275
Learning outcome 5: Be able to monitor a care plan by:	(5.1) agreeing methods for monitoring the way a care plan is delivered See Evidence activity 5.1, p. 275

Learning outcomes	Assessment Criteria
Learning outcome **5**: Be able to monitor a care plan by:	(5.2) collating monitoring information from agreed sources See Practice activity 5.2, p. 276
	(5.3) Recording changes that affect the delivery of the care plan See Evidence activity 5.3 on p. 276
Learning outcome **6**: Be able to facilitate a review of care plans and their implementation by:	(6.1) seeking agreement with the individual and others about: <ul><li>who should be involved in the review process</li><li>criteria to judge effectiveness of the care plan</li></ul>See Evidence activity 6.1 on p. 277
	(6.2) seeking feedback from the individual and others about how the plan is working See Practice activity 6.2, p. 277
	(6.3) using feedback and monitoring/other information to evaluate whether the plan has achieved its objectives See Practice activity 6.3, p. 278
	(6.4) working with the individual and others to agree any revisions to the plan See Evidence activity 6.4, p. 279
	(6.5) documenting the review process and revisions as required See Evidence activity 6.5, p. 280

Good luck!

Web links

Action for Advocacy	www.actionforadvocacy.org.uk
Makaton	www.makaton.org
Photosymbols	www.photosymbols.com
World Health Organisation (WHO)	www.who.int/en
York University	www.york.ac.uk/inst/spru/pubs/rworks/nov2000outc1.pdf

Support individuals to live at home

For Unit HSC 3022

What are you finding out?

There is the saying 'one's home is one's castle', which highlights that individuals can view their homes as invaluable, priceless. Various places can be a 'house', 'shelter', 'accommodation', but having a 'home', somewhere to call your own, is something many people value highly. If an individual needs care and support to meet their needs, then for many, the best option is to assist them to remain at home for as long as possible. Moving a person away from their own home is often the last resort. However, any care organised to support individuals to live at home must be coordinated in a formal structure, with the individual leading the process.

The reading and activities in this chapter will help you to:

■ Understand the principles of supporting individuals to live at home

■ Be able to contribute to planning support for living at home

■ Be able to work with individuals to secure additional services and facilities to enable them to live at home

■ Be able to work in partnership to introduce additional services for individuals living at home

■ Be able to contribute to reviewing support for living at home.

LO1 Understand the principles of supporting individuals to live at home

1.1 Describe how being supported to live at home can benefit an individual

An individual living at home can have many benefits.

Physical benefits include:

■ There are facilities to meet physical needs – bathrooms, kitchens, bedrooms etc.

■ Individuals may have all the physical comforts they like around them.

Intellectual benefits include:

■ Individuals are more likely to know where everything can be found in the home.

■ The individual knows their way around the house.

■ The individual knows the geographical area better, so is more likely to know how to get around.

Emotional benefits include:

■ feeling proud that they are remaining at home

■ improved self-esteem and self worth

■ feeling happy and content that they are in their own home.

Social benefits include:

■ sharing a home with parents, siblings, children etc.

■ friends and family are more likely to live locally

■ they are able to invite friends and family to their home for social events.

Time to reflect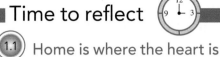

(1.1) Home is where the heart is

Think about your home.

- Why do you like it?
- How would you feel if you had to leave it?

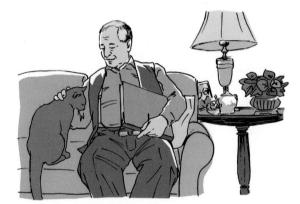

Figure 14.1 Home comforts

It is usually preferable for an individual to remain living in their own home rather than moving them to residential care. Most people want to live where they feel safe and secure. The saying 'Home is where the heart is' means that home is where a person experiences happiness, love or well-being the most. It may be a place where someone has lived most of their life, where their family has lived or still do, where they have memories and experiences. Moving to another setting could be upsetting, distressing and may lead to a lot of anxiety and fear. It may mean moving away from their friends, family and local networks.

Staying at home may be the preferred option regardless of a person's age and ability. Individuals are more likely to feel happy and secure in their own home, surrounded by their loved ones.

Evidence activity

(1.1) How living at home can benefit an individual

Describe the benefits of living at home.

(1.2) Compare the roles of people and agencies that may be needed to support an individual to live at home

There are many people and agencies that may be needed to support an individual to live at home, from a range of health, social and early years services. Often the service classifications can be blurred due to provision increasingly being delivered in multidisciplinary teams and funded through a 'mixed economy of care'.

People or agencies who may be needed to support an individual to live at home include

- GP
- district nurses
- dietician
- optician
- physiotherapist
- chiropodist
- dentists
- psychiatric nurses
- occupational therapists
- social worker
- care assistants
- domiciliary care worker
- housing officers
- counsellors
- home tutors
- educational welfare officers.

Research & investigate

(1.2) Mixed economy of care

- Find out what 'mixed economy of care' means.
- What are the benefits of services being delivered in this way?

These people and agencies are often coordinated by one care worker, who may be a social worker, but increasingly roles are being created solely to coordinate care. This role may be referred to as key worker, care coordinator, facilitator, care manager and case manager or similar, but for ease, key worker will be used throughout this chapter.

There are many roles that people and agencies can take:

■ **Supporting** – some roles, like **advocates**, may support individuals with services and benefits they are entitled to. They may help individuals to organise their finances, education or support. Individuals may need supports regarding rights, benefits, electoral roll forms, insurance, tax, etc. The care worker's role is not usually to advise, but to provide the information, outline advantages and disadvantages and assist individuals to make their own informed decisions. This will help to empower individuals.

Key term

Advocates represent individuals or speak on their behalf to ensure their rights are supported.

■ **Educating** – some roles involve helping individuals to gain knowledge or experience. For a child, this could be at school. For an adult, this could be through training or courses. It could, however, be education in life skills, such as how to manage finances, use a cash machine etc. It could also be educating an individual about their condition or the equipment they now need to use.

■ **Health care** – some roles may involve delivering medical care to individuals. This could be pain relief, dressings, medication, immunisations, treatments, health education, etc.

■ **Social care** – some roles may involve providing social care. This could be providing them with company, preparing meals, domestic support, travel assistance, counselling, welfare, etc.

■ **Planning** – some roles may involve the co-coordination of care. This may mean no actual delivery or provision of care, but managing an individual's care so that the people who are delivering, provide the best quality care.

■ **Adapting/decorating** – some roles may involve adapting the home to make it more accessible for the individual, e.g. putting in ramps, hand rails, stair lifts, lowering cupboards or switches. Some roles may help people with any tasks involving the upkeep of the home, e.g. painting and DIY.

The roles of these people and agencies will not always be performed in the individual's own home, but could be delivered in another setting.

Case Study

 Peter

Peter has spent most of his life being cared for by the women in his life. As a child his mother looked after him, and when his mother was at work his older sister looked after him. He married at 19 and then his wife cooked, cleaned, washed and ironed for him. Peter did his share of the chores in the home, but tended to do traditional gender-specific roles, so he did the manual work like DIY, gardening, decorating, etc. When his wife passed away last year, Peter struggled. He lived on sandwiches and cold food. He became unkempt and his clothes became soiled. The house became increasingly dirty. Neighbours called social services as they thought 'Peter needs to go in a home'.

On assessment, it was clear to all Peter was a bright, able man. He would benefit from being educated and receiving support on skills to live in his own. He is shown how to use the washing machine, microwave and cooker. Some support is organised so that he always gets some hot meals a week. Once a week a care worker visits Peter to check on him and give him any extra help and support he needs.

1. How has this support benefited Peter?

2. Do you think Peter should have 'gone into a home'? Justify your answer.

Evidence activity

 Supporting an individual to live at home

Write a report comparing the role of a selection of people and agencies that could support an individual to live at home.

1.3 **Explain the importance of providing information about benefits, allowances and financial planning which could support individuals to live at home**

On 25 June 2009, the BBC reported on the annual report by the Department of Work and Pensions, which claimed that in 2007/2008 £10.5bn of benefits that people were entitled to were unclaimed. The fact that each year there is such a huge amount of unclaimed benefits, when so many people are living in poverty and disadvantage, is not only ironic but is also tragic. Resources matter to everyone, but if an individual is vulnerable, every resource can contribute to helping their care needs to be met.

A small change to an individual's resources, allowances and financial planning could make a significant difference to their independence if they are then able to organise resources to do more

things for themselves. It can also make a difference to **autonomy**, as individuals will have more control over their life. It can be **empowering**.

Key terms

Autonomy means having personal freedom and the ability to be independent.
Empowering means giving someone control over their life and decisions.

It can be difficult to discuss money as it is an area about which individuals might be embarrassed, reserved or private. Some people may even find it vulgar to discuss finances. It is vital that care workers discuss the subject with sensitivity and tact so that they do not cause any offence.

Benefits and allowances

There is a whole range of benefits that could be claimed or monies reimbursed.

Table 14.1 Possible benefits and allowances available

In retirement	• Pensions: state (payments dependent on whether married or single pension allowance) • Pension Credit and Savings Credit • Cold Weather Payments
Employed on a low income or looking for work	• Income Support • Job Seeker's Allowance • Housing Benefit • Council Tax Benefit • Tax credits • Heating and insulation improvements from the Warm Front scheme
Ill or injured	• Statutory Sick Pay • Employment and Support Allowance • Healthcare Travel Costs Scheme • Prescription Assistance
Expecting or bringing up children	• Maternity Allowance • Statutory Maternity Pay • Child Benefit • Child Maintenance
Disability	• Disability Living Allowance • Attendance Allowance • Independent Living Fund • Carer's Allowance
Bereavement	• Funeral Payments • Bereavement Benefits • War Widow's or Widower's Pension
In education	• EMA • Student loans • Bursaries

These are correct at time of going to press, but names of benefits and eligibility criteria may alter due to any changes in government policy. For up-to-date information on benefits and allowances, Directgov is an excellent website.

Other sources that could be drawn from are any inheritance, savings and private pensions, and individuals could take advantage of discounts on goods or services for older or disabled people, those on low incomes etc.

Financial planning

If an individual has resources, they may need guidance as to how best to use them. Individuals may have savings, stocks or shares or, if not, this may be something they would like to start. They may also like guidance on what tax they should be paying. It is also worth considering how they pay for services, e.g. utilities. Direct debits and standing orders can be simpler and often cheaper than paying bills by cheque or cash, but some people are cautious about setting them up. If an individual is struggling with debt, support should also be offered to help reduce it. Also, there should be guidance on how to spread costs, using monthly payments etc. Helping individuals to save to prepare for any unexpected costs or future care needs is also good practice.

Sources of help could be:

- Citizen's Advice Bureau
- local debt organisations
- credit card companies
- financial advisors
- National Debtline
- Consumer Credit Counselling Service.

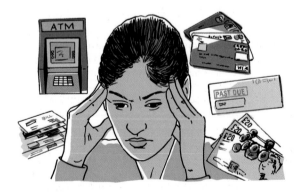

Figure 14.2 In debt and unhappy

Case Study

(1.3) Pound Avenue

There are two individuals on Pound Avenue who are receiving support to assist them to live at home. They have just divulged their financial situations to their care workers.

Rich has been saving up for many years. He doesn't trust banks or anyone else with his money – he keeps it 'safely' secured around his house in tins, under floorboards, under his mattress and in suitcases. He estimates there is around £20,000. He has seen local youths hanging about close to his house and is worried.

Paul lives next door. He was made redundant a few years ago, but never found another job due to his poor health. He never really saved any money when younger and then mismanaged some of his money in his 50s. He struggles to get by every week and is sure he doesn't get the benefits he is entitled to. He recalls putting money into a pension when he worked as a miner in his 20s. He has numerous credit cards which he depends on to get by each week, because, 'Well, everyone does, don't they?' But he is worried. He estimates that he is around £20,000 in debt.

1. In what ways are Rich and Paul each putting themselves at risk?

2. What support would you offer to Rich and Paul?

Evidence activity

(1.3) The importance of providing financial information

Produce a report for a key worker starting work, explaining why it is important to provide information on benefits, allowances and financial planning.

Explain how risk management contributes to supporting individuals to live at home

Risk management is examining a care setting to recognise and redress any potential risks that may occur, in the hope that the risk is either removed or reduced. Apart from being best practice, it is also a legal requirement under the Health and Safety at Work 1974 Act to make sure that individuals and their carers are kept free from risk.

Under the Act, an 'employer' must still carry out risk assessments and take action if the care is being delivered in an individual's own home. Sometimes, however, the hazard cannot be removed, as it is in the individual's home. In this case, making the individual aware of the risk and suggesting and supporting them in how it could be removed is all that can be done. Care workers cannot go into an individual's home and start replacing, changing or moving their possessions without their permission.

In simple terms, risk management is:

1. Identifying risks and hazards.

2. Implementing changes or measures to reduce or eliminate those risks. This could be analysis by

   ■ area, as particular areas have particular hazards, e.g. the kitchen, the bathroom, the bedroom, the garden, etc.

   ■ activity, as particular activities have particular hazards, e.g. personal hygiene, climbing stairs, housework, clothes (washing, drying and ironing), etc.

   ■ hazard, e.g. fire, falls, burns, scalds, electrocution, intruders, security etc.

Having identified the risks, it is vital to apply risk control measures.

By removing risks, which may only require simple changes, individuals are more likely to be able to remain in their own home and be safer. If this is explained to them, and they understand

how it will not only assist them to remain in their own home, but also to allow them to do so safely and more independently, they are more likely to accept and welcome action.

 Evidence activity

1.4 Risk management in the home

Provide a statement for an individual explaining how risk management will contribute to supporting them to live at home.

LO2 Be able to contribute to planning support for living at home

2.1 Identify with an individual the strengths, skills and existing networks they have that could support them to live at home

Identifying with an individual the strengths, skills and existing networks they have will not only allow any support to be person centred, it will also help individuals to keep their autonomy and independence.

Strengths and skills – what an individual can do competently

Different people are good at different things, and a good care worker will recognise and encourage the things that someone is good at. These could be part of their character, for example, an individual may be articulate, able, organised, energetic, positive thinking. Or they could be practical accomplishments, such as sewing, dressmaking, cooking, DIY, gardening, decorating, painting, being creative, etc.

Care workers must recognise what an individual *can* do, not what they *can't* do, as is too often the focus. Value individuals – they should never be undermined. Everyone needs to be proud of their successes and accomplishments. Disregarding someone's strengths and skills doesn't value the person, and if care workers 'take over' and perform these tasks instead, this could lead to increasing dependence and loss of autonomy.

  Research & investigate

1.4 Further details

For further details on risk management and health and safety in general, look at and research the Health & Safety Executive website.

Existing networks – networks an individual may already be part of

People may belong to many networks based on their neighbourhood, religious groups, day centres they attend, public houses they visit, clubs, their medical condition or support groups they belong to, trade unions, past employment, etc.

It is a waste of resources if care is planned to support the individual when the same support is already available and provided elsewhere. Furthermore, it is likely to be less effective if the support is arranged as an 'add on'. The care that is already in place may be more relevant and appropriate for the individual as they have arranged it themselves.

Case Study

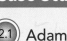 **Adam**

Adam is a young man in his mid 30s who lives at home. He has used a wheelchair since an accident. His carer has arranged for him to have a Christmas meal with a local support group, where Adam doesn't know anyone. Adam is disappointed, as it is the same evening he has arranged to go out with his old football team for a Christmas meal. He knows lots of people who will be there and is looking forward to it. His care worker gets cross with Adam, explaining that he has arranged this now and it is paid for! The care worker has also arranged for the Access Bus to pick Adam up to take him there and return him home, whereas Adam often books taxis for his evenings out as he likes the flexibility they offer.

1. Explain where the care worker has failed Adam in this situation.

2. What should the care worker do in future to support Adam?

Practice activity

2.1 An individual's strengths, skills and existing networks

Choose an individual you know. With their permission, identify with them all the strengths, skills and existing networks
they have which could support them to live at home.

2.2 Identify with an individual their needs that may require additional support and their preferences for how the needs may be met

Just as anyone moving into a new residential setting would have their needs assessed, an individual residing in their own home must also have their needs assessed. This can be done using many methods and formats, but assessment of the following is essential:

- personal
- physical
- financial
- social
- environmental
- safety.

In each of these areas, individuals will need to assess their abilities on a spectrum similar to that shown in Figure 14.4.

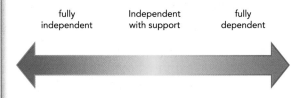

Figure 14.3 Ability spectrum

Clearly a full assessment with an individual will be more detailed and will fully document all the reasons why they feel they are in that position. The whole process has to be person centred and led by the individual themselves. Care workers should not assume anything. All assessment needs to empower an individual. Individuals should lead discussions about how these needs should be met.

Some of the support required may be from:

- training
- adaptations
- equipment
- social interactions
- professional support
- respite care
- transport.

Decisions have to focus around:

■ what individuals feel comfortable with

■ how intrusive it may be in their life

■ how significantly, or soon, it may need adapting if future needs change

■ what can be afforded

■ how it ties in with any informal care or existing networks of support.

All the options need to be discussed with the individual, allowing them to state which ones they prefer. Then a 'package' of support for them to live at home can be drawn up.

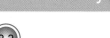

Practice activity

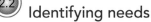

2.2 Identifying needs

For the same individual you used for Practice activity 2.1, identify their needs which may require additional support and their preferences for how the needs may be met.

2.3 Agree with the individual and others the risks that need to be managed in living at home and ways to address them

Living in one's own home may be the most preferred option, but it can have accompanying risks. Once a home has been assessed, individuals need to be made aware of risks so that they can either be dealt with or so the individual can make informed decisions about whether to remain safely in their own home.

Table 14.2 Explains some of the risks associated with living in your own home. Many of these risks may increase if the individual lives on their own, or if they live with another person who is also vulnerable.

Key term

Accentuated means emphasised.

Table 14.2 Potential risks associated with living at home

Risk	Examples
Inappropriate care	Equipment in the own home may not be sufficient.
	Individuals may have to use equipment themselves and they may make mistakes.
Isolation or depression	There could still be a risk of isolation and depression from being alone in one's own home.
Medical care	Care may not be available 24/7 and so the individual may need support when it isn't there.
	When support is arranged, it may be rushed and unsupervised.
Security	Potentially more vulnerable to intruders or crime as on their own.
	Less extensive security systems and maybe less secure windows and doors.
Forgetfulness	Individuals, especially if they have memory issues, may forget to take medication, fulfil daily chores or turn off equipment.
	There may be risks of forgetting to secure the property.
Abuse	If individuals are on their own, there may be less supervision and protection so there may be more opportunity for abuse to occur.
Accidents involving the individual	As more likely to be performing daily activities on their own, more likelihood that their condition or age may lead to an accident.
	Consequences of an accident could be accentuated as it may take longer to get support or treatment.
Accidents involving the accommodation	Equipment and resources may not be professionally monitored, and therefore may be more at risk from electrical fault, fire, failure, food or breakage.

Case Study

 Edward

Edward has early onset dementia. He sometimes forgets to heat up food, and will often eat cold baked beans, for example. Sometimes he forgets to turn the heating up when it is cold or down when it is hot. The wiring throughout the house is loose and the fire alarm has not been checked for years. One day, Edward starts to run the bath, but then gets sidetracked by the snooker on the television. He is only made aware of the flooding when a neighbour comes into his house and alerts him to water dripping through the overflow. On examination, his whole bathroom is flooded and it is leaking through to the kitchen.

1. List the hazards which you feel Edward is at risk from.

2. Start to think about any measures that could be put in place to ensure that Edward can stay in his own home.

Research & investigate

 Abuse

Unfortunately, abuse could happen to anybody, including in an individual in their own home.

- Research the type of abuse that can occur and possible symptoms.

- What systems could be put in place to prevent abuse?

Once all risks have been identified, it is vital that this information is shared with individuals so that they can agree, along with others, the risks that need to be managed and ways to address them. The others involved in this process could be:

- family

- friends

- advocates

- others who are important to the individual's well-being.

These could all be people either living in the same home, providing informal care, or who care about the individual and whose support and involvement is therefore vital.

All the options need to be discussed, in detail, along with the consequences such as costs, disruption, etc. Some risks may be less significant, or can be addressed as soon as they are highlighted, for example, purchasing a multi-way plug to deal with any overloaded sockets.

Many of these hazards will also be reduced by which systems care organisations have in place, including:

- police checks, protocols and supervision

- named wardens and supervisors

- regular safety audits

- regular checks of equipment.

Practice activity

 Risk

Risk assess your home – identify the potential risks and identify ways to address them.

LO3 Be able to work with individuals to secure additional services and facilities to enable them to live at home

3.1 Support the individual and others to access and understand information about resources, services and facilities available to support the individual to live at home

Accessing and understanding information is key if an individual and others involved are to feel any sense of ownership over the support. If necessary, documents must be adapted – if there is any doubt, check whether this needs to be done.

Key term

Accessing means finding and using.

There are a variety of ways to make information accessible and easier to understand.

- Use communication aids

  - For individuals with visual impairments, larger type, Braille and putting the information into an audio format could be beneficial.

  - For individuals with hearing impairments, hearing aids, sign language, signers, lip reading and the written word could be used.

  - Electronic and technological developments are also increasingly effective at aiding communication and should be employed where appropriate.

- Use a simple format

  - Ensure that language is appropriate to the age, ability and understanding of the individual. It is vital that individuals are clear and not confused.

  - If the person speaks a language other than English, ensure that interpreters and translators are available, respecting the right of the individual to fully participate.

- Use communication systems

  - For anyone with emotional difficulties, learning difficulties or behavioural issues, picture aids, photographs, visits, plans, flash cards, etc. may be of use.

  - Makaton could be used. This is a system of signs and gestures.

  - Photosymbols, which use images to send a message, could be used.

Essentially, present the plan in a way that is appropriate to the age, needs, ability and preferences of the individual and, if in doubt, confirm with the individual how they would like details of support to be presented. Inclusiveness should be paramount and individuals must be encouraged to fully participate if the support is to be person centred.

Evidence activity

(3.1) **Accessing and understanding information about resources, services and facilities**

Produce a poster to show how information can be made accessible and understandable.

(3.2) **Work with the individual and others to select resources, facilities and services that will meet the individual's needs and minimise risks**

Individuals must decide, with the others involved, which resources, facilities and services will meet their needs and minimise risks. These must be included in a care plan which formalises the decisions that the individual and others make. Individuals may consider whether anything from the following list would be of use to assist them to live at home safely.

- Training – this could be on how to use everyday equipment such as cookers, microwaves or washing machines.

- Training could be on how to use any equipment that has been installed, e.g. hoists.

- Adaptations – it may be necessary to adapt the home to enable a person to live there comfortably and safely. This could be external changes (e.g. ramps), or internal changes (e.g. a stair lift, lowered units, widened doors).

- Equipment – a vast range of equipment could be bought from various outlets online or from shops and catalogues to allow individuals to be as independent as possible.

Table 14.3 Aids to assist living at home

Mobility aids	Walking frames
	Walking sticks
	Scooter
	Wheelchairs
Eating aids	Angled cutlery
	Non-slip plates
	Cups with handles
Cooking aids	Electronic knives and accessories
	Tap turners
	Kettle tipper
Sleeping aids	Raised beds
	Lowered beds
	Adjustable head rests
	Bed trays
	Angled pillows

Bathing aids	Non slip mats
	Rails
	Dry shampoo
	Hair rinsing trays
	Walk in showers and baths
Personal aids	Commodes
	Continence pads
	Raised toilet seats
Memory aids	Alarms
	Tablet boxes
	Thermostats
	Orientation sheets
	Checklists
	Reminders
Dressing aids	Button fasteners
	Velcro
	Shoe horns
	Sock/stocking aids
	Zipper pulls
Transfer aids	Hoists
	Transfer boards
	Monkey pole/lifting handle

■ Social interactions – whether arranged within the home or out of it, social interactions may be needed to ensure that individuals have a good range of relationships and are not isolated. Visits to day centres and clubs, trips out, or visits to the individual's home may all be useful.

■ Professional support – this could be nursing care, social care, education, therapy, counselling, treatment, medication etc. All will deliver specialist support which can ensure that individuals are as physically and emotionally well as possible.

■ Respite care – this type of support can help individuals to live at home, as it allows informal carers to have a 'holiday' from care. Without this break, care for an individual may suffer indirectly because carers may become stressed and tired. Supporting informal carers helps to support individuals.

■ Transport – having transport arranged to allow individuals to access support may be all that is required. Taxis, cars or minibuses could all be arranged to promote an individual's ability to live at home.

Evidence activity

(3.2) Working with the individual and others to select resources, facilities and services

Choose a condition, impairment or illness. Produce a report on the resources, facilities and services which may meet the needs of an individual with that condition, impairment or illness.

(3.3) Contribute to completing paperwork to apply for required resources, facilities and services, in a way that promotes active participation

Active participation allows the individual more control over their support. Examples of paperwork which might need to be completed are:

■ applications

■ assessments

■ requests

■ feedback

■ finance forms

■ agreements (which may need to be read and signed).

It is vital that this is done accurately and speedily, within deadlines. Poor completion of paperwork may lead to refusal of applications. Individuals may need support in this process. Ideally, it should be the individual who applies, however, if they need assistance with either the practicality of completing an application (handwriting, reading, etc.) or the knowledge of what to submit (content, how to answer questions), then the care worker should assist in a way that is empowering. The care worker should not, however, take over and complete the paperwork themselves.

Initially, paperwork can be daunting. However, with time, individuals may become more fluent with terminology, calculations and requirements and become more confident in completing it independently.

Possible ways to involve an individual are:

- read out questions
- explain questions
- fill in the answers the individual gives
- provide a selection of answers which the individual points to
- use audio formats
- use electronic forms
- use magnifiers and other reading and writing aids
- allow sufficient, dedicated time for an individual to be fully involved.

Time to reflect

 3.3 Involved?

Anthony is a busy care worker, with lots of individuals to see in his schedule. Often he has to help individuals to apply for things such as car tax rebate, housing benefit, new equipment or adaptations. There are times when Anthony is so rushed, he just takes the forms and completes them himself. 'No problem,' he says, 'at least they get done!'

Why is Anthony's practice a problem?

Evidence activity

3.3 Contributing to the completion of paperwork

Produce a brochure detailing ten 'top tips' for promoting active participation when contributing to the completion of paperwork.

 3.4 Obtain permission to provide additional information about the individual in order to secure resources, services and facilities

There are times, when organising support for individuals, when care workers may need to divulge information about the individual. This must be discussed with the individual prior to any disclosure, and they must give their permission. A key principle in providing person-centred care is that permission is gained *before* information is shared. Information belongs to an individual; it should not be given out unless they allow it.

Often, individuals share information with care workers as they have a relationship built on trust. They may feel betrayed if they later find out that this information has been shared with others. Discussing the need to share information and how that will 1) remain confidential and 2) assist in getting the required support, should help an individual to make decisions about their information.

Clearly, if an individual is at risk, or putting others at risk, the boundaries of confidentiality become more blurred and the care worker needs to make a judgement about whether to **breach** confidentiality without the individual's permission. However, this would need to be done in line with procedures, and the care worker should privately divulge the information only to their line manager and not to other staff.

Key term

Breach means to break or override a rule or agreement.

Permission should always be gained in writing, once individuals fully understands whom the information may be shared with. This should all be done in line with the Data Protection Act.

Research & investigate

 3.4 Data Protection Act

Find out about the Data Protection Act.

Evidence activity

(3.4) Obtaining permission to provide additional information about the individual

Produce a statement outlining the importance of gaining permission to provide additional information and how this should be done.

LO4 Be able to work in partnership to introduce additional services for individuals living at home

(4.1) Agree roles and responsibilities for introducing additional support for an individual to live at home

Once it has been agreed which resources, services, facilities or support are to be employed to support the individual to live at home, it is important that everyone is clear about their roles and responsibilities. Otherwise, there could be problems, such as duplications and omissions.

Everyone must be clear about what their role is and what responsibilities they have, to ensure that no one has misunderstood. Good care planning, with clear, detailed documents, which are shared with all partners, is best practice.

Time to reflect

(4.1) Problems

What would happen if care workers providing support for an individual living at home do not communicate?

Evidence activity

(4.1) Agreeing roles and responsibilities for introducing additional support

Arthur lives in his own home with support. He is frail, with severe arthritis, and also suffering from depression. He does not enjoy social interactions, preferring his own company. During the week, four people visit him to support him. On a Monday, two people support him: his counsellor and a care assistant (who is there to tidy his house and prepare food). On Tuesday, he is supported by a care assistant (who washes and irons his clothes and prepares food) and a nurse (who helps with his pain relief). Nobody then supports Arthur from Wednesday until the following Monday. All four staff know that Arthur has 'poor social relationships' and all try to converse with him. Arthur moans that they all try to converse with him, and says: 'Damned busy bodies, always asking the same irrelevant questions. Where's that woman I saw at the beginning? She was nice.' One Friday, while upstairs, the nurse brings some of his washing down and puts it in the washing machine. When the care assistant arrives, he is annoyed and starts to argue with the nurse. They have a full-blown argument in front of Arthur, which upsets him greatly.

Identify the areas where support being delivered to Arthur has not been managed correctly.

Produce a detailed, sample plan for those providing care for Arthur, making clear days, times, roles and responsibilities that would support him best.

(4.2) Introduce the individual to new resources, services, facilities or support groups

Individuals use the support which they know about. If they do not know about it, it is unlikely to be used. As people develop needs or recognise that they require support for current unmet needs, they may need to find new resources, services, facilities or support groups.

This may need to be researched but, for many reasons, it is sometimes difficult to know exactly what is available:

■ Support available can change frequently due to governments, funding and policies changing.

■ Different services may only notify people about their own support, e.g. the NHS may only publicise services it provides, and social services may do the same.

■ Some services are provided voluntarily and so are not publicised within the local service frameworks.

■ Support is not always easily found in directories such as the Yellow Pages or Thomson Local.

■ There can often be duplication with other services, so it is not clear where they fall.

In an ideal world, an individual could research support for a condition and have a full, up-to-date and accurate list of services available to them in their local area, but this is not always possible.

The growth of the internet has made this process much easier. The individual may need to be assisted to use the internet to find suitable support. The local library could also be useful, because it is often possible to use the internet there and it may also have information about local services.

Often, once one source of support is found, finding others can become easier, as word of mouth is often one of the best ways to find out about local support available. The care worker can support the individual and help them to lead this and decide which support is right for them, and then support them to apply/attend should the individual wish.

 Time to reflect

(4.2) Where would you go?

Imagine that one day you found out you had dementia.

● Where would you go to receive support?

● How would you find out where support was?

 Evidence activity

(4.2) Introducing the individual to new resources, services, facilities or support groups

Choose one condition, disability or impairment. Produce a directory of all the resources, services, facilities or support groups available in your local area which may help to support individuals with this condition, disability or impairment.

(4.3) Record and report on the outcomes of additional support measures in required ways

If an individual receives or attends any additional support, it is useful to be able to measure its success. If it isn't effective, other support may also be needed. Success does not always have to be measured in a **quantitative** way, it could also be measured in **qualitative** terms.

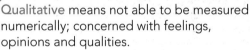 **Key terms**

Qualitative means not able to be measured numerically; concerned with feelings, opinions and qualities.
Quantitative means able to be measured numerically; concerned with quantities.
Anecdotal means based on personal recounts rather than on facts or research.

Quantitative measures of success might be:

■ weight loss or gain (a healthier BMI)

■ improved measures of health – pulse, blood pressure, respiration, cholesterol

■ reduced levels of medication required

■ decreased levels of pain reported on pain assessment scales

■ reduced need for support.

Qualitative measures of success might be:

■ feeling more energetic

■ feeling happier

■ improved self-esteem

- improved social relationships
- improved confidence.

All outcomes need to be recorded and reported (e.g. through reports, charts, graphs, scales, discussions, **anecdotal** evidence, medicals, etc.) so that any support can be reviewed and either finished, adapted or improved. The support can then continue to meet the individual's needs in the best way possible.

Research & investigate

4.3 Scales

Find out about pain assessment scales.

- What are the various formats?
- Why do you think they are useful?

Practice activity

4.3 Recording and reporting the outcomes of additional support measures

While in your real work environment, record and report on outcomes of an additional support measure in the required way.

LO5 Be able to contribute to reviewing support for living at home

5.1 Work with the individual and others to agree methods and timescales for on-going review

Methods

There are various methods for reviewing the support for someone living at home.

Key term

Ad hoc means as and when required.

Timescales

Support can be reviewed according to a variety of timescales:

- ad hoc – situations may occur which need to be shared with all involved as they happen
- periodic – dependent on the nature or severity of the care, reviews may be weekly, monthly, quarterly, half yearly, annually etc.
- final – it may be known at the outset that the care plan will come to an end and needs to be reviewed, for example if care is required when an informal carer is on holiday
- urgent – a situation may occur which is deemed an emergency if the individual is at immediate risk, in which case support may need to be reviewed immediately.

Case Study

5.1 Mr Sandhu

Mr Sandhu is a man in his 50s who has mild mental health issues. With Mr Sandhu's permission, there is a booklet in his kitchen that all his care workers know about. It is carbon copied and so allows for duplicates. Whenever a care worker has supported Mr Sandhu, they report in the book and take a copy back to the office, to put into Mr Sandhu's file. This means a copy is available to all care workers, including the key worker, and one stays with Mr Sandhu. The last entry states:

'Mr Sandhu seemed upset at 9am. He described some nightmares he'd had the previous night, where he was buried alive. After he'd had a cup of tea and got out of bed, he seemed calmer. However, throughout the two hours there, he referred to it four times, saying "that is what you are all going to do to me!" He was not aggressive and I did not feel any threat from Mr Sandhu, but he was clearly upset by this.'

1. Why is this good practice?
2. What would you do next if you were Mr Sandhu's care worker?

Whatever methods or timescale are preferred, it is vital that the individual leads the discussions, and that final decisions are what the individual wants and feels most comfortable with.

Case meetings	Written reports	Telephone calls	Changeover notes
• Set at periodic times or **ad hoc**, where the individual and all involved can discuss support face to face.	• At set periods, it may be required for careworkers to complete formal written reports on how individuals are progressing with living at home.	• More likely to be as and when needed and may be used for more urgent issues. These always need recording somewhere.	• To ensure consistency between staff and everyone is fully aware and there is an overview of care.

Figure 14.4 Methods for reviewing support

Evidence activity

5.1 **Agreeing methods and timescales for on-going review**

Design a role-play showing an interaction between a care worker and an individual. The individual is leading the discussion of the methods and timescales for reviewing their support.

5.2 **Identify any changes in an individual's circumstances that may indicate a need to adjust the type or level of support**

It is hoped that the support arranged will be appropriate and meet the individual's needs to live at home. However, there may be occasions when circumstances dictate that changes need to be made before the set review date.

Circumstances when support may need to be adjusted

■ Health – if an individual's health improves or worsens then support will need to be adjusted to take this into account. Clearly, continuing to support an individual who no longer needs it is inefficient.

■ Social situation – individuals may gain, lose or rekindle friendships, so support may alter accordingly. Informal care may change as people offering informal social support change. Any other people living in the same home may change (people may move in or out), which could lead to changes to an individual's social situation.

■ Financial circumstances – individuals may:

■ be able to purchase support they weren't able to before

■ have to cut back on support they were receiving before, which may mean that the plan needs to be adjusted to make up any shortfall.

■ Legal status – there may be times when an individual's legal status changes. There are five potential statuses an individual could have:

1. An adult, deemed able to do so, has legal rights to decide their own well-being.

2. A minor's parents or guardians hold legal guardianship over their well-being.

3. A child with a care order may be the responsibility of the local authorities, which is legally responsible for their well-being.

4. Adults deemed unfit to make their own decisions may appoint, or have appointed, a legal guardian to represent them.

5. Any individual detained under the Mental Health Act 1983 will have their legal responsibility assumed by the local authorities. If detained in a secure hospital, treatment can be given without their consent.

Evidence activity

5.2 **Identifying any changes in an individual's circumstances**

Your manager informs you of a need to review some of the individuals you are responsible for as their circumstances have changed. Produce a list of sensitive, tactful questions you could ask individuals to find out if their circumstances have changed.

Time to reflect

5.2 Different life

How is your life different to 10 years ago?

How might any support you were receiving have changed since then?

Evidence activity

5.3 Agree revisions to the support provided

Consider Alison in case study 5.3. Describe what best practice would have been here.

5.3 Work with the individual and others to agree revisions to the support provided

There is little point involving an individual from the outset about their support, only to then make revisions without their involvement or support. Individuals need to be involved at all stages. Any revisions need to be formalised and all agencies informed of these, otherwise varying support may occur.

Working with the individual from beginning to end and allowing them to lead the process at every stage will ensure that they are able to remain living at their own home for as long as they feel it is right for them.

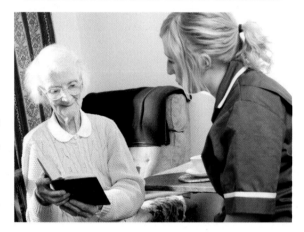

Figure 14.5 Discussing the options

Case Study

5.3 Alison

Alison has just returned home after a long period in hospital due to breast cancer. A package of support has been arranged for her, which she decided upon. It means her staying at her mother's for a month, with the support being delivered there. She is happy with this, as she knows it is just a short-term measure. However, after a week her mother is called into the office at work and informed that she is being made redundant. Alison's care worker hears of this from Alison's mother, and adapts the support offered to Alison to allow her mother to take a full role in her care. The care worker cancels all the support arranged previously.

When the support originally arranged doesn't turn up, Alison is confused. 'Don't worry,' her mother says, 'I'm going to sort everything out now.' Alison is furious. She doesn't always get on with her mother and if she had known this would happen, she would never have agreed to stay with her mother; she would have gone to her own house, to get the support there.

1. What has the care worker failed to do?

2. How would you feel if you were Alison?

Assessment summary

Your reading of this chapter and completion of the activities will have prepared you to be able to engage in personal development in health, social care or children's and young people's settings.

To achieve the unit, your assessor will require you to:

Learning outcomes	Assessment criteria
Learning outcome 1: Understand the principles of supporting individuals to live at home by:	**1.1** describing how being supported to live at home can benefit an individual See Evidence activity 1.1, p. 285
	1.2 comparing the roles of people and agencies who may be needed to support an individual to live at home See Evidence activity 1.2, p. 286
	1.3 explaining the importance of providing information about benefits, allowances and financial planning which could support individuals to live at home See Evidence activity 1.3, p. 288
	1.4 explaining how risk management contributes to supporting individuals to live at home See Evidence activity 1.4, p. 289
Learning outcome 2: Be able to contribute to planning support for living at home by:	**2.1** identifying with an individual the strengths, skills and existing networks they have that could support them to live at home See Practice activity 2.1, p. 290
	2.2 identifying with an individual their needs that may require additional support and their preferences for how the needs may be met See Practice activity 2.2, p. 291
	2.3 agreeing with the individual and others the risks that need to be managed in living at home and ways to address them See Practice activity 2.3, p. 292

Learning outcomes	Assessment criteria
Learning outcome 3: Be able to work with individuals to secure additional services and facilities to enable them to live at home by:	(3.1) supporting the individual and others to access and understand information about resources, services and facilities available to support the individual to live at home See Evidence activity 3.1, p. 293
	(3.2) working with the individual and others to select resources, facilities and services that will meet the individual's needs and minimise risks See Evidence activity 3.2, p. 294
	(3.3) contributing to completing paperwork to apply for required resources, facilities and services, in a way that promotes active participation See Evidence activity 3.3, p. 295
	(3.4) obtaining permission to provide additional information about the individual in order to secure resources, services and facilities See Evidence activity 3.4, p. 296
Learning outcome 4: Be able to work in partnership to introduce additional services for individuals living at home by:	(4.1) agreeing roles and responsibilities for introducing additional support for an individual to live at home See Evidence activity 4.1, p. 296
	(4.2) introducing the individual to new resources, services, facilities or support groups See Evidence activity 4.2, p. 297
	(4.3) recording and reporting on the outcomes of additional support measures in required ways See Practice activity 4.3, p. 298

Learning outcomes	Assessment criteria
Learning outcome 5: Be able to monitor a care plan by:	**5.1** working with the individual and others to agree methods and timescales for on-going review See Evidence activity 5.1, p. 299
	5.2 identifying any changes in an individual's circumstances that may indicate a need to adjust the type or level of support See Evidence activity 5.2, p. 299
	5.3 working with the individual and others to agree revisions to the support provided See Evidence activity 5.3, p. 300

Good luck!

Web links

Directgov   www.direct.gov.uk
Citizen's Advice Bureau   www.citizensadvice.org.uk
National Debtline   www.nationaldebtline.co.uk
Consumer Credit Counselling Service   www.cccs.co.uk
Care standards Act 2000   www.dh.gov.uk
Health and Safety Executive   www.hse.gov.uk

15 Work in partnership with families to support individuals

For Unit HSC 3038

What are you finding out?

Many families provide care and support for their relatives, close friends and neighbours, especially when they are disabled, elderly or chronically ill. This care and support usually arises out of relationships based on love, trust and **obligation**. However, for some people it can become a major responsibility, affecting their paid work and consequently their income, social activities and other family relationships. It is therefore essential that these people are fully supported in order that they can undertake this vital role.

The reading and activities in this chapter will help you to:

■ Understand partnership working with families

■ Be able to establish and maintain positive relationships with families

■ Be able to plan shared approaches to the care and support of individuals with families

■ Be able to work with families to access support in their role as carers

■ Be able to exchange and record information about partnership work with families

■ Be able to contribute to reviewing partnership work with families

■ Be able to provide feedback about support for families.

Key term

Obligation means having to do something because of a legal or moral duty.

LO1 Understand partnership working with families

1.1 Analyse the contribution of families to the care and/or support of individuals

Family carers play a vital role in caring for those who are sick, disabled, elderly, vulnerable or frail. The government recognises that many family members play a very important role in providing care for these individuals across the United Kingdom. In fact, the most accepted source of care and support for individuals in need of care is the family, and the best environment for the person being cared for is often their own home.

Family members are often best placed to provide support for individuals because they:

■ usually have continued and ongoing contact with the individual

■ knew the individual, their preferences and needs prior to their illness

■ often share a **cultural** background and family **value systems** with the individual

■ often have detailed knowledge in relation to the individual's care needs

■ save the health and social care sector a vast amount of money every year

■ provide care and support for individuals which otherwise may not be available.

Key terms

Cultural means related to the customs, ideas and social behaviour of particular people or groups.
Value systems are the principles of right and wrong that are accepted by an individual or a particular group of people.

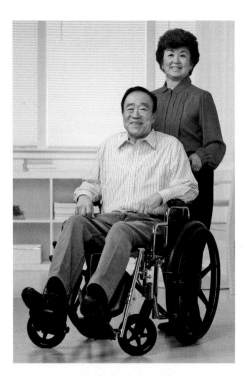

Figure 15.1 Family/informal care

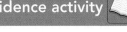

Evidence activity

(1.1) Contribution of families to care and support

Make a note of the qualities that families can bring to the caring role.

How do these qualities differ from the qualities you bring to the role as a health or social care worker?

(1.2) Identify factors that may affect the level of involvement of family members in care and/ or support

There are many people, including parents, daughters, sons, relatives, neighbours and friends who provide care and support in various ways for individuals. However, there are many factors that can affect the level of involvement and support that some of these people can give.

Every family situation is different and will dictate the level of involvement and support the family member can give. Some family members devote a large proportion of their lives to care for their loved ones, often in addition to other responsibilities, such as holding down a job and running a home. Some individuals may have to give up their job in order to care for a family member, and this may impact on their financial circumstances.

There are a number of ways in which the need for family care can arise. For example:

■ An individual's need for care may increase gradually, perhaps as the individual grows older and frailer, or because they develop a **progressive condition** such as motor neurone disease or Alzheimer's disease. Under these circumstances, family carers may find themselves gradually giving more and more time and support as the days go by.

Key term

A progressive condition is one that gets worse over time.

■ Some parents may know prior to giving birth that, perhaps due to a disability, their child's care needs will far exceed the needs of most children. This may continue until the child becomes an adult, and sometimes for even longer.

■ For some family members, the responsibility to provide care may suddenly impact upon their lives, for example following a fall, a stroke, or perhaps a road accident. In these circumstances there will be an immediate, intense and rapid need to adjust to the caring role.

Evidence activity

(1.2) Factors that may affect family involvement

Consider the following two scenarios:

1. Jackie is a 40-year-old working mum of two children aged 13 and 11. She is married, but her husband works away a lot with his job. Jackie is also the main carer for her 65-year-old mother, who has recently had a stroke which has left her with a left-sided weakness. *contd.*

contd.

2. Adam is 19 years old and has started studying full time to become a graphic designer. Adam and his father moved away from the family area following the break-up of his parents' marriage. Adam therefore lives with his father, who has recently been involved in a car accident which has left him with fractured ribs. While he was in hospital, he also suffered a heart attack. Adam is his father's main carer.

Having considered these two scenarios, give a brief outline of the factors that may influence the level of support and care that can be given by Jackie and Adam to their family members.

 Describe dilemmas or conflicts that may arise when working in partnership with families to support individuals

The relationship between health and social care workers, family carers and service users can sometimes be complex and, because of differences in values and opinions, can lead to conflicting situations.

A few of the most common reasons why conflict may occur are:

- an unresolved disagreement that escalates to an emotional level
- a perceived breach of trust
- miscommunication leading to unclear expectations
- clashes of personality or poor relationships
- differences in acquired care values
- competitiveness
- underlying stress and tension
- resentment, guilt
- perceived 'non-caring' or 'interfering'.

Time to reflect

 Conflicting situations

Think about a time when you have been caring for a person in partnership with a family member. Has there ever been a time when a conflicting situation has arisen? Who was the conflict with? Was it between a service user and family member, family member and care worker or service user and care worker?

Evidence activity

 Describe dilemmas or conflicts

Identify dilemmas or conflicts that may arise when working in partnership with families. Give examples of conflicts that may arise between

- service users and their family
- service users and health and social care workers
- a service user's family and the organisation providing care.

1.4 **Explain how the attitudes of a worker affect partnership working with families**

The primary purpose of partnership working is to improve the experience and outcomes of people who use services. This is achieved by minimising organisational barriers between different services. Here we are concerned with the relationship between the organisation and service users' families.

The attitudes of health and social care workers can significantly affect partnership working with families. Health and social care staff who view families as being problematic may be less reluctant to involve the family in all aspects of the individual's care. This could lead to a breakdown in care provision as the family could feel reluctant towards care staff. In turn this could increase the risk of conflict between the care organisation and the service user's family. It is therefore essential that health and social care staff are aware of and welcome the valuable contribution that families can make and encourage their participation in care.

Evidence activity

(1.4) The effects of a worker's attitude

What is the attitude towards partnership working with families within your organisation?

How does this attitude affect partnership working with service users' families?

Think about contrasting attitudes towards partnership working with families:

What effect can a positive attitude have on the provision of care?

What effect can a negative attitude have on the provision of care?

LO2 Be able to establish and maintain positive relationships with families

(2.1) Interact with family members in ways that respect their culture, experiences and expertise

When interacting with service users and their family members, there are many factors that need to be taken into consideration. It is essential that communication takes place in a manner that respects the person's sensory ability, communication needs, culture, experiences and level of knowledge and expertise.

This means that, as a health or social care worker, you ensure that your communication skills meet the needs of the individual when you interact with them. You must never expect the individual to adapt their communication skills to fit in with the organisation, so it is essential to check any specific communication requirements they may have. It may be possible to do this by observation, or by confirming with the individual their preferred method of communication. If you cannot meet the communication needs of an individual, then it is your responsibility to look for extra support if necessary.

It is important to be aware of any cultural differences between yourself and the person you are interacting with in order that you do not offend the person. Within some cultures, for example, it is unacceptable to use a person's first name, and physical contact may be seen as disrespectful. It is also important to be aware of the words you use, as some words can mean different things to different people and within different generations.

Time to reflect

(2.1) Interaction to support the individual

Think about two of your service users and, in particular, think about the way in which you interact with their family members. Try to think of two families that have different communication requirements, for example, an individual who has a sensory impairment and an individual who does not speak English as their first language.

- Are there any differences in the way you communicate with the two families?

- Why do you need to communicate with these individuals in different ways?

- What are the differences?

If you did not meet the needs of these individuals, what could be the consequences?

Practice activity

(2.1) Interact with family members in ways that respect their culture, experiences and expertise

This activity gives you an opportunity to practice interacting with family members in ways which respect their culture, experiences and expertise. *contd.*

Practice activity

contd.

When you are next interacting with relatives, think about the way in which you are interacting with them. Make a note of how you respected their:

- Culture
- Experiences
- Levels of expertise

 2.2 Demonstrate dependability in carrying out actions agreed with families

Dependability is a key aspect of your role as a health and social care worker. It is about being trustworthy and reliable. Demonstrating dependability in carrying out actions agreed with families simply means that we will do what we have said we will do. It is essential that any actions that have been agreed with families are followed through within your care organisation. If actions are not carried out, this could reflect badly on the organisation and will most definitely affect the overall quality of care.

Key term

Dependability is the quality of being reliable and trustworthy.

Practice activity

2.2 Demonstrate dependability

Think about a time when you have demonstrated dependability in carrying out actions that have been agreed with a service user and their family.

Explain the possible consequences of failing to carry out the actions.

2.3 Describe principles for addressing dilemmas or conflicts that may arise in relationships with families

We've already established that there may be times when dilemmas and conflicts arise when supporting service users and their families. It is important to understand that conflict is not always a bad thing, but if not resolved could have detrimental effects on the outcome of care for the service user. The guiding principles behind addressing dilemmas and conflicts are mutual respect, effective communication, an open mind and a desire to understand differing points of view, an enthusiasm to work cooperatively with the family and a willingness to consult, negotiate and compromise.

If a dilemma or conflict arises, it is important that you prevent feelings of **persecution**. Fairness towards the individual, especially if the conflict arises from a complaint, should ensure this. Dealing with conflict is not an easy task; however, there are some guidelines that may help to diffuse conflicting situations.

- Recognise the cause of the conflict and, if you need help to resolve the conflict, speak with your manager.
- Remain calm, speak quietly and clearly and avoid shouting or getting into an argument.
- **Actively listen** to what the person is saying.
- If necessary, make it clear that abuse or violence will not be tolerated
- Try to identify a reasonable compromise. It is essential to be empathetic (show **empathy**) and look for a solution that is in line with common goals.

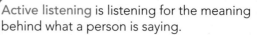

Key terms

Active listening is listening for the meaning behind what a person is saying.
Empathy is the ability to identify with and understand another person's difficulties or feelings.
Persecution is hostility towards and cruel or unfair treatment of someone.

Evidence activity

2.3 Principles for addressing dilemmas or conflicts with families

You are supporting Graham, a service user with a severe learning disability and deteriorating mobility. Graham is being supported in his own home and his parents are partners in his care package. The most recent risk assessment has identified that Graham's mobility has deteriorated and he now needs to be hoisted when being transferred from his bed to his wheelchair. Graham's parents don't like the hoist, and when they are caring for him they use a technique known as a 'drag lift' to transfer him from bed to chair.

When you arrive to support Graham with his personal care, his parents say that they don't want you to use the hoist as they think it is undignified. They are insistent that you use a 'drag lift' to transfer Graham into his chair. You are not happy, as you know this is unsafe and not a recommended practice. Graham's parents are becoming insistent in expressing their unhappiness with the hoist.

Explain why this conflict could have arisen and how you would address this situation.

LO3 Be able to plan shared approaches to the care and support of individuals with families

3.1 Agree with the individual, family members and others the proposed outcomes of partnership working with a family

Agreed and shared outcomes should ensure that individuals, regardless of their underlying care needs, are supported to:

- maintain independence
- remain **autonomous**

Key term

Autonomous means self-governing or independent.

- sustain a family unit which avoids children being required to take on caring roles inappropriately
- participate as equal and active citizens
- maintain the best quality of life
- maintain dignity and respect.

Evidence activity

3.1 Agree the proposed outcome of partnership working

Alice is a 76-year-old woman who cares for her husband Bill. Bill had a stroke three years ago and Alice has cared for him at home since he was discharged from hospital. Bill's care and support package is being coordinated through his local social services and they have commissioned care from a variety of agencies.

Bill needs help with all aspects of daily living, and care workers assist him each morning and evening. In addition, an occupational therapist has had a ramp installed at the entrance to the home, so that Alice can get the wheelchair in and out of the house easily. The neurologist sees Bill every six months to monitor his progress. A speech and language therapist is also involved in his care.

Bill attends a day centre once a week, and he attends a care home for a week once a month, to give Alice a break. Alice receives some support from her local carers organisation (which has offered some training in moving and handling). Getting in and out of the car is now getting more difficult and Alice is seeking support with this.

1. Explain why it is important to agree the proposed outcomes of partnership working with the individual (Bill) the family (Alice) and the other services that are involved in Bill's rehabilitation. *contd.*

Evidence activity

contd.

2. Give an example of how partnership working has been used within your place of work.

3. How are proposed outcomes of partnership working with the individual, family members and others agreed within your area of work?

 Clarify own role, role of family members, and roles of others in supporting the individual

Everything you do as a health and social care worker involves partnership working. You work alongside other people within your workplace, including colleagues, service users and their families. You also work alongside people from other agencies. Each of these people will have different roles, some of which are very clearly defined within codes of practice, contracts and workplace policies. Some health and social care workers provide a supportive role, while others provide services that are more specialised. If partnership working is to be successful, it is important to be sure what role everyone has to play within the partnership and in supporting the service user.

Evidence activity

 Clarify roles in supporting an individual

This activity enables you to demonstrate your understanding of your own role, the role of family members, and the role of others in supporting individuals within your care organisation.

■ Think about a service user who is also receiving support from outside agencies. Identify all of the people who are involved in supporting the individual and outline their role within the partnership.

■ In addition, highlight the role of family members within the support network.

■ How does your role differ from the role of the individuals you have identified above?

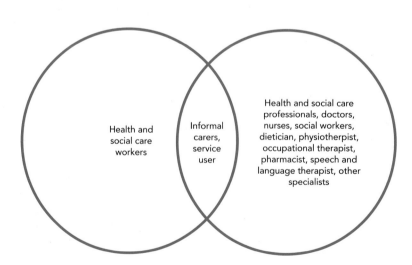

Figure 15.2 Different roles within the team

3.3 Support family members to understand person-centred approaches and agreed ways of working

Social care has been undergoing a radical transformation, moving towards a personalised support and a social care system that engages with people, supporting them to achieve the outcomes they want in their own lives. In 2007 the government made it clear that this transformation needs to be one that is made in partnership, and it demonstrated this through the 'Putting People First' initiative. The ethos of 'Putting People First' is based on **person-centred principles**.

> ### Key term
>
> **Person-centred principles** are principles that ensure that the person is central to all discussions and decisions that are made.

Being person-centred is about seeing things from the perspective of the person and what is important to them. This means listening to each person and helping them to live the life they choose.

Ensuring that services and support are developed in partnership with people and their families is crucial when aiming for person-centredness that truly aims to support people to achieve a good quality of life.

As many family members will be partners in providing care for their loved ones, it is essential that they are aware of the person-centred approach to care.

> ### Practice activity
>
> **3.3 Support family members to understand person centred approaches and agreed ways of working.**
>
> This activity enables you to demonstrate your knowledge of how to support family members to understand person centred approaches and agreed ways of working.
>
> Design a leaflet that explains what person centred care is. The leaflet should be written in a way that is understandable to family members.

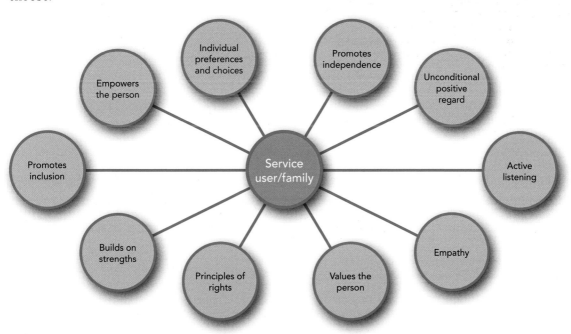

Figure 15.3 Person-centred approaches

3.4 Plan ways to manage risks associated with sharing care or support

Dictionaries define risk as the possibility of suffering harm or loss. In the case of sharing care with others, the risk of harm or loss will be to the detriment of the service user who, if the service is not properly managed, could miss out on treatment, care or support. This may have detrimental effects on the person and their family.

The best way to avoid harm is prevention. This means anticipating problems before they happen. Good communication between all parties is imperative. By sharing information about potential risk, safeguards can then be considered and included at the earliest opportunity.

Partnerships can range from small two-party partnerships to complex multi-agency partnerships.

Although each partnership is unique, and different approaches need to be taken with different types of partnerships, there are some common themes. These are the key principles that make partnership working more effective. The more effective a partnership is at sharing care, the lesser the risks associated with a breakdown in care provision. Here are some top tips for effective partnership working.

■ Shared goals – partners should share the same vision/aims.

■ Trust – partners need to be able to trust in each other's abilities and skills.

■ Clarity of the purpose of the partnerships – clear information about the partners is important. This includes defining boundaries in order that the contribution of each partner is made clear.

■ Shared language – remember, not everyone will understand the jargon used in your organisation. Keep your language clear, simple and understandable.

■ Good communication – talk to each other and establish clear communication links to ensure that each partner understands what they need to contribute.

■ **Equity** between partners – partnership is about understanding the value that everybody brings.

Key term

Equity is the quality of being fair and impartial.

■ Forward thinking – some forethought is required about how conflicts might be resolved should they arise.

Good relationships between partners, a common vision and understanding of expected achievements and what outcomes need to be delivered are critical. Good risk management is also an essential component to successful partnership working.

 Evidence activity

3.4 Plan ways to manage risks

Explain how risks associated with sharing care or support are minimised within your organisation.

3.5 Agree with the individual and family members processes for monitoring the shared support plan

Monitoring of the shared support plan is important in order to ascertain whether planned aspects are proceeding according to the plan. If care is to be person centred, it is essential that individuals and their family members take an active part in the monitoring process. This includes collecting and analysing information that will assist timely decision making, ensure accountability and provide a basis for evaluation and learning. The collection of data could take the form of a questionnaire, or a meeting could take place during which the information is collected verbally and recorded.

 Evidence activity

3.5 Agree processes for monitoring the shared support plan

Explain how the process for monitoring shared support plans is agreed with the individual and key members of their family within your organisation.

LO4 Be able to work with families to access support in their role as carers

4.1 Work with family members to identify the support they need to carry out their role

In order to be able to work with families to access support, you will need to communicate with them to determine their requirements for support. It is essential that you don't impose your views of what you think would be of benefit to the family. What is important here is that you can give the family information that will help them to meet their needs. It is also important to be aware that not all individuals have the ability to ask for support, because they do not always know what is available. You might, therefore, have to ask quite a few questions to establish the needs of the family. You will need to call upon your communication skills and actively listen to what the person is telling you. Prompting questions will also be a useful tool here, for example:

■ What support do you think might help you?

■ Would it help if you could have someone to talk to?

■ Would you like some time to yourself?

■ Would it be helpful to speak to someone about how you are feeling?

Asking questions in this way will help the family to think about the types of support they may need.

Every family and every caring situation is different. Like all service users, their family and carers have individual needs too. Some families will require more or less support than others.

Carers who provide a significant amount of care and on a regular basis are legally entitled to an assessment of their needs when the person they are looking after is being assessed for community care services. A **carers' assessment** gives carers the opportunity to say what could help them with their caring role. The assessment is undertaken by social services and will enable the carer to meet with a social or health worker in order to:

■ identify what help they need to support them as a carer

■ find out what help and support may be available

■ facilitate decisions about the future

Key term

A carers' assessment is an assessment of carers' needs.

Health and social care workers/professionals who are in contact with carers, or who meet new carers, should ensure that they are given the option to have this formal opportunity to talk about their needs.

Families may need support with many aspects of the caring role, and the support may take the form of emotional, psychological, physical or social support. It is essential that carers are fully supported in order to ensure their own health and well-being and to ensure that they are fully supported to carry out the caring role.

Evidence activity

4.1 Work with family members to identify the support they need

Using available resources, find out more information about the 'carers' needs assessment'. Make a note of the areas that are covered within this assessment.

■ Explain the mechanisms that are in place within your organisation that enable you to work with family members to identify the support they need to carry out their role as a carer.

■ Identify the possible consequences of failing to address the family's support needs.

4.2 Provide accessible information about available resources for support

When providing information, careful thought will need to be given to the needs of the person receiving the information and the format of the information.

In order to fully meet the support requirements of service users and families, it is important that any information you provide is in a format that is understandable to them. In order to provide accessible information, it will first be necessary to

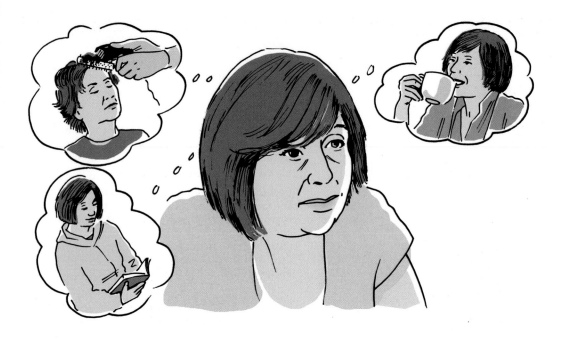

Figure 15.4 Family carers have needs too!

establish the communication requirements of each individual. If you do not have the skills to communicate with the individual, you may have to look for guidance and support from another source. For example, if a family does not speak English, it will be necessary to engage the support of an interpreter.

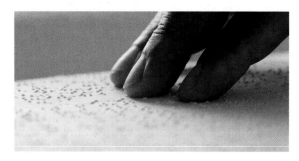

Figure 15.5 Ways of making information accessible

Practice activity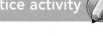

(4.2) Provide accessible information

Talk with your manager about any resources that your organisation has available to support families who are providing care, and the accessibility of these resources. *contd.*

Practice activity

- In addition to the information you have gained from this discussion, undertake a search for other available resources that can be used to support families.

- Put together a folder of all available resources that can be used to inform and support individuals and their families within your organisation.

- Is this information in formats that make it accessible? If so, what formats does the information come in? If not, how can you make this information accessible to your target audience?

(4.3) Work with family members to access resources

No one will expect you to be able to provide an answer to every question a family asks you, or to be able to solve every problem. However, it is important that you know where you can find the information in order that families can access available resources. It will also be helpful to know how best to keep information relating to resources in order that it can be updated and instantly accessed.

There are many places where resources can be accessed, for example through:

■ local organisations such as the library, Citizens Advice Bureau, leisure centre

■ special interest groups such as Mind, Age Concern, the Stroke Association.

In addition, resources can be accessed via the internet. It is, however, essential to bear in mind that some of the resources may not have been verified and so may be inaccurate. It is always best, therefore, to ensure that resources come from official websites.

Careful thought will also need to be given to any difficulties the individual may encounter in attempting to access the required information. For example, the resources may not be in a format that is easy for the person to interpret. The family may not have direct access to a computer, or may not have the skills necessary to access online information. Further information may therefore need to be given in order to ensure that families can access the resources they require.

Practice activity

 4.3 **Work with family members to access resources**

This activity gives you an opportunity to practice demonstrating how you work with families to access resources.

What facilities are in place within your organisation relating to supporting families to access resources?

Think about a particular family who you have worked with to access resources. Maintaining confidentiality, explain the resources the family needed to access and how you supported them to do this.

Where did the family access the resources from?

Did the family experience any difficulties in accessing the resources? If so, how were the difficulties resolved?

LO5 Be able to exchange and record information about partnership work with families

5.1 Exchange information with the individual and family members about the implementation of the plan and changes to their needs and preferences

When exchanging information about the individual it is essential that you have their consent from the individual before discussing anything with their family in order to uphold the principle of confidentiality.

The exchange of information with the individual and their family members is important in ascertaining whether the plan is being effective and whether there are any changes in needs and preferences that need to be taken into consideration.

The exchange of information may take place as part of a review process. The review process ideally should involve everyone who is involved in providing support for the individual. However, the most important people at the review are the individual and their carers and/ or family.

It is essential that changes in needs and preferences are discussed in order that the needs of the person and their family can be fully supported. When exchanging information, it is essential that the method of communication can be understood by the individual and their family. Remember, this is a two-way process and a person-centred approach must be adopted at all times.

Evidence activity

5.1 **Exchanging information about changes to needs and preferences**

■ What factors do you need to take into consideration prior to exchanging information with the individual and their family? *contd.*

Evidence activity

contd.

- What kind of information might you need to exchange with the individual and their family in relation to the implementation of the plan?

- Why is it important to communicate changes in the person's needs and preferences?

5.2 Record information in line with agreed ways of working about progress towards outcomes and the effectiveness of partnership working

Your workplace will have policies and procedures which give guidelines on agreed ways of working when recording information, and it is essential that you follow these guidelines at all times.

Having obtained information from the individual and their family, it is important that the information is recorded within the relevant documentation.

Partnership working involves working in partnership with other people in order to support service users and their families in a joined-up way. In order to guarantee that support is efficient and effective, it is important to ensure that records are completed, up to date, accurate and legible.

When recording information, it is also important to be aware of the implications of the Data Protection Act 1998. This piece of legislation governs the processing and handling of information, and sets out principles that are designed to protect people's rights.

It is important that an individual's progress towards agreed goals is monitored and recorded in order that changes in needs and circumstances can be detected. People's needs do change, sometimes in a positive way, and sometimes in a negative way, and this could have an overall effect on the provision of services a person requires.

Case Study

5.2 Elsie

When Elsie was discharged from hospital six months ago following a broken hip, she was assessed as needing support with various aspects of her personal and social care. The local social services commissioned a care package which consisted of physiotherapy, as mobility was a problem, day care and home care to assist with personal hygiene and dressing requirements and shopping. Elsie's daughter also cares for her, but works full time, so finds she is juggling her personal life a lot of the time.

Within two months, Elsie was feeling much stronger and no longer needed her walking frame. She was also able to get out to do her shopping, but had difficulty bending down to put on her stockings. She enjoys going to the day centre as she gets to play bingo and talk to other people. Elsie's daughter can help out around the home more now as she has changed her working hours to part time.

We can see from this case study that an individual's needs do change over time. It is therefore essential that information is recorded in order to reflect the changes in the individual's circumstances. This will help everyone in the partnership to provide the level of care and support that is needed. A service that is frequently evaluated and updated is more likely to be one that is responsive to the needs of the individual and considers the effective use of commissioned resources.

Practice activity

5.2 Recording information

This activity gives you an opportunity to demonstrate that you are able to record information, in line with agreed ways of working, about progress towards outcomes and the effectiveness of partnership working. *contd.*

Practice activity

contd.

- Identify your workplace procedures for recording information and use these guidelines to evaluate the progress one of your service users is making towards their agreed goals.

- Explain the effect that recording this information has on partnership working.

LO6 Be able to contribute to reviewing partnership work with families

6.1 Agree criteria and processes for reviewing partnership work with families

Reviewing partnership work with families is a two-way process. It is important to ensure that families do not feel excluded from the planning of care. Family members are an integral part of the process and they must feel included. It is also important to establish any changes in relationships that may affect partnership working.

The documents 'Putting People First' and the 'Carers Strategy' have both recognised the importance of respecting family carers as expert care partners with a need to be able to access the integrated and personalised services which will help support them in their caring role. A major key to treating family and carers as partners in care is ensuring that they are equipped with the information relevant to the care and needs of the person they support. It is therefore vital that families are fully involved in the review process.

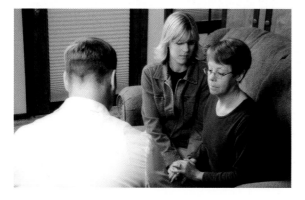

Figure 15.6 Reviewing partnership work

Evidence activity

6.1 Agreeing review criteria and processes

We know how important it is to ensure that families are involved throughout the process of delivering care. Explain how you agree the criteria and processes for reviewing partnership work with families within your organisation.

6.2 Agree criteria and processes for reviewing support for family members

In addition to reviewing the needs and preferences of service users it is essential that support for family members is reviewed on a regular basis. This should be built into the review process and is integral to the health and well being of the carer and in ensuring their needs continue to be met. If carers' needs are not met, they will be ill equipped to continue in their role.

Evidence activity

6.2 Agree criteria and processes for reviewing support for family members

This activity gives you the opportunity to demonstrate your knowledge in agreeing the criteria and processes for reviewing support for family members.

Explain how you agree the criteria and processes for reviewing support for family members within your workplace.

6.3 Encourage the individual and family members to participate in the review

Reviewing partnership work with individuals and families is an important part of the care process because situations, needs and preferences change over time. As circumstances change, the individual's package of care may need to be reviewed in order to ensure those changes are catered for. At agreed regular intervals, all of the parties involved in the partnership should meet to reflect on whether or not the care package is continuing to be effective in meeting the individual's identified needs. The process of review will also assist in gathering information about the circumstances of the individual, the service provided and the service providers. This will then provide all those involved in the provision of care with the opportunity to express their professional views and opinions, to be involved in discussion about how effective the provision of care has been and to recommend any changes that may need to be made.

The process for review should be agreed at the beginning of the partnership, and the regularity with which the review takes place will depend on the complexity of the needs of the service user.

The most important people at a review meeting are the individual and their family, who must be encouraged to participate in the review. The level of participation will depend on the individual's ability to communicate, but the review meeting should be conducted in such a way that the person and their family are able to participate. The individual and their family must be the central focal point around which care is reviewed.

Evidence activity

6.3 Encouraging participation in the review

Explain how individuals and their family are prepared and encouraged to participate in review meetings within your organisation.

6.4 Carry out your own role in the review of partnership working

Your role in the review of partnership working will be dependent upon your level of skill and experience. You may have a key role to play in organising and preparing for the meeting, especially if you are in a senior position or a key

worker position, in which case you will also be central to the review process. It is important throughout the review that everyone gets the chance to have their say. You will be key to ensuring that the team is aware of how the service provision meets the present needs of the individual and what may need to change for future provision. You may also need to support the service user to recognise the impact of any significant changes.

Evidence activity

6.4 Your role in the review of partnership working

- Explain your own role in the review process of partnership working.

- Reflect on a review meeting that you have attended. Who was at the meeting and what were the roles of these people?

- What was your role at the meeting?

LO7 Be able to provide feedback about support for families

7.1 Provide feedback to others about the support accessed by family members

It is important that any information about the support accessed by family members is passed on to other appropriate members of the care team. This will ensure continuity of care and will also ensure that families access available support appropriate to their requirements. Resources can then be directed appropriately and duplication may be prevented. Providing feedback will also ensure that all members of the team are aware of the support provided in order that gaps in service provision can be identified. However, when providing feedback to other members of the team it is essential that you follow your workplace policies and procedures. You must be aware of the need to maintain confidentiality and ensure that any feedback is given on a need-to-know basis.

Evidence activity

7.1 Providing feedback to others

Think about a time when you have had to provide feedback to other members of the team in relation to support accessed by family members.

- What factors did you need to take into consideration?

- Were there any members of the team who did not need to know the information?

- What were the determining factors for those who needed to know?

- How was the feedback presented?

7.2 Report on any gaps in the provision of support for family members

Your organisation should have a policy which stipulates the procedure that should be followed if gaps in the provision of support for family members are detected. Reporting these gaps is essential in order to enable family members to access support. Some families may not be aware of the support that is available to them and so may not be aware of the gap. In fact, carers may be overlooked if they:

- come from a minority group

- care for someone with a stigmatising long-term condition, for example a mental health problem, a substance misuse problem, or HIV/AIDS

- care for a neighbour or friend rather than a family member, or for a same-gender partner

- care for someone who lives in a different local authority area

- have a disability or long-term condition themselves.

7.3 Describe ways to challenge information or support that is discriminatory or inaccessible

Information can be **inaccessible** to some people because of the format in which it is presented. For example, the format may not be appropriate to the functional requirements of the individual. Formats include: the spoken word; sign language; print; Braille; audio tape; videotape; electronic media, such as email. If a person is presented with information which is inaccessible, that individual may be denied the right to make informed choices and this will seriously affect the individual's package of care.

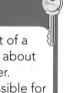

Key terms

Discrimination is the unfair treatment of a person, usually because of prejudice about race, ethnicity, age, religion or gender. Inaccessible means difficult or impossible for a person to reach or understand.

Discrimination relates to a denial of an individual's rights. Information or support that is discriminatory may be based on ethnicity, disability, age, gender or sexual orientation. The main pieces of legislation which relate to these rights are the:

- Disability Discrimination Act 1995

- Race Relations Act 1976

- Sex Discrimination Act 1975

- Equality Act 2010

Your place of work must have systems in place to enable staff to report and challenge information or support that is discriminatory or inaccessible. It is important to realise that a failure to report or challenge under these circumstances could affect the safe delivery of care. It is important, therefore, that you follow your workplace's policies and procedures for reporting and recording your concerns.

Evidence activity

7.2 Reporting gaps in provision of support

What is the procedure within your organisation if you realise there are gaps in the provision of support for family members?

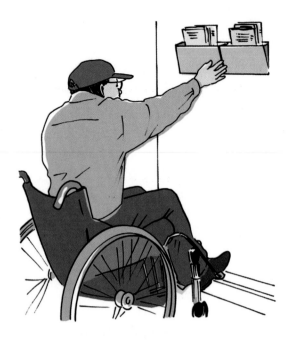

Figure 15.7 Challenging discriminatory practice

Evidence activity

(7.3) Challenging information or support that is discriminatory or inaccessible

Explain the procedure you would follow if you came across information or support which you felt was misleading, discriminatory or difficult to access.

Assessment summary

Your reading of this chapter and completion of the activities will have prepared you to be able to engage in personal development in health, social care or children's and young people's settings.

To achieve the unit, your assessor will require you to:

Learning outcomes	Assessment Criteria
Learning outcome 1: Understand partnership working with families by:	(1.1) analysing the contribution of families to the care and/or support of individuals See Evidence activity 1.1, p. 305
	(1.2) identifying factors that may affect the level of involvement of family members in care and/or support See Evidence activity 1.2, p. 305
	(1.3) describing dilemmas or conflicts that may arise when working in partnership with families to support individuals See Evidence activity 1.3, p. 306
	(1.4) explaining how the attitudes of a worker affect partnership working with families See Evidence activity 1.4, p. 307

Learning outcomes	Assessment Criteria
Learning outcome 2: Be able to establish and maintain positive relationships with families by:	(2.1) interacting with family members in ways that respect their culture, experiences and expertise See Practice activity 2.1, p. 307
	(2.2) demonstrating dependability in carrying out actions agreed with families See Practice activity 2.2, p. 308
	(2.3) describing principles for addressing dilemmas or conflicts that may arise in relationships with families See Evidence activity 2.3, p. 309
Learning outcome 3: Be able to plan shared approaches to the care and support of individuals with families by:	(3.1) agreeing with the individual, family members and others the proposed outcomes of partnership working with a family See Evidence activity 3.1, p. 309
	(3.2) clarifying own role, role of family members, and roles of others in supporting the individual See Evidence activity 3.2, p. 310
	(3.3) supporting family members to understand person-centred approaches and agreed ways of working See Practice activity 3.3, p. 311
	(3.4) planning ways to manage risks associated with sharing care or support See Evidence activity 3.4, p. 312
	(3.5) agreeing with the individual and family members processes for monitoring the shared support plan See Evidence activity 3.5, p. 312

Learning outcomes	Assessment Criteria
Learning outcome 4: Be able to work with families to access support in their role as carers by:	(4.1) working with family members to identify the support they need to carry out their role See Evidence activity 4.1, p. 313
	(4.2) providing accessible information about available resources for support See Practice activity 4.2, p. 314
	(4.3) working with family members to access resources See Practice activity 4.3, p. 315
Learning outcome 5: Be able to exchange and record information about partnership work with families by:	(5.1) exchanging information with the individual and family members about: • implementation of the plan • changes to needs and preferences See Evidence activity 5.1, p. 315
	(5.2) recording information in line with agreed ways of working about: • progress towards outcomes • effectiveness of partnership working See Practice activity 5.2, p. 316
Learning outcome 6: Be able to contribute to reviewing partnership work with families by:	(6.1) agreeing criteria and processes for reviewing partnership work with families See Evidence activity 6.1, p. 317
	(6.2) agreeing criteria and processes for reviewing support for family members See Evidence activity 6.2, p. 317
	(6.3) encouraging the individual and family members to participate in the review See Evidence activity 6.3, p. 318

Learning outcomes	Assessment Criteria
Learning outcome 6: Be able to contribute to reviewing partnership work with families by:	(6.4) carrying out own role in the review of partnership working See Evidence activity 6.4, p. 318
Learning outcome 7: Be able to provide feedback about support for families by:	(7.1) providing feedback to others about the support accessed by family members See Evidence activity 7.1, p. 319
	(7.2) reporting on any gaps in the provision of support for family members See Evidence activity 7.2, p. 319
	(7.3) describing ways to challenge information or support that is discriminatory or inaccessible See Evidence activity 7.3, p. 320

Good luck!

Web links

Department of Health	www.dh.gov.uk
Princess Royal Trust for Carers	www.carers.org
Care Quality Commission	www.cqc.org.uk
Community care website	www.communitycare.org

Support individuals at the end of life

For Unit HSC 3048

What are you finding out?

Many people think that end of life care is only concerned with supporting people through the process of dying. This is certainly not the case. End of life care is aimed at helping those with advanced, progressive and incurable illness to live as well as possible until they die. It focuses on preparing for the anticipated death and managing the end stage of a terminal medical condition, and includes care during and around the time of death, and immediately afterwards.

There has been a growing recognition of the need to enable people nearing the end of their life to experience a 'good death', and as the public has become more aware of the principles of end of life care, there is now a greater expectation of the delivery of high-quality end of life care.

End of life care is not confined to specialist services, but includes services provided by any health and social care worker in any setting. It is therefore essential that every person who works in an environment that provides end of life care is aware of the requirements aimed at ensuring that a person nearing the end of life can make the most of their life until the very end.

The reading and activities in this chapter will help you to:

■ Understand the requirements of legislation and agreed ways of working to protect the rights of individuals at the end of life

■ Understand factors affecting end of life care

■ Understand advance care planning in relation to end of life care

■ Be able to provide support to individuals and key people during end of life care

■ Understand how to address sensitive issues in relation to end of life care

■ Understand the role of organisations and support services available to individuals and key people in relation to end of life care

■ Be able to access support for the individual or key people from the wider team

■ Be able to support individuals through the process of dying

■ Be able to take action following the death of individuals

■ Be able to manage your own feelings in relation to the dying or death of individuals.

LO1 Understand the requirements of legislation and agreed ways of working to protect the rights of individuals at the end of life

1.1 Outline legal requirements and agreed ways of working designed to protect the rights of individuals in end of life care

Within a document entitled 'Treatment and care towards the end of life: good practice in decision making', the General Medical Council identified that some groups of people can experience inequalities in getting access to healthcare services and in the standard of care provided. It is in fact well known that some older people, people with disabilities and people from ethnic minority groups sometimes receive poor standards of care towards the end of their life. This can be because of:

- physical barriers

- communication barriers

- mistaken beliefs about what end of life care involves

- lack of knowledge among care providers due to lack of training

- lack of knowledge about the service user's needs and interests.

Evidence activity

1.1 Protecting the rights of individuals in end of life care

Think about the guidelines, legislation and codes of practice that are relevant to your job role. Which of these are relevant to end of life care?

Explain why these guidelines, codes of practice and pieces of legislation are important when caring for a person who is nearing the end of their life.

The Mental Capacity Act 2005

This is an important part of the existing legal framework aimed at protecting the rights of individuals throughout end of life care, and governs decision making on behalf of adults who lack capacity to make some or all decisions for themselves.

The Act has three broad objectives:

1. To support people who have impaired capacity so that they can make decisions for themselves

2. To provide them with a protective framework for decision making when an individual is unable to make decisions for him or herself

3. To provide a framework for those who have to make and implement decisions in relation to individuals who do not have the capacity to make decisions for themselves.

The Act is underpinned by five underlying principles. These are:

1. **A presumption of capacity** – Everybody has the right to make their own decisions, and so a person must be assumed to have capacity, unless it is established that the person lacks capacity to make the decision in question.

2. **The right for individuals to be supported to make their own decisions** – Individuals must never be treated as being unable to make a decision unless all practicable steps to help the person to do so have been taken, without success.

3. **The right to make decisions which may seem eccentric or unwise to other people** – Individuals must not be treated as unable to make a decision merely because the decision appears unwise.

4. **Best interests** – Acts done or decisions made on behalf of a person established to be lacking capacity must be in the person's best interests.

5. **Least restrictive interventions** – People's rights and freedoms must be restricted as little as possible.

The Mental Capacity Act therefore has major implications in relation to **end of life care** and **advance care planning**. It also addresses the rights of individuals to make advance refusals associated with care. These relate to the refusal of certain treatments, for example a wish not to be resuscitated or mechanically ventilated. The Act is aimed at protecting the rights of all vulnerable adults, and protects against health care professionals and others making decisions for the person and overriding previous choices. In addition, it takes into account the need for the person to be involved in decisions about their care, and is underpinned by five key principles:

- A presumption of capacity.

- The right for individuals to be supported to make their own decisions.

- Unwise decisions.

- Best interest.

- Least restrictive intervention.

Key terms

Advance care planning is a process of discussion between the health care team, the service user and their family. It enables the people to make plans for their future.

Key terms

End of life care is an important part of palliative care, and usually refers to the care of a person during the last part of their life, from the point at which it has become clear that the person is in a progressive state of decline.

The Mental Capacity Act 2005 is also backed up by a Code of Practice which sets out best practice and covers an extensive range of guidance relating to specific scenarios.

There are also other pieces of legislation and guidelines that relate to people who may either lack capacity or need to make decisions, and it is important for health and social care workers to be aware of how these pieces of legislation may influence their practice when caring for people at the end of their life

The Human Right Act 1998

This Act requires public authorities to act compatibly with the rights set out in the European Convention of Human Rights. This Act came into effect in October 2000 and outlines 16 rights and freedoms that all individuals are entitled to. The Act makes it unlawful for any public body to act in a way that contravenes the rights and freedoms of people.

Disability Discrimination Act 1995

This Act is important in ensuring that every person can access and actively participate in a high standard of end of life care, regardless of their ability. Within health and social care this has implications in relation to accessing services and ensuring that information is provided in a format that the person can understand.

Data Protection Act 1998

The primary purpose of the Data Protection Act is to protect people's right to privacy when personal information about them is processed. This Act relates to the collection, use, storage, disclosure and destruction of personal information and applies to information that is held on computer as well as written media, images and recordings.

Access to Health Records Act 1990

Deceased people have the same rights to confidentiality as when they were alive. The Access to Health Records Act 1990, however, makes provision for someone who may be entitled to compensation to access records relating to the cause of death. This gives emphasis to the importance of robust and accurate documentation.

Key term

Deceased means dead. The term can also be used to mean the person who has died.

The National End of Life Care Strategy

This Strategy is a comprehensive framework aimed at promoting a high standard of care for all adults approaching the end of their life. It was published in 2008 and identified a **care pathway** approach for the delivery of integrated care. The End of Life Care Pathway was developed to help care providers providing health and social care to people nearing the end of life. The care pathway identified in the strategy involves the following steps:

Key term

Care pathways are used to systematically plan and follow up a specific programme of care.

- discussions as the end of life approaches
- assessment and care planning
- coordination of care
- service delivery
- last days of life
- care after death.

The Nursing and Midwifery Council Standards of conduct, performance and ethics for nurses and midwives

The Nursing and Midwifery Council sets out the standards of conduct, performance and ethics which nurses and midwives must adhere to and apply within their work.

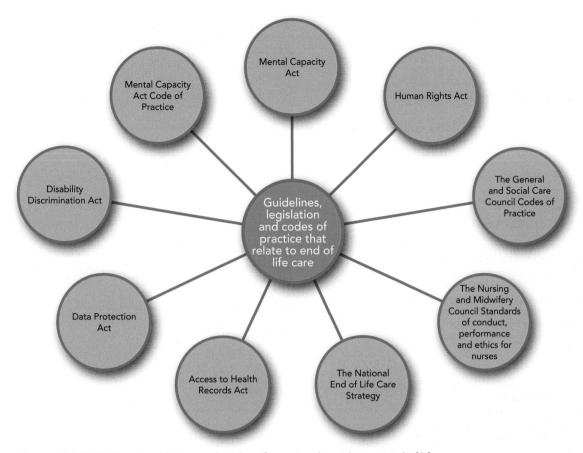

Figure 16.1 Guidelines, legislation and codes of practice that relate to end of life care

The General Social Care Council Codes of Practice

These codes of practice for social care workers set out the standards of practice that everyone who works in health and social care should meet.

1.2 How does legislation designed to protect the rights of individuals in end of life care apply to your job role?

Your workplace will have policies and procedures aimed at protecting the rights of individuals who are nearing the end of life. The policies should set out the arrangements your workplace has for complying with the legislation, and the procedures will describe the ways of working which must be followed for the policies to be implemented.

You must provide individuals who are approaching the end of their life with the same standard of care as any other service user. You must therefore treat the person and those close to them with dignity, respect and compassion, especially when they are facing difficult situations and decisions about care. You must also respect their privacy and right to confidentiality.

Key term

Compassion is sympathy and concern for another person's suffering, and the wish to relieve it.

Evidence activity

1.2 Legislation that applies to your job role

Explain how you ensure that you are working in line with current and up-to-date legislation and why it is important that you follow the guidelines, legislation and codes of practice when caring for service users who are nearing the end of their life.

LO2 Understand factors affecting end of life care

2.1 Outline key points of theories about the emotional and psychological processes that individuals and key people may experience with the approach of death

It may be tempting to assume that grief is a process which only begins following the death of a person. There are occasions when this does happen, for example when a person dies suddenly or unexpectedly. However, it is important to realise that grief can begin as soon as it is known that a person is living with a life-limiting condition. You may have heard the term **'anticipatory grief'. Grief** is a term used to describe the emotional and psychological reaction that a person may feel in response to loss. 'Anticipatory grief' refers to the feelings that the individual and their loved ones may experience prior to death (in anticipation of it). It can help the person who is dying and their loved ones to prepare for death by allowing them to mourn the various losses that occur as a result of death. We will further explore some of these losses within section 2.4.

Key terms

Anticipatory grief is the sense of loss and grief that occurs before a person dies, as the loss is anticipated.

Grief is the sadness a person feels, usually as a result of loss.

There are many theories that explain the emotional stages a person goes through when nearing the end of their life, but the most famous theorist on this subject is Dr Elisabeth Kübler Ross. According to Kübler Ross, there are five stages a dying person goes through when faced with a life-limiting diagnosis. These progress from denial through to acceptance. The work of Kübler Ross related to the experiences of people who are dying, but it has been adapted by other authors and used as a means of describing grief more generally.

■ **Stage 1 Denial and isolation** – denial can manifest itself through emotions of shock and disbelief. There may be feelings associated with numbness. The person may feel as though this is a dream and that what they are experiencing is not true.

■ **Stage 2 Anger** – following the denial stage, the individual will come to terms with the reality of what is happening to them, and the feelings associated with denial may lead to intense feelings of anger. Anger can manifest itself in several ways. The person may feel resentful and rage at what they are faced with. They may ask 'Why me?'

■ **Stage 3 Bargaining** – this is a stage where individuals begin to adjust their goals, hopes and expectations. The person may attempt to negotiate the situation either with another person or with God. This stage often involves promises of better behaviour or significant life change which will be made in exchange for the reversal of the loss.

■ **Stage 4 Depression** – once the realisation that the situation is not reversible sinks in, the individual often becomes depressed. It is within this stage that the individual realises the inevitability of what is happening to them, the reality of the impending loss and its irreversibility. It is within this stage that grieving people begin to cry and experience difficulties with sleeping or eating.

■ **Stage 5 Acceptance** – this is the stage where the individual comes to terms with what is happening. Kübler Ross acknowledges that if a person has enough time, and has been given support in working through the stages of grief, they will reach a stage where they can finally come to terms with what is happening to them.

These stages are not rigid, they are guidelines, and Kübler Ross emphasises the fact that they can occur in any order and at any time. They can also happen simultaneously.

Elisabeth Kübler Ross (1969) On death and dying.

Evidence activity

2.1 Emotional and psychological processes

Explain what is meant by the term 'anticipatory grief' and how this relates to a person who is facing the end of their life.

Research & investigate

2.1 Theories

In addition to the theory identified by Kübler Ross, research another theory related to the emotional and psychological processes that individuals may experience with the approach of death. *contd.*

Research & investigate

contd.

How does the theory compare with that of Elisabeth Kübler Ross?

2.2 Explain how the beliefs, religion and culture of individuals and key people influence end of life care

Culture and **religion** play an important role in the lives of many individuals, but it is important to remember that people will vary in the strictness of their religious observance. Adopting a multi-faith approach to care is essential if health and social care workers are to fully support every individual's religious and cultural beliefs throughout the end of their life. Religious and cultural beliefs can influence an individual's end of life care in many ways.

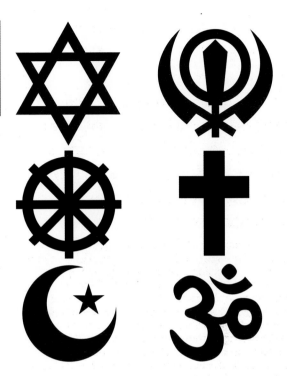

Figure 16.2 Religious and cultural beliefs

Key terms

Culture refers to the customs, ideas and social behaviour of particular people or groups. It is about their way of life.

Religion refers to a particular system of faith or worship.

Understanding each service user, and their religious and cultural needs and preferences, is essential to providing end of life care in a manner that is acceptable to their individual values and ideals. A person's religious and cultural beliefs may even prevent them from accessing end of life care.

Time to reflect

2.2 Religious and Cultural care

Think about how your care setting demonstrates that it is meeting the religious and cultural needs of people who are being cared for there.

Is there anything that could be done to better meet the religious and cultural needs of individuals?

Evidence activity

2.2 How the beliefs, religion and culture influence end of life care

Explain why it is important for health and social care workers to be aware of people's religious and cultural differences when supporting an individual who is nearing the end of their life.

2.3 Explain why key people may have a distinctive role in an individual's end of life care

The Government's End of Life Care Strategy recognises the important role of family, close friends and informal carers for people who are approaching the end of their life. Family members and close friends are a vital part of the care team and often derive satisfaction from knowing that they can help with the care and comfort of their loved ones. A person-centred approach to caring for individuals who are nearing the end of their lives must involve family and close friends.

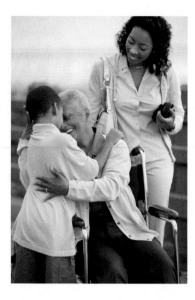

Figure 16.3 The importance of family and friends

Maintaining relationships with family and friends is an essential element of positive care.

Evidence activity

2.3 Why key people have a distinctive role in end of life care

This activity allows you to demonstrate your knowledge of the importance of involving the individual's family and friends in end of life care.

■ Explain why it is important to involve family and close friends in an individual's end of life care.

■ What role do these people play?

2.4 Explain why support for an individual's health and well-being may not always relate to their terminal condition

When a person is faced with dying, it is not just the loss of life they are faced with. They will also experience many other losses, all of which could impact on their health and well-being. For example, a person may lose their:

■ sense of independence

■ sense of security

■ sense of identity

■ aspirations, hopes, dreams and plans for the future

■ social role

■ earnings

■ employment status

■ important relationships

■ sexual function

■ self-esteem.

This list is not exhaustive; there are many other losses that an individual may experience. We do not always think of loss in this way, especially when caring for people who are nearing the end of their life, because the ultimate loss we focus on is the actual loss of life. It is, however, essential to bear in mind that a person facing death will most certainly be facing loss in other areas of their life, all of which could contribute to their 'total pain'. The concept of 'total pain' was first used by Dame Cicely Saunders to emphasise the fact that pain is much more than a physical phenomenon.

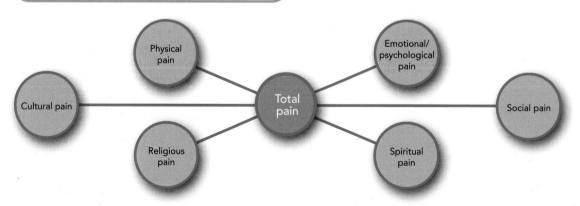

Figure 16.4 Total pain

reduce the risk of conflicting decisions later in the care process.

In addition, everyone deserves the best quality of care when they are faced with life-limiting conditions and death. Involving service users and giving them control over their end of life care will also ensure that they receive care which is **person centred** and dignified in approach. It is essential that the individual and the people who matter to them are actively involved in decisions concerning their end of life care.

Evidence activity

(2.4) Other aspects of health and well-being

Health and well-being may not always relate to the terminal condition. When supporting a person who is nearing the end of their life, what other elements do you need to take into account in order to ensure that they are supported in a holistic manner?

LO3 Understand advance care planning in relation to end of life care

(3.1) Describe the benefits to an individual of having as much control as possible over their end of life care

Autonomy and choice over health care decisions are major features within the field of end of life care. The advance care planning process allows individuals to exercise control over their end of life care and can provide a number of benefits for the person nearing the end of their life.

Key term

Autonomy is an individual's ability to remain independent and make decisions. Approaches that are person centred focus on what is important to the person. The person is the focal point around which everything else is geared.

For example, advance care planning ensures that the individual can:

- express their priorities, which can be considered at a future time
- identify where they wish to die
- identify issues which they feel need to be dealt with sooner rather than later
- make professionals aware of their wishes
- where appropriate, promote important discussions between family members

Evidence activity

(3.1) Benefits of an individual having as much control as possible over their care

- Explain why it is important to ensure individuals who are nearing the end of their life have as much control over health care decisions as possible.
- Why is this of benefit to the person and their family?
- What could be a possible consequence if individuals are not given the ability to exercise control?

(3.2) Explain the purpose of advance care planning in relation to end of life care

Advance care planning has been defined within The National Council for Palliative Care guidance 'Advance Care Planning: A guide for health and social care staff 2007' as:

'A process of discussion between an individual and their care providers irrespective of discipline. If the individual wishes, their family and friends may be included. With the individual's agreement, the discussion should be documented, regularly reviewed, and communicated to key persons involved in their care.'

We can therefore assume that advance care planning is a process that is used to discuss and plan ahead. It involves the discussion and documentation of service users' wishes. Family members and friends can be involved if the service user wishes.

The types of wishes and preferences that are commonly discussed include:

■ where the individual would like to be cared for towards the end of their life – this is supported through the **Preferred Priorities for Care (PPC)**.

■ choices about the type of treatment and care they wish to receive

■ choices about the type of treatment and care they would not wish to receive

■ arrangements in relation to the individual's funeral.

> ### Key term
>
> Preferred Priorities for Care (PPC) is a document in which individuals can record their wishes and preferences for the last years or months of their lives.

There are two specific areas within advance care planning. These are:

1. Advance statement of wishes and preferences – this relates to the formalisation of what service users *do* wish to happen to them in the future.

2. Advance decisions – this clarifies what service users *do not* wish to happen to them in the future. The Mental Capacity Act (2005) gives people in England and Wales a statutory right to refuse treatment, through an 'advance decision'.

Once an advance care plan has been drawn up, it is essential that it is reviewed on a regular basis in order to identify any changes in wishes.

Evidence activity

 The purpose of advance care planning

■ What is the purpose of advance care planning in relation to end of life care?

■ How does this differ from general care planning?

■ How does your workplace incorporate advance care planning into the care of service users?

 Describe own role in supporting and recording decisions about advance care planning

Your role in supporting and recording decisions relating to advance care planning will depend upon your experience, level of skill and any training you have received to prepare you for this role. In all instances it is essential that you work within your own sphere of competence and follow your workplace policies and procedures at all times.

The process of advance care planning can be broken down into four broad areas:

■ the opening conversation

■ exploring the options

■ identifying wishes and preferences

■ recording and communicating.

The opening conversation

Advance care planning may be started by either an individual or the provider of care at any time. However, it may be triggered by certain events, for example:

■ the death of a spouse or close friend

■ a diagnosis of a life-limiting condition

■ a change in progress of an existing condition

■ the consideration of new treatment options

■ a need to consider a different care setting

■ a change in personal circumstances

■ changes within the dynamics of the family.

Careful consideration must be given to individuals who cannot communicate their needs because of disability or some other reason.

Exploring the options

An individual may have strong views about things they would or would not like to happen as they near the end of their life. These decisions may range from where the individual wishes to be cared for to the names of people who they wish to represent them.

Identifying wishes and preferences

An individual's wishes and preferences will be unique to them. It is essential to use a whole-person approach to assessment and explore the physical, psychological, social, spiritual, cultural and environmental wishes and preferences of each service user.

Recording and communicating

Once an individual has made their wishes and preferences known, a statement of their wishes will need to be made. This could be communicated in writing or through recorded conversations. The statement could contain both medical and non-medical information, for example:

- preferred place of care
- beliefs and values
- religious needs
- organ donation
- treatment options.

Health and social care workers cannot make a record of the discussion without the permission of the service user. Consent to share the advance care plan with anybody else, including the service user's family and health or social care professionals, must be obtained before any information can be shared.

Evidence activity

 3.3 Supporting and recording decisions about advance care planning

- Describe the role you play in supporting and recording advance care plans within your area of care.

- What sort of information must be recorded within an advance care plan?

3.4 Outline ethical and legal issues that may arise in relation to advance care planning

Ethical dilemmas arise when there is a perceived conflicting duty to the person who is nearing the end of life. For example, a conflict between a duty to preserve life and a duty to act in an individual's best interests, or when an ethical principle such as respect for autonomy conflicts with a duty not to harm.

Key term

Ethical dilemmas are dilemmas relating to the principles of right and wrong.

Ethical and legal issues can arise within end of life care surrounding the subject of advance decisions to refuse treatment. These decisions can include 'Do not attempt resuscitation' orders, refusal of mechanical ventilation and artificial feeding. Very often, these advance decisions do not come to light until a person has lost the capacity to make decisions. In such cases, health care professionals must start from the presumption that the individual had capacity when the decision was made.

Ethical issues may arise if health care professionals are not aware of an individual's advance decisions to refuse treatment. At present, there is no national registration system to help professionals establish whether an advance decision has been made, and the service user may not be well enough to inform the team that they have made an advance decision.

The relatives of the individual may not agree with the content of the advance decision and, when faced with a loved one's imminent death, may plead with health care professionals to ignore an advance decision.

Currently in the UK, it is recognised that where death is unavoidable, life-sustaining treatments such as, resuscitation, artificial ventilation, dialysis or artificial feeding may be withdrawn or withheld. In such cases the goal of care becomes the relief of symptoms. Basic care and comfort must be provided and can never be withheld.

Evidence activity

 3.4 Ethical and legal issues that may arise

Explain the types of ethical and legal issues that could arise in relation to advance care planning, and outline the steps that are taken within your organisation to minimise the risk of these ethical and legal issues from occurring.

LO4 Be able to provide support to individuals and key people during end of life care

 Support the individual and key people to explore their thoughts and feelings about death and dying

'Quality of life' is a term that is frequently used within care organisations, and it is something that carers strive to ensure when providing care for and supporting service users. 'Quality of death', however, is something that we rarely discuss, yet death is as inevitable a part of life as being born.

A good end of life experience is the ultimate aim of **palliative care**, and involves preserving dignity and autonomy. In order to enable service users to have a good end of life experience, it is essential to actively involve the person who is dying, and their family, in all decision making. This may include decisions about treatment options, end of life care and where the person wishes to die.

Key term

Palliative care aims to enhance the quality of life of service users who are faced with a life-limiting illness and their families. It focuses on increasing comfort through prevention and treatment of suffering.

Achieving a good end of life experience for most people will involve some or all of the following:

■ Maintaining control over what is happening.

■ Knowing when death is imminent and understanding what can be expected throughout the process of dying.

■ Ensuring that family and friends are around when this is the service user's wish – but be mindful that some service users may not want lots of visitors.

■ Having time to say goodbye to the people who are important to the service user.

■ Ensuring the individual can choose where they wish to die.

■ Being able to issue advance directives which ensure that their wishes are respected.

■ Ensuring that the individual can die peacefully and at ease with dignity and privacy.

■ Having control over pain relief and other symptom control, but not having to take unnecessary medication.

■ Being able to access expert information, advice and support as and when necessary.

■ Ensuring that the spiritual, cultural and religious preferences of the individual are recognised and respected.

■ Being able to die when it is 'time to go', without unnecessarily prolonging the individual's life.

■ Not being alone at the end, unless that is what the individual wants.

Time to reflect

 Individual experiences

Think about a time when you have supported a person who is nearing the end of their life.

● Would you consider the experience as a good outcome for the person and their family?

● Were there any aspects of the experience you think were not handled particularly well?

● What do you feel could have been done differently in order to change the outcome of the experience?

Evidence activity

4.1 Supporting people to explore their thoughts and feelings about death and dying

Explain the steps that are taken within your organisation to support individuals and their family and close friends to explore their feelings about death and dying.

4.2 Provide support for the individual and key people that respects their beliefs, religion and culture

Adopting a multi-faith approach to the delivery of end of life care is essential if health and social care workers are to fully support service users and their loved ones with their cultural and religious beliefs.

It is important to realise that, although individuals may share the same religion, within each faith there may be different schools of thought. For example, within Christianity there are different churches (e.g. Catholic, Church of England, Pentecostal and Anglican). It is therefore important to consult with the individual and their family on matters concerning their particular cultural and religious requirements.

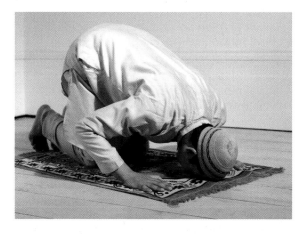

Figure 16.5 Respecting beliefs, religion and culture

People of different religions will have unique requirements relating to prayer, diet and routines of personal hygiene. It is essential that health and social care workers are aware of these in order that the individual can be fully supported.

An important part of a person's culture and religion may include sacred practices or rituals. These could relate to prayer, anointing with oils or personal care. It is important that provision is made in order that these practices can be carried out in private.

Some religions have dietary requirements, for example forbidding certain foods or preparing food in a specific way.

Different cultures and religious groups hold differing beliefs in relation to life and death, and these may be evident both before and after a person has died. The person's **religious rites** must be upheld following death, and every effort must be made to ensure that the body is handled in line with the person's cultural and religious beliefs.

Key term

Religious rites are the established practice of ceremony that must be performed following the death of a person.

Evidence activity

4.2 Respecting people's beliefs, religion and culture

Choose three service users who have different faiths. Explain the factors you would need to take into account when providing support for these people and their families in relation to their beliefs, religion and culture.

4.3 Demonstrate ways to help the individual feel respected and valued throughout the end of life period

It is very important that people who are nearing the end of their life feel respected and valued. Health and social care staff have a major role in ensuring that this happens. First and foremost, it is essential to realise that the person is a **multifaceted** being with unique experiences, qualities, values and needs.

Key term

Multifaceted means having many different qualities or features.

People who are nearing the end of their life have the same basic human rights as other people. In addition, throughout the end of life care period, these people also have a right to:

■ a high standard of care

■ make choices

- be given explanations in order that they can make informed choices
- be treated with dignity and afforded their privacy
- have their cultural and religious beliefs respected
- have their physical and psychological needs addressed in the course of their daily care
- be as independent as possible
- be safe and secure
- enjoy freedom of movement.

Considering the rights of individuals is one of the core concepts of delivering person-centred care.

Practice activity

4.3 Helping individuals feel respected and valued

Observe a colleague throughout the course of your shift. Make a note of all the actions the member of staff takes to help service users feel respected and valued.

What did they do well? Are there any aspects of care that could be improved?

Ask your colleague to observe you, throughout the course of your shift, while caring for a person who is nearing the end of their life. Your colleague can then provide you with feedback about the ways you help individuals to feel valued and respected.

Are there any aspects that you do particularly well? Are there any areas where improvements could be made?

4.4 Provide information to the individual and/or key people about the individual's illness and the support available

When providing individuals with information, it is important that it is presented in a format that is understandable to them. Not everyone can communicate in the same way, and it is important that you are able to communicate with the individual in a way which is suitable for them.

Confidentiality is also important when communicating with service users and the people who are important to them. Ensure that privacy is afforded and that the service user is happy for you to discuss information in the presence of their loved ones.

Evidence activity

4.4 Providing information about the illness and the support available

This activity enables you to demonstrate your knowledge of the factors that need to be taken into consideration when providing information about the individual's illness and the support available to the individual and their family and close friends.

Stanley has been diagnosed with motor neurone disease. He and his family are aware of the diagnosis, but need some more information about how the disease progresses and where they can receive further support. Stanley has a hearing impairment and his speech is slurred. You have been asked to support Stanley and give him the information he needs.

Explain how you would prepare to do this and the factors you would need to take into account when communicating the information to Stanley.

4.5 Give examples of how an individual's well-being can be enhanced

Environmental factors

The environment can have an enormous impact on a person's well-being as they approach the end of their life. An environment which is clinical and cold is likely to reinforce to the person that they are living with an illness, while an environment which is homely and warm is more likely to enhance the person's well-being. For some people it may be particularly important that they can get outside. A sensory garden can provide the senses with different colours, smells, sounds and textures.

Non-medical interventions

Non-medical interventions will depend on the individual and their abilities. For some people, just having someone there can have an enormous impact on their sense of well-being. Holding the person's hand, if this is acceptable to them, can be soothing. There are many ways in which symptoms can be relieved using non-medical interventions, for example, a person who is experiencing difficulty with breathing can be supported to reposition themselves – sitting upright can alleviate the distress that comes with being breathless.

Equipment and aids

The use of equipment and aids can help a person to maintain their independence, for example assistive technology can be used to remind a person that it is time to take their medication.

Alternative therapies

Alternative therapies are also referred to as unconventional therapies. These therapies are used instead of conventional treatments. There are many reasons why people choose alternative therapies, for example, some people fear the side effects of conventional treatments.

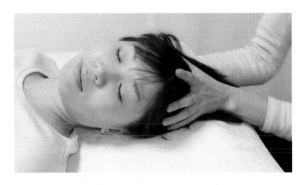

Figure 16.6 Alternative therapies

> ### Evidence activity
>
> **Give examples of how an individual's well-being can be enhanced**
>
> Think about your service users and in particular a person who is nearing the end of their life. Give examples of factors which have been accessed to enhance the life of the individual, taking into account:
>
> *contd.*

> ### Evidence activity
>
> ■ the environment
>
> ■ non-medical interventions
>
> ■ equipment and aids
>
> ■ alternative therapies.

(4.6) Contribute to partnership working with key people to support the individual's well-being

Partnership working is an essential aspect in supporting people who are nearing the end of their life. The partners that you work with may include:

■ the individuals you support, their carers, family and friends

■ your colleagues and other members of the immediate care team

■ members of the specialist palliative care team

■ hospital staff

■ the individual's GP

■ advocacy services.

The most important people in partnership working are the individuals you support and the people who are important to them. If these people feel they are actively participating in the partnership, this can have a dramatic effect on their overall health and well-being.

> ### Evidence activity
>
> (4.6) **Contribute to partnership working to support well-being**
>
> Explain how you contribute to partnership working within your care environment.
>
> Make a note of the other members of the team within the partnership and give a brief account of their role in supporting the person who is nearing the end of their life.

LO5 Understand how to address sensitive issues in relation to end of life care

 5.1 **Explain the importance of recording significant conversations during end of life care**

The wishes of people approaching the end of life are not always known by members of the wider healthcare team or the service users' families. This can lead to situations where service users are denied the care that is important to them or in the setting where they would want to receive it. This could lead to a situation where service users' wishes and advance decisions are not taken into consideration. Significant conversations could relate to the advance care planning process and may lead to a review of the advance care plan. It is therefore essential that any significant conversations are appropriately recorded, with the consent of the service user.

 Evidence activity

5.1 The importance of recording significant conversations

Explain why it is important to record significant conversations during end of life care.

 5.2 Explain factors that influence who should give significant news to an individual or key people

Your workplace will have policies and procedures which will indicate who should give significant news to the individual and/or their loved ones. In some instances, especially surrounding a diagnosis, the individual's doctor will be the one to break significant news to them. However, much more recently this process has involved a range of health care professionals such as clinical nurse specialists.

It is important to remember that significant news may not just relate to a diagnosis, it may also relate to issues such as changes in treatment or the place where treatment will take place. It may be that a physiotherapist tells a service user that they can't go home because the equipment they need has not yet been delivered to their home.

Evidence activity

5.2 Factors that influence who should give significant news

Identify the types of significant news that may need to be communicated with service users, and explain the factors that influence who gives significant news to service users, their family and close friends within your workplace.

 5.3 Describe conflicts and legal or ethical issues that may arise in relation to death, dying or end of life care

We discussed in section 3.4 some of the legal and ethical issues that can arise in relation to advance care planning. As a person nears the end of their life, there are often difficult decisions to be made. Some of the decisions surround aspects associated with treatments. Other conflicts that may arise relate directly to issues surrounding confidentiality. When a life-limiting diagnosis has been made, the service user may not want to tell other members of the family. Equally, family members may be aware of the diagnosis and wish the service user not to be told. This raises enormous issues in relation to planning and making advance decisions.

One of the most common issues concerns whether to stop or withhold potentially life-prolonging treatment. Decisions about medical treatments and the withdrawal of treatments can cause conflict between health professionals and the family of the person who is dying, especially if the expectations of the family are different from the expectations of the care team.

5.3 Conflicts and legal or ethical issues that may arise

This activity enables you to demonstrate your understanding of conflicts and legal issues that may arise in relation to death, dying and end of life care.

Susan, a 68-year-old lady, has been undergoing investigations to find out whether she has bowel cancer. The test results have come back and Susan has indicated to you that she does not want her husband to know if the results are positive. She would prefer to lie to him and tell him that everything is clear.

Explain the ethical issues and possible conflicts which could arise from this scenario.

Research & investigate

5.3 Ethical issues

Talk with your colleagues and use available media sources (e.g. newspapers, internet and textbooks) to research a case study relating to ethical issues in end of life care. Two examples are those of Dianne Pretty and Debbie Purdy.

Identify the ethical dilemmas presented by the case study and explain how the dilemmas have come about.

5.4 Analyse ways to address such conflicts

Advance care planning can go a long way to avoiding conflicts of interest, because it enhances a discussion of end of life issues between the service user, the family and the people who are providing care. Perhaps even more importantly, it provides reassurance that the service user's wishes will be upheld even when they have lost capacity to make decisions. Advance care planning can therefore prevent confusion and conflict when end of life decisions need to be made. It is easy to see how lack of advance care planning could lead to conflicting situations. Effective advance care planning, good education and clear channels of communication between the service user, care staff, family and the specialist palliative care team can help in avoiding such conflict.

5.4 Analyse ways to address such conflicts

From the ethical issues and conflicts that you identified in Evidence activity 5.3, explain the actions that could be taken in order to address the conflicts.

LO6 Understand the role of organisations and support services available to individuals and key people in relation to end of life care

6.1 Describe the role of support organisations and specialist services that may contribute to end of life care

It is important to realise that a person's care needs cannot be met by one individual alone. When an individual is diagnosed with a life-limiting condition it is essential that all steps are taken in order to meet their individual needs. Following a thorough assessment, an individual care package, which will call upon the skills and knowledge of a wide range of people, will be drawn up in partnership with the individual.

In addition to the support that can be provided by health and social care workers, there are a number of supportive organisations and specialist services that can make valuable contributions to supporting a person who is nearing the end of their life.

When a person is diagnosed with a life-limiting condition, their GP will usually inform their local social services department. Although social services do not provide specialist palliative care services, they may be able to fulfil a number of roles and offer a range of services which, when combined with palliative care services, can contribute significantly to an individual's total care package within their own home. They can provide and refer individuals to a range of services which may include one or more of the following:

■ Provision of a needs assessment – social services have a legal obligation to assess care needs and to provide any services that have been highlighted as necessary.

■ Provision of a carers' assessment – carers providing informal care are entitled to have their needs assessed.

■ Home care – this is the care provided within the person's home.

■ Support and advice through community support teams – community care teams assess the needs of the individual within their home and help the individual to sustain independent living skills.

■ Day centre services – these can provide social stimulation as well as involving the individual in a range of activities, such as hobbies and crafts.

■ Hospital social work teams – if an individual is admitted to hospital, their needs must be assessed before they return home in order that necessary services can be put in place prior to discharge.

■ Assistance and advice regarding benefits – many people who are diagnosed with a life-limiting condition may not realise that they may be entitled to benefits.

■ Provision of specialist equipment – this may be needed in order to ensure that the person remains as independent as possible.

■ Provision of housing adaptations – adaptations to the home include items such as grab rails, wheelchair ramps or specially designed showers.

■ Care home facilities – if a person's condition deteriorates, it may become necessary to consider the need to move into a residential care home.

Hospice care

Dame Cicely Saunders was the founder of the hospice movement. She used the term to refer to a place providing specialist care for dying people, building St Christopher's Hospice in London, the world's first purpose-built hospice. A hospice provides person-centred medical, nursing and emotional care free of charge for individuals who are being treated for a life-limiting condition and their families. It is important to point out that hospices are not places where people go to die. The average length of stay in a hospice is one to two weeks, after which many people return to their own homes.

Hospices can provide respite care, and can also provide palliative care to help alleviate pain and other distressing symptoms that can be experienced by people as they near the end of their life.

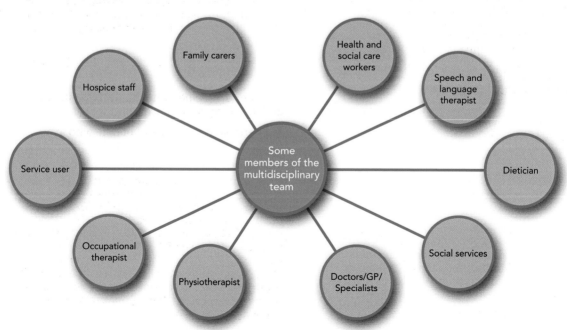

Figure 16.7 Members of the multidisciplinary palliative care team

Volunteers and voluntary groups

Volunteers and voluntary organisations play a very important role in supporting people who are nearing the end of their life. Voluntary organisations are formally structured, non-profit making, independent organisations.

Grant making charities

The Association of Charity Officers is a national umbrella body for benevolent charities. These are charities that provide aid and advice to needy individuals. The association links individuals who are in need with national and local grant making charities that may be able to help them. Grant making charities are charities that can give financial assistance in certain circumstances.

Organisations that can help with aids equipment and adaptations

Aids, equipment and adaptations may be essential in ensuring that an individual can remain as independent as possible for as long as possible. Social services may be able to help with these if they are identified through the assessment process.

National organisations for specific health conditions

There are some organisations that provide information relating to specific conditions, for example, The Alzheimer's Society is a charity that works to improve the quality of life of people living with dementia. National organisations for specific health conditions can provide information about the individual's condition, support for the person and their family and may also be able to give guidance on specific issues.

 Evidence activity

 6.1 The role of support organisations and specialist services

Annie is a 56-year-old lady in the end stages of motor neurone disease. She has a **tracheostomy tube** in situ as she cannot easily clear secretions from her chest. She is married and her main carer is her 60-year-old husband. Annie lives in her own home

contd.

 Evidence activity

and, in her advance care plan, she expressed a wish to die at home. She does not wish to be admitted to hospital.

Which support organisations and specialist services do you think would be required to ensure that Annie can continue to be cared for at home?

 Key term

A tracheostomy tube is a tube which is inserted into a surgically created opening in the wind pipe (trachea) to keep it open.

6.2 Analyse the role and value of an advocate in relation to end of life care

The word advocacy is derived from the Latin *advocare* which means 'to call to one's aid'. It relates to standing up for an individual or group who are unable to do this themselves. An advocate therefore helps service users to express their needs and wishes.

If a person needs support with making choices about their care or expressing their views, they should be able to use a free advocacy service. Advocates:

■ are independent of health and social care services

■ support the person with decision making and speaking for themselves

■ represent the views of people who are unable to represent their own views.

The Mental Capacity Act also set up the Independent Mental Capacity Advocate (IMCA) service. This service helps vulnerable people who cannot make some (or all) important decisions about their lives. The IMCA service means that certain people who lack capacity will be helped to make difficult decisions, for example in relation to medical treatment choices, or where they live and choose to die. It is aimed at people who do not have relatives or friends to speak for them. A lack of mental capacity could be due to:

- a stroke or brain injury
- a mental health problem
- a dementia-related condition
- a learning disability
- unconsciousness.

 Evidence activity

 6.2 The role and value of an advocate

Explain the role of the advocate in end of life care.

6.3 Explain how to establish when an advocate may be beneficial

Advocacy services are crucial when people are more vulnerable because, for example, they have learning difficulties or are being treated under a section of the Mental Health Act. Advocacy services may need to be called upon when a person has been assessed as lacking capacity. Health and social care workers must always assume that a person has capacity to make decisions unless an assessment has proven that it is lacking.

According to the Mental Capacity Act, there are two questions that need to be answered in order to assess capacity.

1. Is there an impairment of or disturbance in the functioning of a person's mind or brain?

If so:

2. Is the impairment or disturbance sufficient that the person lacks the capacity to make a particular decision?

 Evidence activity

6.3 Establishing when an advocate may be beneficial

- Explain the circumstances under which a person nearing the end of their life might require advocacy services.
- What is the procedure you would follow if a service user required the support of an advocate?

 6.4 Explain why support for spiritual needs may be especially important at the end of life

The meaning of the term 'spirituality' is often misunderstood, with many people believing that spirituality and religion are the same thing. However, this is not necessarily true. All over the world, the term spirituality has different meanings, and it means different things to different people. It is something that we can feel, but it is very difficult to describe. In its broadest sense, however, spirituality is what gives meaning, value and purpose to our lives. It is about what makes our thoughts and beliefs unique to us.

A person's spiritual needs in relation to their feelings and culture may not always be obviously apparent and may be overlooked due to poor communication or the intensity of a person's care requirements. In addition, it could be easy to shy away from discussing the service user's fears, due to concerns about upsetting them further or not being able to deal with the consequences of what they may say.

 Evidence activity

6.4 The importance of support for spiritual needs

Explain why is it important to ensure that a person's spiritual needs are addressed as the person is nearing the end of their life.

6.5 Describe a range of sources of support to address spiritual needs

However much support you give, there may be times when service users do not wish to discuss their concerns with you. It is at these times when additional support can be offered. Some specialist nurses within the palliative care team are able to offer support, but consideration should also be given to contacting a chaplain, minister, priest or any requested spiritual representative in order that the individual can address their concerns.

Evidence activity

(6.5) Sources of support to address spiritual needs

■ Explain how you ensure that you are meeting the spiritual needs of service users within your care organisation.

■ Make a note of the sources of support that are available to support spiritual needs, and describe each one.

LO7 Be able to access support for the individual or key people from the wider team

(7.1) Identify when support would best be offered by other members of the team

It is essential that you recognise your boundaries in relation to the provision of end of life care, so that you know when other members of the team may need to be called upon.

Many healthcare professionals can be involved in providing end of life care, and the type of support will depend on the needs of the service user. Hospital doctors and nurses, GPs, community nurses and counsellors, social services, religious ministers, complementary therapists or physiotherapists are only a few of the professionals who may be called upon for support. Most hospitals have specialist palliative care teams that coordinate these services. Working beside general staff, they deliver end of life care to service users and their families in many care environments including hospitals, care homes, hospices and within the person's own home.

Evidence activity

(7.1) When support would best be offered by other members of the team

Think about your service users.

■ While maintaining confidentiality, identify any service users who are accessing support outside of the immediate care team. *contd.*

Evidence activity

■ Under what circumstances are these individuals receiving specialist support?

■ What factors triggered the referral?

(7.2) Liaise with other members of the team to provide identified support for the individual or key people

It is important that you are aware of the services that are available to your service users and that you know when these services should be accessed. The appropriate professional will assess the service user's needs and ensure that appropriate care is put in place. The team will take a holistic approach to care, which means they will take into account all aspects of the service user's well-being, including their:

■ physical symptoms – for example pain, nausea, vomiting, difficulties with eating and drinking, constipation and breathlessness

■ psychological symptoms – for example anxiety or fear

■ spiritual issues – for example examining feelings and considering questions such as, 'Why is this happening to me?' 'What will happen after I die?'

■ social issues – for example looking at the best place to support the person, whether this be at home or in a care home, and also considering practical issues such as deciding where the person wishes to die.

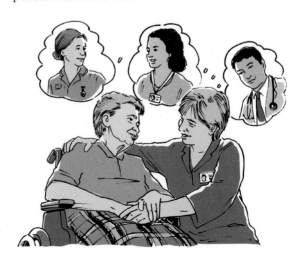

Figure 16.8 You are not alone!

7.2 Providing identified support for individual

Explain the processes that are in place within your workplace that allow timely communication with other members of the team and to ensure a person centred approach is used to caring for people who are nearing the end of their life.

LO8 Be able to support individuals through the process of dying

8.1 Carry out own role in an individual's care

When supporting individuals who are nearing the end of their life, it is essential that you work within your sphere of competence and provide care in accordance with your workplace policies and procedures. Within your role, you will be responsible for providing supportive care in order to support the individual and their family to live with their condition and the treatment of it, and to enter the dying phase with dignity. In providing end of life care you must remember that you are part of a wider team and any care provided must be in accordance with the plan of care which has been agreed through partnership decisions.

 Practice activity

8.1 Your role in an individual's care

Maintaining confidentiality, make some notes about the individual to create a case study. Within the case study, explain the aspects of care that you have been involved with.

Explain the boundaries of your role when providing care for people who are nearing the end of their life.

8.2 Contribute to addressing any distress experienced by the individual promptly and in agreed ways

One of the aims of palliative care is to prevent or relieve any distress a person may be experiencing. The manifestation of distress and its causes will vary from person to person. Distress can be physical or emotional, and can be related directly to the psychological aspects of living with a life-limiting condition or to the physical symptoms that can occur as a person is nearing the end of their life.

When a person has numerous symptoms, it is important to work with them to establish which symptom needs to be addressed first. Distressing symptoms may include:

- pain
- weakness
- fatigue
- skin irritations, e.g. itching
- pressure ulcers
- anorexia (loss of appetite)
- mouth problems (ulcers and sores).

When caring for service users who are experiencing distressing symptoms, it is important first to determine the cause of the symptom. If a person is experiencing pain, it is likely that they will be prescribed medication and, in some instances, very strong analgesics. A side effect of these types of medication is constipation. This could lead to further distress as the person struggles to defecate.

If the cause of the symptom is known, steps can be taken to alleviate the distress. Often it is not knowing what the problem is that can cause more distress than the symptom itself. Not all symptoms can be alleviated with medication. Some symptoms can be relieved by simple measures such as supporting a person with their oral hygiene, which can go a long way to prevent and alleviate a sore mouth.

Evidence activity

8.2 **Addressing distress promptly and in agreed ways**

Think about a service user who is receiving end of life care. Identify any distressing symptoms you have observed them experiencing. Explain how you have supported the person to alleviate their symptoms and any associated distress.

- What were the symptoms?
- What measures did you take?
- How effective were the measures?
- Did you need to involve any other services, for example physiotherapist, doctor, palliative care nurse?

8.3 Adapt support to reflect the individual's changing needs or responses

In order to fully support a person with distressing symptoms, it is crucial that they are observed for changes in their needs. Some symptoms may improve, but others may appear. It is essential that health and social care workers fully observe individuals in order that appropriate support can be offered, thus minimising the extent of any distress caused.

How do we know if a person's needs change?

Observations can be invasive or non-invasive in approach. Invasive monitoring is likely to take place in a hospital environment, whereas non-invasive monitoring is more likely to take place in a care home environment. It is here that health and social care workers play a crucial role in being vigilant in order to identify changes and act upon them at the earliest opportunity.

The person-centred nature of palliative care demands a multidisciplinary team approach and often involves the coordination of input from different health and social care workers with differing levels of skill and knowledge. It is important that care workers have core skills in providing care to people who are nearing the end of their life in order that they can provide ongoing support and reassurance. However, it is important that care workers only work within their level of experience and expertise.

Evidence activity

8.3 **Adapt support to reflect changing needs**

This activity enables you to demonstrate how you would adapt support to reflect an individual's changing needs or responses.

Harold is a 76-year-old gentleman who has received a diagnosis of bowel cancer two months ago. The doctor told Harold that the cancer was inoperable, and that care would focus on making his quality of life as good as it could be. Up until now, Harold has been relatively pain free and has been able to eat small amounts of food. You have noticed that his pain has got much worse and he is only prescribed paracetamol. He has also lost his appetite and cannot keep any food down as he feels sick a lot of the time. He is now starting to become distressed with his symptoms and keeps expressing that he 'just wants to die.'

Explain the steps you would now take.

8.4 Assess when an individual and key people need to be alone

Although death and dying are universal, every person's experience of death will be unique. There are no hard and fast rules here and it is important to assess each situation as it arises. Some families will want to spend time alone with their loved one, but there will be other families who clearly do not want to spend time alone. It is important that care staff remain non-judgmental. Every person copes with their emotions in different ways, which will also be influenced by their cultural beliefs.

Evidence activity

8.4 **Assess when people need to be alone**

Explain the circumstances under which service users and their family may wish to be left alone.

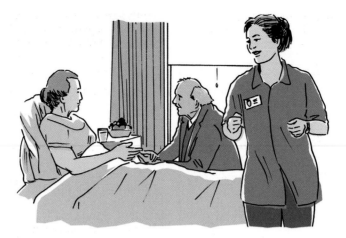

Figure 16.9 Give me some space

LO9 Take action following the death of individuals

 9.1 Explain why it is important to know about an individual's wishes for their after death care

It is important to recognise that end of life care does not stop at the point of death. The period following the death of a service user can be a very emotional time for all concerned, including the individual's family and friends, other service users and other members of the care team.

It is essential to be aware of the person's wishes following their death in order that they can be upheld. Some people may determine all aspects of their care following their death, including the specifics of their funeral. Some may express a wish to donate their organs following death, and it is important that care staff are aware of this in order that the wish can be fulfilled.

Evidence activity

9.1 The importance of an individual's wishes for their after death care

Think about your service users and identify any particular after death wishes that have been requested by them.

Explain why it is important to ensure that these wishes are respected following the person's death.

9.2 Carry out actions immediately following a death that respect the individual's wishes and follow agreed ways of working

Your place of work will have its own policies and procedures in relation to what to do when a service user dies, and it is important that you follow these guidelines. The first thing to remember is that there should be no rush to move the body. Relatives and friends should be given as much time as they need to say goodbye to their loved one. First and foremost, relatives will require your support immediately following the death. It is important that their wishes are taken into consideration when tending to the deceased person.

■ The death will need to be verified – you must follow your workplace guidelines which will give you guidance on who needs to be contacted. Usually this will be the deceased's GP. However, where the death was expected and there are 'do not resuscitate' orders in place, some senior nurses can verify the death.

■ The time of death and the individuals present should be documented in the service user's care notes.

■ If the next of kin is not present then contact will need to be made.

■ Support will need to be given to any family and friends who are present.

■ **Last offices** should be performed according to the individual's personal beliefs, religious beliefs and following any special requirements.

■ Arrangements will need to be made for the deceased to be transported to the mortuary or to the agreed place of rest.

> ## Key term
>
> The term last offices refers to the care given to a body after death. It is a process that demonstrates respect for the deceased and is focused on respecting their religious and cultural beliefs, as well as health and safety and legal requirements (Dougherty and Lister, 2004).

Providing practical information

When a person dies, the family will have many decisions and arrangements to make. Some of the decisions may have been made before the service user dies, but the bereaved family will need information before they leave on what will happen next. There is little point in trying to provide information when the family is still saying goodbye to the individual. It is better to wait until the family asks what they should do next, or you could ask at an appropriate time if they have any questions.

Because the family may be distressed, they may have difficulty in retaining verbal information, so it may be useful to give them written information on how and where to register the death.

Most registrar offices have an appointment system, so you will need to advise the family to telephone the office in advance. If the death was expected, the person's GP will be able to issue a death certificate fairly quickly. The certificate will state the cause of death and will be needed before the death can be registered.

If the person dies in their own home, or in a care home, their death must be registered within five days in the district where the home is located. Following the registration, the registrar will issue a certificate to authorise burial or cremation.

Presenting the deceased person's belongings

It is not just the deceased person who needs to be treated with respect; thought also needs to be given to the way in which the deceased person's belongings are presented to their loved ones.

Last offices

Following death, the body must be prepared for transfer to the mortuary or funeral directors in a way that does not compromise health and safety.

Health and social care workers must work in line with their organisation's policies, which should have been developed to ensure that the body is treated with dignity and respect while ensuring that health and safety are not compromised.

Last offices should always take into account:

■ compliance with policies, procedures and legal requirements

■ dignity and privacy of the deceased person and their family

■ respect for the deceased person's religious and cultural beliefs

■ protection of health and social care workers. Standard precautions must be applied as any infectious risk present before death will also be present after death.

Family members may wish to help with the last offices procedure – this may support religious or cultural beliefs. Clear communication is vital in order to minimise unnecessary distress and to provide support and reassurance. The procedure should not expose the family to any risk, and guidance and advice should be offered to reduce any known risks.

> ## Evidence activity
>
> ### 9.2 Carrying out actions immediately following a death
>
> Following the death of a service user, certain procedures need to be undertaken. You can think about a specific service user for whom you have provided after death care, or you can discuss the procedure with your manager/supervisor. Make a note of the procedure for:
>
> ■ reporting the death
>
> ■ explaining the process of registering the death
>
> ■ carrying out last offices
>
> ■ ensuring that the person's cultural and religious needs are taken into consideration
>
> ■ arranging for the deceased to be transported to the mortuary/undertakers
>
> ■ ensuring that health and safety issues are addressed
>
> ■ presenting the deceased's belongings to relatives.

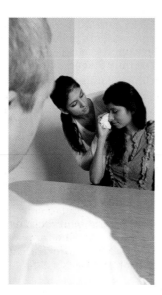

Figure 16.10 Providing comfort

 Describe ways to support key people immediately following an individual's death

The period immediately after the death of a service user can be a highly emotional time for family and friends, other service users and care staff. It is not surprising that health and social care workers sometimes feel unsure how to react or what to say to the family.

Supporting the family's wishes

Some families may choose to be with their loved one as they approach death. However, not everyone will choose to be present as the person dies. Some people may find the situation too painful and may have previously expressed that they would prefer to be contacted when the person dies. It is vital to establish the family's wishes before death occurs.

For some people, the act of visiting the deceased may be too painful, and they may wish to remember the person as they were. For this reason, some families may choose not to spend time with the body. It is essential that health and social care workers remain non-judgmental and respect the wishes of the family.

Ensure that the family has access to a quiet area if possible, perhaps somewhere where they can access facilities to make a drink.

Other people who may be affected

In addition to caring for the deceased and their family and friends, it is also important to remember others who may be affected by the death. These people could include other members of staff or other service users. There is no right or wrong way to tell other service users, but what is important is that the death is not 'hushed up'. Some service users may want to pay their respects or may want to attend the funeral, and they should not be denied this right.

Evidence activity

 9.3 Supporting key people immediately following an individual's death

Describe the ways in which you can support the family and close friends of an individual immediately following their death.

What factors would you need to take into consideration?

LO10 Managing your own feelings in relation to the dying or death of individuals

 Identify ways to manage your own feelings in relation to an individual's dying or death

Evidence activity

 10.1 Managing your own feelings

Identify the actions you take in order to ensure that you are able to manage your own feelings when caring for a person who is dying.

It's not just family and friends who experience feelings associated with loss and grief. End of life care is an area of health care that places unique demands on health and social care workers who, very often, have not received any formal training in this field. Therefore, there may be times when health and social care workers also experience the feelings associated with loss and grief, and this can happen either before or after a person has died.

Unfortunately, however, within an organisation which provides care for many people, there often isn't time to grieve, as there are other service users who need to be cared for. Some health and social care workers may attempt to conceal their personal grief in an effort to uphold a professional appearance and remain strong for the deceased, the person's family and others in their care.

10.2 Utilise support systems to deal with own feelings in relation to an individual's dying or death

Feelings associated with grief among health and social care workers can be common following the death of a service user, and it is important that the care organisation is one which encourages the expression of grief in order to ensure that staff are able to come to terms with loss within their workplace.

Health and social care workers who deal with death on a regular basis, and are not given the opportunity to express their feelings, may also be more at risk of developing **cumulative grief**.

Key term

Cumulative grief is when a person experiences several losses or several deaths close together, making it difficult for them to recover from one loss because another loss occurs.

Depending on where you work, there may be a dedicated person who is responsible for particular areas relating to bereavement. If this is the case, it may be helpful to make an appointment to discuss your feelings with this person. It is only by adopting these practices that we will change the 'stiff upper lip' culture that exists within some care environments.

Evidence activity

 10.2 Support systems to deal with your feelings

Explain the systems that are in place within your organisation to help you and your colleagues deal with your feelings when caring for people who are dying.

Assessment summary

Your reading of this chapter and completion of the activities will have prepared you to be able to engage in personal development in health, social care or children's and young people's settings.

To achieve the unit, your assessor will require you to:

Learning outcomes	Assessment Criteria
Learning outcome **1**: Understand the requirements of legislation and agreed ways of working to protect the rights of individuals at the end of life by:	**1.1** outlining the legal requirements and agreed ways of working designed to protect the rights of individuals in end of life care See Evidence activity 1.1, p. 325
	1.2 explaining how legislation designed to protect the rights of individuals in end of life care applies to own job role See Evidence activity 1.2, p. 327

Learning outcomes	Assessment Criteria
Learning outcome **2**: Understand factors affecting end of life care by:	(2.1) outlining key points of theories about the emotional and psychological processes that individuals and key people may experience with the approach of death See Evidence activity 2.1, p. 328
	(2.2) explaining how the beliefs, religion and culture of individuals and key people influence end of life care See Evidence activity 2.2, p. 329
	(2.3) explaining why key people may have a distinctive role in an individual's end of life care See Evidence activity 2.3, p. 330
	(2.4) explaining why support for an individual's health and well-being may not always relate to their terminal condition See Evidence activity 2.4, p. 331
Learning outcome **3**: Understand advance care planning in relation to end of life care by:	(3.1) describing the benefits to an individual of having as much control as possible over their end of life care See Evidence activity 3.1, p. 331
	(3.2) explaining the purpose of advance care planning in relation to end of life care See Evidence activity 3.2, p. 332
	(3.3) describing your own role in supporting and recording decisions about advance care planning See Evidence activity 3.3, p. 333
	(3.4) outlining ethical and legal issues that may arise in relation to advance care planning See Evidence activity 3.4, p. 333

Learning outcomes	Assessment Criteria
Learning outcome 4: Be able to provide support to individuals and key people during end of life care by:	(4.1) supporting the individual and key people to explore their thoughts and feelings about death and dying See Evidence activity 4.1, p. 334
	(4.2) providing support for the individual and key people that respects their beliefs, religion and culture See Evidence activity 4.2, p. 335
	(4.3) demonstrating ways to help the individual feel respected and valued throughout the end of life period See Practice activity 4.3, p. 336
	(4.4) providing information to the individual and/or key people about the individual's illness and the support available See Evidence activity 4.4, p. 336
	(4.5) Giving examples of how an individual's well-being can be enhanced by: • environmental factors • non-medical interventions • use of equipment and aids • alternative therapies. See Evidence activity 4.5, p. 337
	(4.6) contributing to partnership working with key people to support the individual's well-being See Evidence activity 4.6, p. 337
Learning outcome 5: Understand how to address sensitive issues in relation to end of life care by:	(5.1) explaining the importance of recording significant conversations during end of life care See Evidence activity 5.1, p. 338

Learning outcomes	Assessment Criteria
Learning outcome 5: Understand how to address sensitive issues in relation to end of life care by:	(5.2) explaining factors that influence who should give significant news to an individual or key people See Evidence activity 5.2, p. 338
	(5.3) describing conflicts and legal or ethical issues that may arise in relation to death, dying or end of life care See Evidence activity 5.3, p. 339
	(5.4) analysing ways to address such conflicts See Evidence activity 5.4, p. 339
Learning outcome 6: Understand the role of organisations and support services available to individuals and key people in relation to end of life care by:	(6.1) describing the role of support organisations and specialist services that may contribute to end of life care See Evidence activity 6.1, p. 341
	(6.2) analysing the role and value of an advocate in relation to end of life care See Evidence activity 6.2, p. 342
	(6.3) explaining how to establish when an advocate may be beneficial See Evidence activity 6.3, p. 342
	(6.4) explaining why support for spiritual needs may be especially important at the end of life See Evidence activity 6.4, p. 342
	(6.5) describing a range of sources of support to address spiritual needs See Evidence activity 6.5, p. 343

Learning outcomes	Assessment Criteria
Learning outcome 7: Be able to access support for the individual or key people from the wider team by:	7.1 identifying when support would best be offered by other members of the team See Evidence activity 7.1, p. 343
	7.2 liaising with other members of the team to provide identified support for the individual or key people See Evidence activity 7.2, p. 344
Learning outcome 8: Be able to support individuals through the process of dying by:	8.1 carrying out your own role in an individual's care See Practice activity 8.1, p. 344
	8.2 contributing to addressing any distress experienced by the individual promptly and in agreed ways See Evidence activity 8.2, p. 345
	8.3 adapting support to reflect the individual's changing needs or responses See Evidence activity 8.3, p. 345
	8.4 assessing when an individual and key people need to be alone See Evidence activity 8.4, p. 345
Learning outcome 9: Be able to take action following the death of individuals by:	9.1 explaining why it is important to know about an individual's wishes for their after-death care See Evidence activity 9.1, p. 346
	9.2 carrying out actions immediately following a death that respect the individual's wishes and follow agreed ways of working See Evidence activity 9.2, p. 347

Learning outcomes	Assessment Criteria
Learning outcome **9**: Be able to take action following the death of individuals by:	**9.3** describing ways to support key people immediately following an individual's death See Evidence activity 9.3, p. 348
Learning outcome **10**: Be able to manage own feelings in relation to the dying or death of individuals by:	**10.1** identifying ways to manage own feelings in relation to an individual's dying or death See Evidence activity 10.1, p. 348
	10.2 utilising support systems to deal with own feelings in relation to an individual's dying or death See Evidence activity 10.2, p. 349

Good luck!

Web links

Alzheimer's Society	www.alzheimers.org.uk
Care Quality Commission (CQC)	www.cqc.org.uk
Cruse Bereavement Care	www.crusebereavementcare.org.uk
Department of Health	www.dh.gov.uk
Huntington's Disease Association	www.hda.org.uk
Macmillan Cancer Support	www.macmillan.org.uk
Marie Curie Cancer Care	www.mariecurie.org.uk
Multiple Sclerosis Society	www.mssociety.org.uk
National Council for Palliative Care	www.ncpc.org.uk
National End of Life Care Programme	www.endoflifecareforadults.nhs.uk
Parkinson's Disease Society	www.parkinsons.org.uk
The Motor Neurone Disease Association	www.mndassociation.org
Princess Royal Trust for Carers	www.carers.org

GLOSSARY

Accentuated Emphasised.

Access To see, obtain or retrieve.

Accessing Finding and using.

Acronyms Words formed from the initial letters of several words, e.g. NHS.

Active listening Listening for the meaning behind what a person is saying.

Active participation When a person takes an active rather than a passive role in their own care and support.

Advisory, Conciliation and Arbitration Service (ACAS) Provides confidential and impartial advice to assist workers in resolving issues in the workplace.

Accountable Having to answer to someone for your actions.

Ad hoc As and when required.

Advance care planning A process of discussion between the health care team, the service user and their family. It enables the person to make plans for their future.

Advocate Someone who speaks up on behalf of an individual so that their views are heard, their rights promoted and any problems they have can be solved.

Allied health professionals Clinical healthcare professionals as distinct from medicine, dentistry and nursing, who work in a healthcare team to make the healthcare system function.

Alzheimer's disease A progressive disease that affects the brain and causes dementia.

Ambient In the surrounding environment.

Ancillary workers Staff who do not provide hands-on care in health and social care settings.

Anecdotal Based on personal recounts rather than on facts or research.

Anticipatory grief The sense of loss and grief that occurs before a person dies, as the loss is anticipated.

Apathy Lack of motivation or 'get up and go'.

Archiving Storing records, documents, or other materials of historical interest.

Articulation The formation of clear and distinct words when communication through speech.

Aseptic Free of disease-causing micro-organisms.

Autonomous Self-governing or independent.

Autonomy Being independent and self-reliant.

Back up To copy saved information so that it is preserved in the event of equipment failure.

Barrier hand cream A cream that helps reduce the effects of skin contact with harmful substances.

Body fluids These include blood, plasma and cerebrospinal fluid.

Body language Conscious and unconscious communication through movements or attitudes of the body.

Braille A system of writing and printing for blind or visually impaired people. Varied arrangements of raised dots representing letters and numerals are identified by touch.

Breach To break or override a rule or agreement.

Bronchi The large airways that carry air from the trachea into the lungs.

Carcinogenic Capable of causing cancer.

Care episode One of a series of care tasks in the course of a continuous care activity.

Care pathways Ways to systematically plan and follow up a specific programme of care.

Care plan Also known as a support plan, individual plan or care delivery plan, it is the document in which day-to-day requirements and preferences for care and support are detailed.

Carer Someone who, without payment, provides help and support to a partner, child, relative, friend or neighbour, who could not manage without their help.

Carers' assessment An assessment of carers' needs.

Catheter A plastic tube inserted into the body to drain fluid.

CCTV Closed circuit television.

Chronologically In order of time or occurrence.

Clinical waste Any material that has the potential to put health at risk, e.g. soiled dressings, incontinence pads and colostomy bags.

Closed questions Questions that result in set answers, e.g. yes/no, true/false.

Coaching A method of directing, instructing and training a person or group of people, to help them achieve some goal or develop specific skills.

Cognitive impairment Difficulty in carrying out intellectual functions, such as learning, thinking and remembering.

Comatose Unable to exhibit any voluntary movement or behaviour and unable to understand what is happening.

Communication cycle This involves having an idea, expressing it such that others can understand, and receiving and understanding others' responses.

Compassion Sympathy and concern for another person's suffering, and the wish to relieve it.

Compensate To give something, such as money, as payment or reparation for a service or loss.

Competence The ability to do something successful due to having the right knowledge, understanding and capabilities.

Competent An individual is deemed competent when they have a clear appreciation and understanding of the facts, and the implications and consequences of an action.

Complementary and alternative medicine (CAM) The term for health care products and practices that are not part of standard, scientific care.

Confidential Refers to private information intended to be kept secret.

Criminal Records Bureau (CRB) Holds information about individuals, such as convictions, cautions, reprimands and warnings.

Critique A critical discussion of a specified topic.

Cross-infection The spread of pathogens, harmful bacteria, viruses, fungi or parasites from one person, object, place or part of the body to another.

Cultural Related to the customs, ideas and social behaviour of particular people or groups.

Culture The customs, ideas and social behaviour of particular people or groups. It is about their way of life.

Cumulative grief A type of grief that occurs when a person experiences several losses or several deaths close together, making it difficult for them to recover from one loss because another loss occurs.

Deceased Dead. The term can also be used to mean the person who has died.

Delict A concept of civil law in which a wilful wrong or an act of negligence gives rise to a legal obligation between parties, even though there has been no contract between the parties.

Dependability The quality of being reliable and trustworthy.

Direct payments Local council payments to people who have been assessed as needing help from social services, and who would like to arrange and pay for their own care and support services instead of receiving them directly from the local council.

Discrimination The unfair treatment of a person, usually because of prejudice about race, ethnicity, age, religion or gender.

Distance learning Study that allows you to learn in your own time while being supported by a tutor by telephone, email etc.

Diversity Variety, particularly in relation to people. You must understand that each individual is unique.

Domiciliary carers Sometimes referred to as 'home carers', these are carers who provide support in an individual's own home.

Duty of care Acting in the very best interests of the people you work with.

E-learning The use of technology to enable people to learn at their convenience. Usually learning that takes place electronically, over the internet.

Empathy The ability to identify with and understand another person's difficulties or feelings.

Empowering Allowing people to have control over their own lives.

Empty-nest syndrome The array of feelings experienced by some parents after their children have grown and left home.

End of life care Usually refers to the care of a person during the last part of their life, from the point at which it has become clear that the person is in a progressive state of decline.

Episode of care One of a series of care tasks in the course of a continuous care activity.

Equity The quality of being fair and impartial.

European Economic Area (EEA) An economic association of European countries.

Ethical Principled, moral.

Ethical dilemmas Dilemmas relating to the principles of right and wrong.

Evidence-based policies Policies that have been proved to work.

Exudate Fluid that seeps out of injured tissues.

Fitting Any item that is free standing or hung by a nail or hook.

Fixture Any item that is bolted to the floor or walls.

Fractured Broken.

Gene The basic biological unit of inheritance.

Ginkgo biloba A herb used for its medicinal properties.

Green Paper A consultation document issued by the government, which contains policy proposals for debate and discussion before a final decision is taken on the best policy option.

Grief The sadness a person feels, usually as a result of loss.

Haemoglobin The protein in red blood cells that carries the oxygen needed by the body to create energy.

Health and Safety Executive (HSE) The national independent watchdog for work-related health, safety and illness, working to reduce workplace death and serious injury.

Health Protection Unit (HPU) A local centre of the Health Protection Agency (HPA).

Hearing loop Provides information on an induction loop system, to assist the hearing impaired by transmitting sound from a sound system, microphone, television or other source, directly to a hearing aid.

Holistic Acknowledging the 'whole'.

Holistic approach An approach that meets all aspects of an individual's care needs, including physical, intellectual, emotional, social and spiritual.

HRT An acronym for hormone replacement therapy.

Inaccessible Difficult or impossible to reach or understand.

Inaccuracies Things that are not accurate, containing mistakes/errors.

Incidence Occurrence.

Indwelling device A device that is inserted into the body, such as a catheter.

Infinite Never ending, without a limit.

Ingestion Taking something into the body through eating or drinking.

Integrity The quality of being morally upright, credible, trusting. Integrity of data is to do with its accuracy and completeness.

Inter-agency working When two or more agencies or organisations that have a shared interest in supporting people who have care needs work together.

Interdependence Dependence between two or more people.

Interpersonal skills The positive people skills that nurture effective communication and relationships.

Interventions Measures whose purpose is to improve health or alter the course of disease.

Introspection Examining you own thoughts and feelings.

Isolation The physical separation of an infected patient from others.

Jargon The specialist or technical language of a trade or profession.

Lasting Power of Attorney The responsibility an individual gives to someone they trust to make financial and health decisions on their behalf at a time in the future when they lack the mental capacity to make decisions or no longer wish to make those decisions themselves.

Last offices The care given to a body after death.

Learning style The way a person takes in, understands, expresses and remembers information, in other words, the way they learn best.

Legible Clear, readable, understandable.

Liability The state of being legally obliged and responsible.

Ligament A band of tissue that connects bones, typically to support a joint.

List 99 A list of teachers who are considered unsuitable or banned from working with children in school.

Logistics The full management of a task or procedure, from beginning to end.

Makaton A system that uses signs and symbols to enable people with communication and learning difficulties to communicate.

Maladministration Incompetent management.

Manual Done with the hands or controlled by hand, using human effort, skill, power, energy.

Media The means of communication, such as radio and television, newspapers and magazines, that reach or influence people widely.

Mediator An intermediary third party, who is neutral and helps negotiate agreed outcomes.

Medical model of disability Views disability as a 'problem' that belongs to the disabled individual.

Mentoring A developmental relationship in which a more experienced person helps someone who has less experience.

Micro-organisms Organisms such as bacteria, parasites and fungi that can only be seen with the use of a microscope.

Mucous membranes Mucous-secreting membranes lining the body cavities and canals that connect with the external air, such as the alimentary canal and respiratory tract.

Multidisciplinary teamwork When members of different professions work together.

Multifaceted Having many different qualities or features.

Musculoskeletal system The system of muscles and tendons, bones, joints and ligaments that move the body and maintain its form.

Muscle tone The tension or resistance to movement in a muscle that enables us to keep our bodies in a certain position.

Needle stick injury A skin puncture by a hypodermic needle or other sharp object.

Neurological disease A disease of the nervous system.

Neurotransmitters Chemicals that are involved with the transmission of messages between nerve cells.

Non-verbal communication (NVC) Body language.

Obligation Having to do something because of a legal or moral duty.

Open questions Questions that can, in theory, result in any answer and can be better for getting people's opinions than closed questions.

Optimum The best or most favourable point, degree or amount – the ideal.

Ostracised Excluded or ignored.

Outcome-based performance indicators A method of measuring the degree to which outcomes are achieved.

Palliative care Care that aims to enhance the quality of life of service users who are faced with a life-limiting illness and their families. It focuses on increasing comfort through prevention and treatment of suffering.

Paraphrasing Rephrasing in your own words what someone else has said.

Pathogen A disease-producing bacterium, fungus, virus, infestation or prion.

Pathogenic Able to cause disease.

PEG feeding Feeding via a tube inserted through the skin and into the stomach.

Perceiving Understanding.

Periphery The edge of something.

Persecution Hostility towards and cruel or unfair treatment of someone, usually because of prejudice about race, ethnicity, age, religion or gender.

Perseveration To use the same words and behaviours over and over again, without any specific purpose.

Personal or sensitive data Information about ethnic origin, religious and political beliefs, health, disability, criminal offences or alleged offences, sexual life and trade union membership.

Personalisation agenda Promotes individual choice and control over the shape of client support in all care settings.

Person-centred approaches/principles Approaches/principles that ensure that the person is central to all discussions and decisions that are made.

Plaques Insoluble protein deposits that build up around nerve cells.

PoCA Protection of Children Act. This, with the PoVA, replaced by the Vetting and Barring Scheme in October 2009.

Point of care The location where care is given.

PoVA Protection of Vulnerable Adults. This, with the PoCA, replaced by the Vetting and Barring Scheme in October 2009.

Preferred Priorities for Care (PPC) is a document in which individuals can record their wishes and preferences for the last years or months of their lives.

Prevalence The proportion of individuals in a population having a disease.

Prevalence rate Frequency.

Professional registration Demonstrates that you have met standards of competence. It is a requirement for employment for a number of professionals.

Prognosis A prediction about how something will develop.

Progressive condition A condition that gets worse over time.

Qualitative Not able to be measured numerically; concerned with feelings, opinions and qualities.

Quantitative Able to be measured numerically; concerned with quantities.

Religion A particular system of faith or worship.

Religious rites The established practice of ceremony that must be performed following the death of a person.

Reportable injuries Injuries that keep someone away from work or unable to do their normal duties for more than three days.

Reservoir An environment in which a micro-organism can live and reproduce.

Respite care Care that gives families a short break from the duties of constant care.

Responsible Being accountable for your actions and being prepared to improve.

RIDDOR Reporting of Injuries, Diseases and Dangerous Occurrences Regulations.

Risks When related to information, these are things that may cause loss of or damage to the information. Risk in general is the possibility of suffering harm or loss; danger.

Royal College of Nursing (RCN) Represents nurses and nursing, promotes excellence in practice and shapes health policies.

Sector Skills Councils (SSC) Employer-led organisations that work to boost the skills of their sector workforces.

Sharps Items of equipment that can cause cuts or puncture injuries.

Single-use equipment Items that can only be used once.

Slipped disc Occurs when one of the discs of the spine is ruptured and the jelly-like substance inside leaks out, putting pressure on the spinal cord. It causes intense back pain as well as pain in other areas of the body.

Spore A temporary, dormant structure into which a bacterium changes when conditions for its survival become hazardous.

Stakeholder A person or group having an interest in the success of an activity, enterprise etc.

Standard precautions Precautions based upon a set of principles designed to minimise exposure to and transmission of a wide variety of micro-organisms.

Syndrome A group of related symptoms.

Tangles Insoluble twisted protein fibres that build up inside nerve cells.

Tendon A band of tissue that connects a muscle with a bone.

Tort Any wrongdoing for which an action for damages may be brought.

A tracheostomy tube A tube which is inserted into a surgically created opening in the wind pipe (trachea) to keep it open.

Tracking A process that highlights any alterations made to a document.

Unethical Not right, moral or honourable.

Uniform Clothing of a distinctive design worn by members of a particular group or organisation as a means of identification.

User group A group of people who have similar health and social care needs.

Username and password The names that someone uses for identification purposes when logging on to a computer.

Value systems The principles of right and wrong that are accepted by an individual or a particular group of people.

Vertigo A reeling sensation, a feeling that you are about to fall.

Viable Alive and able to reproduce.

Visual system The eyes, optic muscles, retinas and optic nerve.

Waste products These include urine, faeces, tears and mucous.

Wilfully Deliberately, intentionally.

Work sector A division of the national economy, for example the manufacturing sector, the private sector.

Work shadowing Observing a professional in their workplace to get a taste of what their job involves.

Index

Bettws Library & Information Centre

30/9/14